Emerging, Reemerging, and Persistent Infectious Diseases of Cattle

Guest Editors

SANJAY KAPIL, DVM, MS, PhD

D. SCOTT McVEY, DVM, PhD

VETERINARY CLINICS OF NORTH AMERICA: FOOD ANIMAL PRACTICE

www.vetfood.theclinics.com

Consulting Editor
ROBERT A. SMITH, DVM, MS

March 2010 • Volume 26 • Number 1

SAUNDERS an imprint of ELSEVIER, Inc.

W.B. SAUNDERS COMPANY

A Division of Elsevier Inc.

1600 John F. Kennedy Boulevard • Suite 1800 • Philadelphia, PA 19103-2899

http://www.vetfood.theclinics.com

**VETERINARY CLINICS OF NORTH AMERICA: FOOD ANIMAL PRACTICE Volume 26, Number 1
March 2010 ISSN 0749-0720, ISBN-13: 978-1-4377-1885-0**

Editor: John Vassallo; j.vassallo@elsevier.com
Developmental Editor: Donald Mumford

Veterinary Clinics of North America: Food Animal Practice (ISSN 0749-0720) is published in March, July, and November by Elsevier Inc., 360 Park Avenue South, New York, NY 10010-1710. Subscription prices are $179.00 per year (domestic individuals), $265.00 per year (domestic institutions), $89.00 per year (domestic students/residents), $208.00 per year (Canadian individuals), $346.00 per year (Canadian institutions), $263.00 per year (international individuals), $346.00 per year (international institutions), and $135.00 per year (international and Canadian students/residents). To receive student/resident rate, orders must be accompanied by name of affiliated institution, date of term, and the *signature* of program/residency coordinator on institution letterhead. Orders will be billed at individual rate until proof of status is received. Foreign air speed delivery is included in all *Clinics* subscription prices. All prices are subject to change without notice. **POSTMASTER:** Send address changes to *Veterinary Clinics of North America: Food Animal Practice*, Elsevier Health Sciences Division, Subscription Customer Service, 3251 Riverport Lane, Maryland Heights, MO 63043. Customer Service (orders, claims, online, change of address): Elsevier Health Sciences Division, Subscription Customer Service, 3251 Riverport Lane, Maryland Heights, MO 63043. Tel: 1-800-654-2452 (U.S. and Canada); 314-447-8871 (ouside U.S. and Canada). Fax: 314-447-8029. E-mail: journalscustomerservice-usa@elsevier.com (for print support); journalsonlinesupport-usa@elsevier.com (for online support).

Reprints. For copies of 100 or more, of articles in this publication, please contact the Commercial Reprints Department, Elsevier Inc., 360 Park Avenue South, New York, NY 10010-1710. Tel.: 212-633-3812; Fax: 212-462-1935; E-mail: reprints@elsevier.com.

Veterinary Clinics of North America: Food Animal Practice is covered in *Current Contents/Agriculture, Biology and Environmental Sciences, MEDLINE/PubMed (Index Medicus),* and *Excerpta Medica.*

Printed and bound by CPI Group (UK) Ltd, Croydon, CR0 4YY
Transferred to Digital Print 2011

Contributors

CONSULTING EDITOR

ROBERT A. SMITH, DVM, MS
Diplomate, American Board of Veterinary Practitioners; Veterinary Research and
Consulting Services, LLC, Greeley, Colorado

GUEST EDITORS

SANJAY KAPIL, DVM, MS, PhD
Diplomate, American College of Veterinary Microbiology (Virology and Immunology);
Virologist, Oklahoma Animal Disease Diagnostic Laboratory, Center for Veterinary
Health Sciences, Stillwater, Oklahoma; Professor of Virology, Department of Veterinary
Pathology, Oklahoma State University, Stillwater, Oklahoma

D. SCOTT McVEY, DVM, PhD
Professor of Clinical Microbiology, School of Veterinary Medicine and Biomedical
Sciences, University of nebrasica Lincoln, Lincoln; Director and Professor, nebraska
Animal Diagnostic Center, Lincoln, nebraska

AUTHORS

JOHN A. ANGELOS, DVM, PhD
Diplomate, American College of Veterinary Internal Medicine; Associate Professor,
Department of Medicine and Epidemiology, School of Veterinary Medicine, University
of California, Davis, California

MÉLANIE J. BOILEAU, DVM, MS
Diplomate, American College of Veterinary Internal Medicine (Large Animal);
Assistant Professor, Food Animal Medicine and Surgery, Department of Veterinary Clinical
Sciences, Oklahoma State University Center for Veterinary Health Sciences, Stillwater,
Oklahoma

RONALD FAYER, PhD
Environmental Microbiology and Food Safety Laboratory, US Department of Agriculture,
Beltsville, Maryland

DEE GRIFFIN, DVM, MS
Professor, Department of Veterinary and Biomedical Sciences, Great Plains Veterinary
Educational Center, University of Nebraska – Lincoln, Clay Center, Nebraska

SANJAY KAPIL, DVM, MS, PhD
Diplomate, American College of Veterinary Microbiology (Virology and Immunology);
Virologist, Oklahoma Animal Disease Diagnostic Laboratory, Center for Veterinary
Health Sciences, Stillwater, Oklahoma; Professor of Virology, Department of Veterinary
Pathology, Oklahoma State University, Stillwater, Oklahoma

N. JAMES MACLACHLAN, BVSc, MS, PhD
Diplomate, American College Veterinary Pathologists; Department of Pathology, Microbiology and Immunology, School of Veterinary Medicine, University of California, Davis, California

D. SCOTT McVEY, DVM, PhD
Professor of Clinical Microbiology, School of Veterinary Medicine and Biomedical Sciences, University of Nebraska Lincoln, Lincoln; Director and Professor, Nebraska Animal Diagnostic Center, Lincoln, Nebraska

RODNEY A. MOXLEY, DVM, PhD
Professor, School of Veterinary Medicine & Biomedical Sciences, University of Nebraska-Lincoln, Lincoln, Nebraska

JEROME C. NIETFELD, DVM, PhD
Professor, Department of Diagnostic Medicine/Pathobiology, College of Veterinary Medicine, Kansas State University, Manhattan, Kansas

STEVEN OLSEN, DVM, PhD
Veterinary Research Officer, Infectious Bacterial Diseases Research Unit, United States Department of Agriculture, Agricultural Research Service, National Animal Disease Center, Ames, Iowa

JACK RHYAN, DVM, MS
Veterinary Medical Officer, US Department of Agriculture, Animal and Plant Health Inspection Service, Veterinary Services, Fort Collins, Colorado

JULIA F. RIDPATH, PhD
Ruminant Diseases and Immunology Research Unit, National Animal Disease Center, USDA, Agricultural Research Service, Ames, Iowa

MICHAEL W. RIGGS, DVM, PhD
Diplomate, American College of Veterinary Pathologists; Associate Professor, Department of Veterinary Science and Microbiology, University of Arizona, Tucson, Arizona

JISHU SHI, DVM, PhD
Associate Professor of Immunology, Department of Anatomy and Physiology, College of Veterinary Medicine, Kansas State University, Manhattan, Kansas

DAVID R. SMITH, DVM, PhD
Diplomate, American College of Veterinary Preventive Medicine (Epidemiology); Professor, School of Veterinary Medicine & Biomedical Sciences, University of Nebraska-Lincoln, Lincoln, Nebraska

MICHAEL T. SWEENEY, MS
Veterinary Medicine Research and Development, Pfizer Animal Health, Kalamazoo, Michigan

FRED TATUM, PhD
Research Microbiologist, Infectious Bacterial Diseases Research Unit, United States Department of Agriculture, Agricultural Research Service, National Animal Disease Center, Ames, Iowa

HANA VAN CAMPEN, DVM, PhD
Associate Professor, Veterinary Diagnostic Laboratory, Department of Microbiology, Immunology and Pathology, Colorado State University, Fort Collins, Colorado

JEFFREY L. WATTS, PhD, RM (NRCM), M(ASCP)
Veterinary Medicine Research and Development, Pfizer Animal Health, Kalamazoo, Michigan

CAROL R. WYATT, PhD
Associate Professor, Department of Diagnostic Medicine/Pathobiology, College of Veterinary Medicine, Kansas State University, Manhattan, Kansas

HANA VAN CAMPEN, DVM, PhD
Associate Professor, Veterinary Diagnostic Laboratory, Department of Microbiology, Immunology and Pathology, Colorado State University, Fort Collins, Colorado

JEFFREY L. WATTS, PhD, RM (NRCM), M(ASCP)
Veterinary Medicine Research and Development, Pfizer Animal Health, Kalamazoo, Michigan

CAROL R. WYATT, PhD
Associate Professor, Department of Diagnostic Medicine/Pathobiology, College of Veterinary Medicine, Kansas State University, Manhattan, Kansas

Contents

shedding of these organisms. However, much less emphasis has been given to their roles as diarrheagenic pathogens of cattle. The goal of this article is to address the question of pathogenicity, with a review that focuses on the results of studies of natural and experimental infections with these organisms. The authors conclude that there is overwhelming evidence that many different serogroups of AEEC are diarrheagenic pathogens of calves.

Despite technological, biologic, and pharmacologic advances the bacterial component of the bovine respiratory disease (BRD) complex continues to have a major adverse effect on the health and wellbeing of stocker and feeder cattle. Overlooked in this disappointing assessment is evaluation of the effects that working with younger, lighter-weight cattle have on managing the bacterial component of the BRD complex. Most problems associated with BRD come from cattle taken from and comingled with cattle operations that have inconsistent or nonexistent cattle health management. This article reviews the biologic, clinical, and management aspects of *Pasteurella multocida, Mannheimia haemolytica, Histophilus somni,* and *Mycoplasma bovis,* primarily as related to current production management considerations of stocker and feeder cattle.

Moraxella bovoculi is a recently described gram-negative coccus that was isolated from eyes of calves with infectious bovine keratoconjunctivitis (IBK, or "pinkeye") in 2002. This organism probably has been associated with IBK for many years and, until it was shown to be distinct from *M ovis,* may have been incorrectly identified as *M ovis, Branhamella ovis, M ovis*–like, or *B ovis*–like by diagnostic laboratories. *M bovoculi* can be isolated from normal calves and cattle with IBK or conjunctivitis. An exact role for *M bovoculi* in the pathogenesis of IBK is uncertain; however, anecdotal evidence of autogenous *M bovoculi* bacterins successfully preventing IBK suggests that it may play a role in IBK pathogenesis. Developers of vaccines against IBK should consider including *M bovoculi* antigens in vaccines to prevent IBK.

The introduction of newer antimicrobial agents over the past two decades has dramatically improved the treatment of bovine respiratory disease (BRD). In the same time period, the implementation of standardized susceptibility test methods and BRD-specific interpretive criteria has substantially improved the ability to detect clinical resistance in the BRD pathogens. Although overall levels of resistance to the newer antimicrobial agents are generally low, recent data have indicated the potential for emergence and dissemination of a resistant clone in cattle. These data indicate the need for long-term surveillance of antimicrobial resistance in the BRD pathogens and a better understanding of the epidemiology of antimicrobial resistance in these pathogens.

> The recent emergence of bluetongue virus (BTV) infection has attracted much interest because of the potential role of climate change and increased ambient temperature in causing the drastic recent alteration in the global distribution of this virus. Although there have been repeated assertions that climate change will alter the distribution of arboviruses and their vectors, specific examples are lacking in which the role of global warming alone has been unambiguously defined in the spread of such infections. This article summarizes recent events in Europe and the current status of BTV in the Americas and elsewhere in the context of potential global emergence of the BTV infection and disease of ruminants.

> Well-designed immunization programs have an important role in the control of disease outbreaks in cattle. The success of these immunization programs depends on the coordinated and effective use of an efficacious vaccine along with other required control measures. Efforts to improve key characteristics of vaccines (such as onset of immunity, duration of immunity, and basic safety and efficacy) will allow greater utility of the vaccines for outbreak control.

THE CLINICS ARE NOW AVAILABLE ONLINE!

Access your subscription at:
www.theclinics.com

Preface

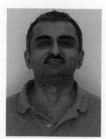 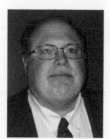

Sanjay Kapil, DVM, MS, PhD   D. Scott McVey, DVM, PhD
Guest Editors

Dear Colleagues, Veterinarians, Diagnosticians, Herdsmen, and Students:

We are delighted to bring this latest issue of the *Veterinary Clinics of North America: Food Animal Clinics* with contributions from the leaders in the field of bovine infectious diseases. We have sought out experts in the fields of treatment, prevention, ecology, and pathology of bovine infectious diseases. Both of us are associated with veterinary diagnostic laboratories in the middle of cattle country in the United States. Making full use of our experience and contacts in the field, we have approached international authorities on topics of interest and asked them to provide articles based on their years of scientific research and experience and on relevant developments gleaned from peer-reviewed scientific literature.

We hope you will enjoy the breadth of topics in this issue, which covers systemic diseases and enteric, respiratory, and localized infections caused by bacteria, protozoa, and viruses. We have covered some of the newly emerged genotypes of infections, such as bluetongue virus-8 in Europe. We have included cryptosporidiosis and brucellosis, which have extreme zoonotic importance. We have covered ecology of bovine infections and the role played by wildlife in livestock infections.

We thank the editors of Elsevier, especially John Vassallo and Dr Robert Smith, for bringing this issue to you. Dr Sanjay Kapil thanks his mentor, Professor Sagar M. Goyal at the University of Minnesota, St Paul, Minnesota; and his colleagues at the Oklahoma Animal Disease Diagnostic Laboratory, especially Dr Bill Johnson, director and pathologist, for interesting case conferences every week that highlight critical issues emerging in United States animal agriculture. Dr Scott McVey thanks his

doi:10.1016/j.cvfa.2009.11.001
vetfood.theclinics.com

mentor, Dr Raymond Loan, and his colleagues at the Nebraska Veterinary Diagnostic Center. Best wishes!

Sanjay Kapil, DVM, MS, PhD
Oklahoma Animal Disease Diagnostic Laboratory
Farm and Ridge Road, Stillwater, OK 74078, USA

D. Scott McVey, DVM, PhD
Nebraska Animal Diagnostic Center
Fair Street & E. Campus Loop, 1900 N. 42nd Street
Lincoln, NE 68583, USA

E-mail addresses:
sanjay.kapil@okstate.edu (S. Kapil)
dmcvey2@unlnotes.unl.edu (D.S. McVey)

Field Necropsy Techniques and Proper Specimen Submission for Investigation of Emerging Infectious Diseases of Food Animals

Jerome C. Nietfeld, DVM, PhD

KEYWORDS

- Bovine • Food animals • Emerging diseases • Necropsy
- Specimen collection

When investigating disease outbreaks, antemortem samples from animals displaying clinical signs typical of the problem are important in arriving at a correct diagnosis, but the systems and tissues that can be readily examined and sampled are limited. In some instances, especially those where animals are found dead without premonitory signs, necropsy is the only method available to determine the cause of death. Consequently, necropsy remains an important tool in investigating disease problems, especially new and emerging diseases.

Usually animals to be necropsied are ones that have recently died. In cases of animals that were chronically ill, extensively treated, or severely decomposed, the causative agent is often no longer present and laboratory tests identify only secondary pathogens or postmortem contaminants. In those cases, it can be more rewarding to euthanize one or more acutely affected animals, if that option is available. With chronic or persistent diseases, however, such as tuberculosis, Johne's disease, bovine virus diarrhea, and others, chronically affected animals can be the specimens of choice. After the animals to be necropsied are positively identified, individual animal identification information, owner's name, animal's location, history adequately describing

Department of Diagnostic Medicine/Pathobiology, Mosier Hall, College of Veterinary Medicine, Kansas State University, Manhattan, KS 66506, USA
E-mail address: nietfeld@vet.k-state.edu

Vet Clin Food Anim 26 (2010) 1–13
doi:10.1016/j.cvfa.2009.10.005
0749-0720/10/$ – see front matter © 2010 Elsevier Inc. All rights reserved.

the problem, clinical signs, and owner's or caretaker's assessment of the likely cause should be recorded. If possible, before moving animals to be necropsied, visually examine them, the other animals in the group, and their environment.

Sometimes the basic problem is apparent, making it possible to concentrate on one or more organ systems. In these cases, a complete necropsy and full set of tissues may not be necessary; however, this increases the risk of overlooking other contributing diseases or failing to correctly identify the cause if it is not what is expected. Generally, if a thorough necropsy is performed and tissues are examined and saved (**Table 1**), there is an adequate set of samples. If there are questions concerning sample collection, call the laboratory to which the samples are sent, explain the situation, and ask for advice. If at any time there is suspicion of a foreign animal disease, contact the US Department of Agriculture area veterinarian in charge, the state veterinarian, or the state department of animal health before removing any samples from the premise. Digital photographs e-mailed to a diagnostic laboratory or regulatory officials can be a help.

Consideration should be given to the necropsy site and disposal of the carcass. If a facility does not have a designated site, look for one that is convenient, does not present a biosecurity risk, and can be disinfected or where the topsoil can be removed and buried or covered by fresh soil.[1] At facilities where dead animals are normally composted or buried, it is usually best to perform a necropsy at or near the disposal site. If animals are to be rendered, the carcasses must be accessible by truck.[1] Animals euthanized with drugs that create a residue, such as barbiturates[2]; cattle with their head or brain removed; and sheep and goats cannot be rendered, and an alternate disposal method must be found.

Before beginning, all materials required to perform a necropsy and to collect and identify samples should be available.[1,3,4] It is important to have a source of clean water, a large plastic bucket, a scrub brush, disinfectant to clean and disinfect gloves, necropsy instruments, and cutting surfaces during a necropsy to keep bacterial contamination of samples to a minimum and between necropsies to prevent cross-contamination of samples from different animals. It also is important to rinse disinfected items with clean water to prevent contamination of samples with disinfectant. An insulated cooler and frozen gel ice packs to chill the fresh samples as soon as possible after collection help maintain specimen quality.

The 2007 American Veterinary Medical Association[2] Guidelines on Euthanasia describe acceptable methods of euthanasia. Descriptions of approved methods and their uses, advantages, and disadvantages are available online for cattle,[5] sheep and goats,[6] and swine.[7] In most cases, barbiturates, penetrating captive bolt, and gunshot are the only practical methods available for on-farm use and if a brain needs to be examined, captive bolt and gunshot are not suitable. If animals are to be euthanized, first collect serum and whole blood.

NECROPSY PROCEDURE

Although necropsy techniques taught at different schools of veterinary medicine differ somewhat, they all provide a systematic process that allows all body systems to be examined and are suitable for investigation of emerging diseases. In-depth reviews describing necropsy techniques for food animals have been published[1,3] and are available online.[4] The method described by Mason and Madden[1] is especially suited for field necropsies because the abdominal and thoracic viscera are left at least partially attached to the carcass, everything removed from the animal can be placed in the abdomen and thorax, and the incision can be closed with twine or rope. This makes disposal of the carcass easier than if parts are scattered about the necropsy area, and the hides of cattle can usually be salvaged by rendering companies.

External Examination and Opening the Carcass

Before opening an animal, perform a quick external examination paying attention to overall body condition, skin, hair coat, eyes, ears, feet, joints, external genitalia, body orifices, mammary glands, and, if there was lactation, mammary secretions. If there are external lesions, such as ulcers, vesicles, draining tracts, and so forth, collect samples, such as fluid from vesicles, swabs, and fixed and unfixed tissue specimens. After positioning the animal on its left side, make a skin incision along the ventral midline from the lower lip to the anus veering to the right of midline lateral to the penis or mammary glands.[1] Without making additional cuts through the skin, reflect both right legs along with the skin covering the trunk, neck, and head to the dorsal midline. As the skin is reflected, examine and collect the mandibular and superficial inguinal lymph nodes. Cut the attachments of the tongue to the mandible and exteriorize it ventrally. Examine the tongue and oral cavity and continue by cutting the soft palate and hyoid bones and dissecting the larynx, trachea, and esophagus from the surrounding tissue to the thoracic inlet. The tonsils can be removed with the larynx or dissected out separately. The retropharyngeal lymph nodes can be removed at this time or after the head is removed.

Opening the Abdominal and Thoracic Cavities

Carefully open the abdominal cavity leaving the abdominal wall attached along the ventral midline to help in closing the carcass when the necropsy is completed.[1] After cutting the diaphragm, cut the ribs near their dorsal attachments to the vertebrae, then reach inside the thorax and partially cut through the ribs at the costochondral junctions.[1] This allows the thoracic wall to be reflected ventrally but remain attached to the body so that it can be replaced when the necropsy is finished. Alternately, the ribs can be cut completely at the costochondral junctions and the entire rib cage removed and replaced when the necropsy is finished. Cut the greater omentum near its dorsal attachments, reflect it ventrally, and pull the small intestines from the pelvis.[1] This allows easy access to all abdominal and thoracic organs, except for the spleen which lies beneath the rumen (**Fig. 1**). The left kidney is easily accessed by reflecting the intestines dorsally over the right flank.

If care has been taken to not cut into the digestive tract, the tissues should be minimally contaminated; this is a good time to collect samples for microbiologic and molecular diagnostic tests. First wash, disinfect, and rinse gloves and necropsy instruments to keep contamination of samples to a minimum. Fresh samples also can be collected as the different organ systems are individually examined, but that usually results in more tissue contamination. Usually the gastrointestinal tract is sampled last, but in cases of primary gastrointestinal disease, especially if an animal was euthanized, examine and sample the gastrointestinal tract before the other systems, because the small intestines of food animals undergo rapid autolysis.

Examination of Thoracic Viscera

Open the pericardial sac and note the quantity, color, and consistency of the pericardial fluid. Normally there is a small amount of clear to amber, serous fluid that can be used for bacterial culture or in place of serum in serologic tests.[8] Dissect the trachea, esophagus, lungs, and heart from their attachments at the thoracic inlet and to the thoracic wall. Cut the aorta but not the esophagus leaving the heart and lungs attached to the carcass. Examine the external and cut surfaces of the tongue, the

Table 1
Necropsy tissues/organs to examine and, if indicated, collect for further tests

Examine	Fixed	Collect
External examination		
Skin	Yes	If Ind
Feet	If Ind	If Ind
Eyes	If Ind	If Ind
Mammary glands	Yes	If Ind
Testes	Yes	If Ind
Genitalia	Yes	If Ind
Oral cavity, neck, and subcutis		
Inguinal LN	Yes	Yes
Mandibular LN	Yes	Yes
Oral mucosa	If Ind	If Ind
Tonsil	Yes	Yes
Nasal cavity/turbinates	If Ind	If Ind
Larynx	If Ind	If Ind
Retropharyngeal LN	Yes	Yes
Trachea	Yes	Yes
Thyroid glands	Yes	If Ind
Esophagus	Yes	Yes
Thoracic cavity		
Lungs	Yes	Yes
Mediastinal LN	Yes	Yes
Tracheobronchial LN	Yes	Yes
Heart	Yes	Yes
Pleural fluid	NA	Yes
Pericardial fluid	NA	Yes
Abdominal cavity		
Kidneys	Yes	Yes
Ureters	If Ind	If Ind
Bladder	Yes	If Ind
Adrenal glands	Yes	If Ind
Liver	Yes	Yes
Gallbladder	If Ind	If Ind
Pancreas	Yes	If Ind
Hepatic LN	Yes	Yes
Ileocecal LN	Yes	Yes
Mesenteric LN	Yes	Yes
Uterus	Yes	If Ind
Ovaries	Yes	If Ind
Forestomachs	Yes	If Ind
Adomasum/stomach	Yes	Yes
Duodenum	Yes	Yes
Jejunum	Yes	Yes
Ileum	Yes	Yes

Cecum	Yes	If Ind
Spiral colon	Yes	Yes
Descending colon	Yes	Yes
Colon contents	NA	Yes
Spleen	Yes	Yes
Skeletal muscles	Yes	If Ind
Joints	If Ind	If Ind
Brain	Yes	Yes
Spinal cord	If Ind	If Ind
Blood and serum	NA	Yes

Abbreviations: If Ind, examine and, if indicated by history or if abnormal, save a sample; LN, lymph nodes; NA, not applicable; Yes, examine and save a sample.

thyroid glands, and the cervical, tracheobronchial, and mediastinal lymph nodes. Open the full length of the esophagus and trachea into the mainstem bronchi and collect the necessary specimens. Collect samples of all lung lobes, and, if there is grossly visible pneumonia, include normal and abnormal lung.

There are several methods for opening the heart[1,3,4] and all work well as long as all parts are inspected. A simple method that is easy to remember is to follow the flow of blood through the heart. Begin by opening the vena cava and follow it into the right atrium, through the right atrioventricular (AV) valve into the right ventricle, and out the pulmonary valve into the pulmonary artery. Turn the heart over, open the pulmonary vein, and follow it into the left atrium and through the left AV valve into the left ventricle. After inspecting the left ventricle, insert a knife or scissors into the aorta lying

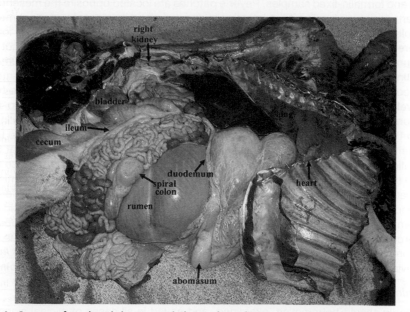

Fig. 1. Carcass after the abdomen and thorax have been opened. This is a good time to collect samples for microbiologic tests before the samples are further contaminated. The left kidney is visible if the small intestines are reflected over the right flank. The spleen lies beneath the rumen between it and the left body wall.

directly beneath the left AV valve and make an incision through the AV valve opening, the aortic valve, and the proximal aorta. If the heart is normal, collect and fix at least one full-thickness section of left ventricle through the papillary muscle. If there is any indication of cardiac pathology, collect and fix full-thickness sections of the free wall of both ventricles, the interventricular septum, the atria, and any abnormal areas. Also, save fresh specimens for microbiologic examination, if needed.

Examination of Abdominal Viscera

Dissect out the kidneys with the ureters to the bladder. Longitudinally incise the kidneys, peel off their capsule, and examine the cut and outer surfaces. Open and collect a sample of the bladder. The adrenal glands can be removed with the kidneys or separately. The genital tract can also be examined and sampled at this time. If desired, the entire genitourinary tract can be removed intact by removing a piece of the right lateral pelvis and dissecting out the pelvic portions of the genitourinary tracts with or without the rectum. The pelvis is opened by making a transverse cut through the shaft of the ilium anterior to the acetabulum and a second cut through the cranial (acetabular) branch of the pubis into the obturator foramen and extending it posteriorly through the ischium and dissecting out the acetabulum and surrounding bone.[1]

Find and examine the hepatic lymph nodes and pancreas. Open the gallbladder, note the color and consistency of its contents, and, if desired, swab it for bacterial culture. Make transverse sections through the liver at 1- to 2-cm intervals and collect representative samples.

When examining a gastrointestinal tract, the important thing is to examine all parts. The order is less important. A good method is to find the cecum and with it the ileum, spiral colon, and the ileocecal and mesenteric lymph nodes. Open the ileum and 2 to 5 meters of the distal jejunum, taking care to examine the Peyer's patches, and collect fresh and formalin-fixed samples. Peyer's patches are located opposite the mesentery and are easier to visualize if the intestine is opened along its mesenteric attachment. Samples of intestine for microbiology should be unopened sections 6- to 10-cm long. If more than one sample is placed in the same container, tie off the ends. Do not fix long unopened pieces of intestine, because formalin penetrates slowly into the lumen, resulting in sloughing of the mucosal epithelium. Also, do not physically scrape intestinal contents from the mucosal surface of sections for histopathology, because that severely damages the mucosa. Instead, cut sections 1- to 2-cm long, grasp the sections by their edges with a forceps, and swish them around in the formalin to wash the contents from the mucosal surface and to help the formalin penetrate into the lumen. You can also open the sections halfway or completely to insure that the formalin contacts the mucosal surface. In most cases it is not necessary to open the entire small intestine, but the remaining jejunum and duodenum should be examined and sampled in several locations so that all regions and any areas that appear different or abnormal are examined. Areas of intestine that are dilated, green, and thin-walled are decomposed and rarely diagnostic.[9] Open and sample the cecum, multiple loops of spiral colon, the descending colon, and the rectum. Open and examine the abomasum, the forestomachs, and their contents and, if desired, collect rumen contents. After removing its contents, lift up the rumen and examine and collect samples of the spleen.

Examination of the Central Nervous System

The brain should be removed, examined, and saved in all cases of clinical signs of central nervous system disease and when necropsy and antemortem clinical signs have not identified other systems as the cause of illness or death. Remove the head by disarticulating it at the atlanto-occipital joint. A sample of cerebrospinal fluid can

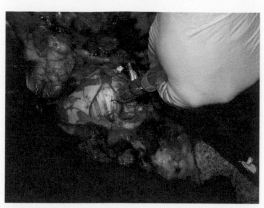

Fig. 2. Collection of cerebrospinal fluid from the ventral aspect of the allanto-occipital joint. Insert the needle to one side of midline until hitting bone, retract slightly, and aspirate.

be obtained by cutting down to and opening the ventral atlanto-occipital membrane and inserting a needle attached to a syringe through the dura until it hits bone, retracting the needle slightly and aspirating (**Fig. 2**).[1,3] If the needle is inserted just lateral to the midline, aspirating blood is less likely. The retropharyngeal lymph nodes are most easily found after the head is removed. The brain can be removed from food animals by one of several similar methods, using a small axe, cleaver, hatchet, or saw.[1,3,4] One method is to complete the cuts shown in **Fig. 3** with a hatchet, small axe, or cleaver. To remove the top of the skull, it is necessary to cut the attachment between the dura mater and the calvarium. After removing the top of the skull, cut the dura covering the cerebral cortices, the cerebellum, and brainstem, including the tentorium cerebelli between the cerebral hemispheres and the cerebellum (**Fig. 4**). Tip the head back on the occipital condyles, cut the ofactory nerves, and continue cutting cranial nerves until the brain comes free.

In cases of suspected central nervous system disease, the first priority is to collect and submit samples that, if needed, are suitable for rabies testing. The Centers for

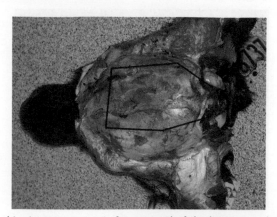

Fig. 3. Skull after skinning to prepare it for removal of the brain. Cut along the black lines with a hatchet, axe, or cleaver so that the bones of the calvarium are cut and then use something like the tip of the hatchet or cleaver to pry upward on the calvarium. The attachment between the dura mater and the calvarium has to be cut to remove the calvarium. The same cuts can be made with a saw or a combination of saw, wood chisel, and mallet.

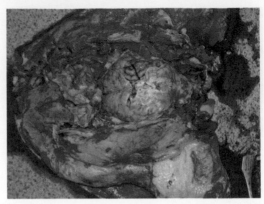

Fig. 4. Skull with the calvarium removed and the brain exposed. The dura covering the cerebrum, cerebellum, the space between the two, and the brainstem has to be cut before the brain can be removed.

Disease Control and Prevention require that an unfixed complete cross section of brainstem and the cerebellum or both hippocampuses be examined, with the cerebellum preferred over the hippocampuses (**Fig. 5**). The second priority for ruminant brains is obex for transmissible spongiform encephalopathy testing (see **Fig. 5**). Submit obex from cattle unfixed and from sheep and goats fixed. For other tests, save pieces of cerebral cortex, cerebellum, and brainstem unfixed and place the remainder in formalin. If uncertain about what to fix and not to fix, submit the entire brain unfixed.

The spinal cord can be removed by chopping away the bone lateral to the spinal cord with an axe or cleaver until the spinal canal is exposed enough to remove the cord.[1,3] In most cases involving infectious diseases, short segments of spinal cord yield results comparable to the entire cord. To do this, make transverse cuts through the spinal column two vertebrae in length and remove the segments from the carcass. Using a forceps and a thin scissors, cut the spinal nerves and remove the spinal cord

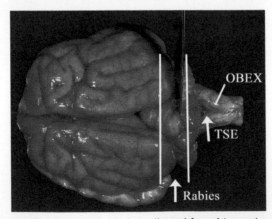

Fig. 5. Brain demonstrating the samples to be collected for rabies and transmissible spongiform encephalopathy (TSE) tests. A complete cross section of cerebellum and underlying brainstem submitted unfixed is the sample preferred by the Centers for Disease Control and Prevention for the rabies test. Submit the obex from cattle fresh and from small ruminants fixed. If in doubt, submit the entire brain unfixed.

and dura from each segment (**Fig. 6**). Open the dura and save a portion of each segment fresh and in formalin.

Examination of Muscles and Joints

To examine muscles and joints, it is necessary to skin the legs and areas over muscles to be examined. After removing the skin, cut through the muscles and connective tissue over the medial surface of the joints. Joint fluid can be obtained by aspiration with a needle and syringe. Open and inspect the joints and save pieces of joint capsule and synovial membranes. Skin the areas over muscle groups to be examined and make serial cuts through the muscles 1- to 2-cm apart and collect samples.

When completed, place the head and any other tissues or organs removed from the carcass into the abdomen or thorax, replace the abdominal wall flap, the right rib cage, and the reflected legs to their original positions, and tie the edges of the skin together along the midline with rope or twine.[1] Do not use wire if an animal is to be rendered.

COLLECTING SAMPLES
General Considerations

For the best laboratory results, collect samples for microbiologic tests as aseptically as possible, chill them as soon as possible, and keep them chilled until they arrive at the laboratory. If samples cannot be delivered to a laboratory on the day of collection, ship them so that they arrive the next day. Individually label all sample containers so that they can be identified if they are mixed with other samples or separated from their paperwork at any stage of the process. It is best not to freeze the samples but if a delay of more than 2 or 3 days is expected, frozen is better than decomposed. Freezing at −70°C and delivering on dry ice is better than freezing in a conventional freezer.

Samples for Histopathology

For proper fixation, cut tissue 5- to 7-mm thick and fix in 10% buffered neutral formalin using a ratio of 10 volumes of formalin to 1 volume of tissue. Several tissues can be fixed in the same container. In cold weather, ethanol can be added at 1 part ethanol to 9 parts 10% buffered formalin to prevent the formalin from freezing in transit.[9] To reduce the amount of formalin shipped, allow tissues to fix 24 hours, pour off the formalin, and ship with just enough formalin to keep the samples moist or, with formalin, moisten gauze pads.

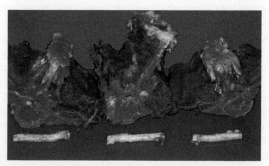

Fig. 6. Cross sections of vertebral column with each corresponding portion of spinal cord and dura removed. Open the dura and submit a portion of each spinal cord section fresh and fixed in formalin.

Samples for Bacteriology

Tissues and organs should be 3 to 5 cm on each side so that the surfaces can be seared when cultured. It is best to place each sample in an individually labeled sterile plastic bag, but if several samples are placed in the same container, never mix gastrointestinal samples with other tissues. Do not submit fluids in syringes, especially if they have an attached needle. Transfer the contents to blood collection tubes without additives or to sterile plastic tubes. Fluids and tissue surfaces can be sampled using bacterial culturettes with transport media. Special culturettes are available for anaerobic bacteria, but those with Amies gel, but not liquid, are suitable for aerobic and anaerobic bacteria. Clear Amies gel, but not Amies with charcoal, is also suitable for *Mycoplasma* spp.

If it is more than 2 days before samples arrive at a laboratory or if there is considerable autolysis or bacterial contamination at necropsy, it is sometimes recommended that swabs be taken from the tissues and the swabs submitted.[4] To do this, heat a spatula with a propane torch until it is red hot, sear the surface of the tissue, make an incision in the seared surface with a sterile scalpel, insert a swab, and place the swab into a culturette with bacterial transport medium.

Samples for Virology and Molecular Diagnostics

Postmortem autolysis, drying, heat, and pH fluctuations inactivate many viruses and can degrade nucleic acid, especially RNA. Cool temperature, moisture, and protein have a stabilizing effect. Pools of small pieces (<1 cm^3) of chilled tissues are suitable for virus isolation and molecular diagnostics; however, it is best to submit samples individually and allow diagnostic laboratory personnel to select samples for pooling. Always submit contaminated samples, such as intestines and tonsils, in separate containers. Do not pool samples from several animals for virus isolation, because neutralizing antibodies from one animal can prevent isolation of viruses from the entire pool. Samples from several animals can often be pooled for tests, such as ELISA or polymerase chain reaction, but let laboratory personnel do the pooling so that if a pool is positive they can test individual animal samples. Many viruses have a viremic phase and whole blood and serum are often excellent samples.

Swabs in viral transport media can be used for virus isolation, ELISA, polymerase chain reaction, and other tests. Some viruses can be isolated from swabs transported in culturettes containing liquid media designed for bacteria, but bacterial overgrowth can lead to pH changes that inactivate some viruses. Brain-heart infusion broth[10] and sterile saline can be used as transport media, especially if gentamicin (50 µg/mL) is added to help prevent bacterial overgrowth. Because it contains protein and some buffering capacity, brain-heart infusion broth should maintain viability of fragile viruses longer than saline. Commercially available viral transport media contain protein to stabilize viruses, buffers to prevent pH fluctuation, and antibiotics to prevent bacterial overgrowth and are also suitable for mycoplasmas and chlamydiae. Many diagnostic laboratories supply tubes of transport medium. To prevent excessive dilution, do not use more than 2 to 3 mL of transport medium per tube. Use Dacron, rayon, or polyester swabs with plastic or metal shafts. Do not use calcium alginate swabs or swabs with wooden shafts. Transport media containing agar (such as Amies gel) or charcoal inhibit many molecular tests and virus isolation and should not be used.

Samples for electron microscopy should be kept chilled and not placed in transport medium or frozen.

Samples for Parasitology

Submit samples, such as skin, tissues, organs, or feces (≥ 5 mL), individually in sterile plastic containers. Fix parasites for identification in 10% formalin.

Samples for Serology, Serum Biochemistry, and Hematology

Collect samples for hematologic and serum biochemistries from live animals. Serologic tests are best performed on serum from live animals, but pericardial fluid and serum from blood taken from the heart or a large vein of dead animals can be used if the animals are minimally decomposed. Fluids from decomposed animals can give false-positive serum neutralization results at low dilutions. Hemolysis can interfere with some tests; therefore, separate sera from the blood clots before shipment. Sera can be frozen if a delay in shipment is expected, but do not freeze until after the sera have been removed from the clots. If complete blood counts or blood parasite examinations are anticipated, prepare and air dry two blood smears at the time the blood is collected.

SHIPPING AND PACKAGING DIAGNOSTIC SAMPLES

Specimens that contain or might contain infectious agents are classified as category A or B by the US Department of Transportation and the International Air Transport Association.[11,12] Samples suspected of containing highly virulent agents that can cause death or permanent disability of healthy individuals, and pure cultures of many animal and zoonotic pathogens are classified as category A infectious substances and require special training, permits, and shipping methods. Before shipping pure cultures of infectious agents, check with the diagnostic laboratory or shipper. Animal diagnostic samples that might contain infectious agents from North America are classified as category B infectious substances and can be shipped by common carriers if packaged and labeled properly. Diagnostic samples must be triple-packaged with enough absorbent and cushioning material to prevent leakage in case of accidents. The samples are placed in primary containers that can be plastic, glass, or metal with a positive means of ensuring a leak-proof seal. Wide-mouthed plastic containers with screw-on lids or latches to hold snap-down lids in place and Whirl-Pak bags (Nasco, Fort Atkinson, WI) are acceptable. Avoid shipping formalin in glass containers. Lids on plastic containers and the tabs on Whirl-Pak bags should be secured with tape to prevent loosening and leakage in transit. Ziplock-type plastic bags are not suitable primary containers, because the seal frequently fails and they leak. Primary containers must not contain more than 1 L of liquid or 1 kg of solid tissue.

Primary containers are placed inside a leak-proof secondary container with enough absorbent material (such as cellulose wadding, cotton, wool, purchased absorbent packets, paper towels, or baby diapers) to absorb the entire liquid contents of the primary containers. Ziplock-type bags are acceptable as secondary containers. If several fragile containers, such as glass blood tubes, are placed in a secondary container, the primary containers must be individually wrapped or placed in a compartmentalized container so that they do not contact one another. It is best not to mix containers of unfixed tissues and containers with formalin in the same secondary container, to decrease the possibility of contamination of unfixed samples with formalin or formaldehyde gas.

Secondary containers are placed inside a rigid outer container with enough frozen gel cold packs (ice is not recommended) to keep unfixed samples cold until they arrive at their destination. Surround the specimens and the cold packs with cushioning material to prevent the contents from shifting in transit, to help insulate the contents,

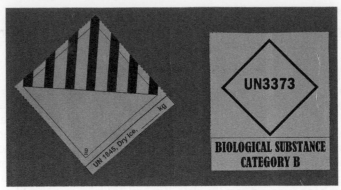

Fig. 7. Labels required to be affixed to packages containing category B biological substances and dry ice.

and to prevent leakage of the primary containers if the package is dropped. The outer package must not contain more than 4 L of liquid or 4 kg of solid material. An exception to the weight limit is if a whole animal or organ is shipped. Place diagnostic laboratory forms and a list of the package's contents in a waterproof plastic bag in the outer container. At least one surface of the outer package must have an outer dimension of at least 10.0 cm by 10.0 cm (4 in × 4 in) and an outer surface must have a clearly visible diamond-shaped UN3373 label and be marked (typed or handwritten), "Biologic Substance, Category B" (**Fig. 7**). The name and telephone number of a person with knowledge concerning the material shipped and emergency response measures in case of an accident are required on the outside of the package. Samples not expected to contain infectious agents, such as serum for serologic or biochemistry tests, do not require a UN3373 shipping label, but the package should be marked "Exempt animal specimen." Other packaging requirements for category B and exempt specimens are the same.

Packages containing dry ice must be constructed so that CO_2 given off by evaporating dry ice can escape, and they must carry a hazardous material label with the words, "dry ice", and the quantity of dry ice (see **Fig. 7**). Before shipping dry ice by air, check with the shipper because some do not accept it. The shipping labels and more detailed shipping regulations are available online[12] and can be downloaded and printed, cut out, and fastened to packages with clear tape, or the labels can be purchased commercially.

If the time, effort, and expense to necropsy one or more animals and to collect and ship samples to a laboratory are expended, it is important to take the extra time to make sure that the samples are packaged and shipped properly. If a diagnostic package leaks and people are exposed to infectious agents or other packages are damaged because of improper packaging, the damages are the responsibility of the shipper.

SUMMARY

This article briefly reviews criteria for selecting animals for necropsy, outlines necropsy procedure, and outlines samples to collect when investigating new or emerging diseases of food animals. It gives recommendations on how to collect samples for submission to a diagnostic laboratory and how to package and ship the samples so that they comply with federal regulations concerning shipment of diagnostic samples that might contain infectious substances.

REFERENCES

1. Mason GL, Madden DJ. Performing the field necropsy examination. Vet Clin North Am Food Anim Pract 2007;23(3):503–26.
2. American Veterinary Medical Association website. AVMA Guidelines on Euthanasia (Formerly Report of the AVMA Panel on Euthanasia), June 2007. Available at: http://www.avma.org/issues/animal_welfare/euthanasia.pdf. Accessed April 10, 2009.
3. Andrews JL, Van Alstine WG, Schwartz KJ. A basic approach to food animal necropsy. Vet Clin North Am Food Anim Pract 1986;2(1):1–29.
4. Cornell University College of Veterinary Medicine website. Virtual vet: bovine necropsy module. Available at: http://www.vet.cornell.edu/bovine/default.aspx. Accessed April 10, 2009.
5. American Association of Bovine Practitioners website. Practical euthanasia of cattle. Available at: http://aabp.org/resources/euth.pdf. Accessed April 10, 2009.
6. California Department of Food and Agriculture website. The emergency euthanasia of sheep and goats. Available at: http://www.cdfa.ca.gov/Ahfss/Emergency_Preparedness/pdfs/Sheep_Euth.pdf. Accessed April 10, 2009.
7. American Association of Swine Veterinarians website. On-farm euthanasia of swine recommendations for the producer. Available at: http://www.aasv.org/aasv/documents/SwineEuthanasia.pdf. Accessed April 10, 2009.
8. Ruth GR. Necropsy of adult cattle. Vet Clin North Am Food Anim Pract 1986;2(1):119–27.
9. Blanchard PC. Sampling techniques for the diagnosis of digestive diseases. Vet Clin North Am Food Anim Pract 2000;16(1):23–36.
10. Killian ML. Avian influenza virus sample types, collection, and handling. Methods Mol Biol 2008;436:7–12.
11. Kansas State Veterinary Diagnostic Laboratory website. Packing Instructions—Class 6—Toxic and Infectious Substances. Available at: http://www.vet.k-state.edu/depts/dmp/service/specimens.htm. Accessed November 2, 2009.
12. Cornell University College of Veterinary Medicine website. Shipping specimens to the animal health diagnostic center. Available at: http://www.diaglab.vet.cornell.edu/pdf/ShippingSpecimens.pdf. Accessed April 17, 2009.

Bovine Brucellosis

Steven Olsen, DVM, PhD*, Fred Tatum, PhD

KEYWORDS

• *Brucella abortus* • Brucellosis • Vaccination • Strain

Infection of cattle caused by *Brucella abortus* (ie, bovine brucellosis) has been of political importance in the United States for many decades. Regulatory programs to control or eradicate brucellosis in cattle were first initiated in the United States in 1934 as part of a recovery program to reduce cattle populations during severe drought conditions.[1] In 1954, the Congress appropriated funds to change the brucellosis control program to an eradication program as a joint effort between federal and state governments and cattle producers.

In the United States, the Animal and Plant Health Inspection Service of the US Department of Agriculture is responsible for managing national eradication or control programs that target livestock diseases of economic or zoonotic importance. Because the brucellosis eradication program has been ongoing for decades, a significant financial investment has been made in an effort to eliminate brucellosis. Although several new infected cattle herds have recently been identified, the United States achieved a milestone in 2008 in that, for the first time, all states were simultaneously declared free of cattle brucellosis.

DISEASE CHARACTERISTICS

The most common clinical manifestation of brucellosis in natural hosts is reproductive loss resulting from abortion, birth of weak offspring, or infertility.[2] In particular, third trimester abortion of dead or weak, nonviable calves is the hallmark of brucellosis. Aborted fetuses are generally fresh with minimal autolysis. Although mammary gland infection may not result in visible clinical symptoms or gross lesions, *Brucella* spp frequently localize in the mammary gland and cause mastitis.[2] Brucellosis can negatively affect lactation as one study demonstrated that a reduction in disease prevalence was associated with increased milk production.[3] Other clinical signs associated with brucellosis in cattle are rare. Occasionally, *Brucella* spp can localize in joints, bones, male reproductive tissues, or other aberrant locations where inflammation and associated pathology induce lesions and clinical signs.

Gross lesions in cattle are not pathognomonic but can include variable necrosis of cotyledons across the placenta and thickening of intercotyledonary areas.[4] Common

Infectious Bacterial Diseases Research Unit, United States Department of Agriculture, Agricultural Research Service, National Animal Disease Center, 2300 Dayton Avenue, Ames, IA 50010, USA
* Corresponding author.
E-mail address: Steven.olsen@ars.usda.gov (S. Olsen).

Vet Clin Food Anim 26 (2010) 15–27
doi:10.1016/j.cvfa.2009.10.006
0749-0720/10/$ – see front matter. Published by Elsevier Inc.

histologic lesions of maternal tissues include necrotic placentitis and lymphosuppurative or lymphohistiocytic interstitial mastitis. The most frequent fetal lesion is a multifocal, histiocytic bronchopneumonia with or without suppurative infiltrates. Fetal lesions may also include variable foci of necrotizing arteritis, necrosis, and granulomas in the lung and other tissues.

THE PATHOGEN

B abortus, like other members of the genus Brucella, is a facultative intracellular pathogen that infects mammalian hosts. Brucellae are small (0.4–3 μm), gram-negative, coccobacillary organisms within Alphaproteobacteria. B abortus has 2 circular chromosomes encoding approximately 3.2 Mb and has been divided into 7 biovars based on biochemical, phenotypic, and antigenic properties.[5] Only biovars 1, 2, and 4 of B abortus have been reported in the United States. Although biotyping is used for epidemiologic purposes, it is somewhat subjective because it is based on subtle differences, including requirements for higher CO_2 tensions for growth, production of hydrogen sulfide, growth on media containing dyes (thionine or basic fuchsin), and agglutination with monospecific A and M antisera.[5,6]

Because brucellae use multiple mechanisms to protect against DNA mutations, there is a 94% identity at the nucleotide level across the genus. The high homology in the Brucella genus has led some scientists to propose that brucellae are actually one species.[7] Because of the stability of Brucella genomes, molecular assays designed to assess genetic relationships between isolates (ie, restriction fragment length polymorphism) are ineffective for epidemiologic investigations or strain comparisons. A recent molecular technique, variable number tandem repeat, which evaluates strings of nucleotide repeats in noncoding areas of the chromosome, has been used to compare genetic relationships among strains.[8]

Transmission of B abortus is primarily through direct or aerosolized mucosal contact with fluids or tissues associated with the birth or abortion of infected fetuses.[9] Because bacterial concentrations in fetal fluids or placenta after abortion can be as high as 10^9 to 10^{10} colony-forming units (CFUs)/g and minimum infectious doses are estimated in the 10^3 to 10^4 CFU range, abortion events can laterally transmit brucellosis to many cattle that have contact with birthing materials. Vertical transmission to offspring can occur through shedding of B abortus in milk. Although Brucella can colonize the male reproductive tract and cause seroconversion, bulls are considered dead-end hosts, as venereal transmission is not considered to be of significance for B abortus.[10] Brucella can temporarily be recovered from environmental samples (ie, soil) associated with infected animals. However, B abortus is not considered to be a commensal bacterium, and environmental persistence is generally accepted to be of no epidemiologic importance because direct or close contact with aborted material or infected animals is required for transmission.[11] Therefore, maintenance of B abortus in cattle requires continual infection of susceptible hosts.

Once B abortus has entered a susceptible host, bacteria initially localize in lymphatic tissues draining the site of entry. After a brief period of bacteremia, brucellae localize in phagocytic and reticuloepithelial cells throughout the body.[9] Bacteremia occurs periodically and transiently in chronically infected cattle, but the number of bacteria in the blood is at low numbers as B abortus is infrequently isolated from blood samples obtained from seropositive cattle. Although controversial, the preferential localization of B abortus in the reproductive tract has been hypothesized to be related to the high concentration of erythritol in fetal placenta because this sugar promotes the growth of B abortus and is metabolically preferred over glucose.[12]

The entry of nonopsonized smooth *Brucella* into phagocytic cells relies on the cyto-skeleton of the host cell for internalization and occurs through interactions of the bacterial lipopolysaccharide O side chain with cholesterol-rich microdomains, termed lipid rafts, within the phagocyte plasma membrane.[13–16] Internalized *Brucella* initially localize within phagocytes in an acidified membrane-bound compartment (phago-some) where they are exposed to free oxygen radicals generated by the respiratory burst.[17] Early localization in an acidified environment is important for the replication and survival of *Brucella*, and it induces the expression of the *virB* operon, a type IV secretion system. Activation of the *virB* operon neutralizes the pH of the phagosome, and other *Brucella* genes modify the phagosomal compartment to prevent phago-some maturation and lysosome fusion.[18] This allows *Brucella* to establish an intracel-lular niche with limited exposure to oxygen- or nitrogen-free radicals but limited in available nutrients. Most brucellae (approximately 70%–85%) are eliminated by phag-olysosome fusion, but creation of the modified phagosomal compartment allows intra-cellular survival of some.[19] *Brucella* uses stationary-phase physiology and siderophores to scavenge iron as a mechanism for long-term survival within the nutrient-poor intracellular environment of the modified phagosome.[11] This unique internal environment is also responsible for limiting antibiotic action and explains some of the discrepancies between in vitro and in vivo studies on the survival of brucellae.[19]

In contrast, opsonization of *Brucella* strains increases the entry 10-fold. However, such an entry is targeted to phagosomes that mature and fuse with lysosomes to form phagolysosomes. Localization within phagolysosome compartments leads to intracellular killing of brucellae by monocytes.

DISEASE PREVENTION/REGULATORY PROGRAMS

Brucellosis regulatory programs were primarily developed as the most efficient way to prevent human infections.[20–23] These programs also assist producers in preventing economic losses that are associated with fetal losses, decreased milk production, and reduced fertility. The brucellosis eradication program in the United States is based on (1) vaccination of prepubescent heifers, (2) serologic testing at the first point of assembly (livestock markets, stockyards), (3) traceback of reactor animals to the herd of origin, (4) quarantine of infected herds, and (5) test and removal of seropositive animals or herd depopulation.[1] Because eradication programs are expensive and require good record keeping and infrastructure, brucellosis programs in some coun-tries may be designed to control brucellosis rather than to eradicate it.

Although antibody responses do not correlate with protection, identifying humoral responses is a valid method to determine if an animal has been exposed to *Brucella* spp. Conventional brucellosis surveillance tests are primarily based on the detection of antibodies against an immunodominant epitope on the *Brucella* lipopolysaccharide, the O side chain (perosamine residue). In the United States, serologic methods that combine screening tests (high sensitivity, lower specificity) with confirmatory tests (high specificity, lower sensitivity) are designed to detect reactor animals economically and accurately. The presence of antibodies against *Brucella* does not necessarily mean that the animal is infected at the time of testing but does indicate that the animal has been previously infected with *Brucella*. Regulations consider any seropositive animal to be infected because brucellae are intracellular pathogens and isolation by noninvasive microbiologic methods is not always reliable. Accurate assessment of *Brucella* infection requires sampling of internal lymphatic tissues, which can only be obtained postmortem at necropsy or during processing at an abattoir.

CATTLE VACCINATION

Vaccination is a critical tool to control or eradicate brucellosis; it primarily prevents clinical effects of the disease (ie, abortions or infected calves) that lead to transmission.[24] In the United States, routine brucellosis vaccination is administered via intramuscular or subcutaneous injection and limited to prepubescent heifers (4–12 months). Vaccination recommendations were originally designed to minimize the retained titers from strain 19 vaccination. Vaccination programs have not included males because they are not considered to have a significant role in disease transmission. In infected herds, vaccination of adult cows with a reduced vaccine dosage has been conducted with regulatory approval.

Long-term protection of cattle against brucellosis is associated with the stimulation of cellular immunity, whereas antibodies are considered to play a minor role in protecting cattle against B $abortus$.[25] Although specific correlates of protective immunity are currently not known in cattle, it is believed that protection is mediated by the T_H1 subset of $CD4^+$ lymphocytes and is associated with the production of interferon-γ.[26] Despite efforts to develop a nonliving brucellosis vaccine, killed vaccines are generally deficient in the stimulation of cellular immune responses and are less efficacious than live vaccines in cattle and other animals.[25] Delivery of brucellosis vaccines by alternative routes (ie, oral and intraconjunctival) has been reported to be efficacious against B $abortus$, but protection is less consistent or repeatable as compared with parenteral vaccination.

Most effective regulatory programs combine vaccination and serologic testing. Vaccination programs are very effective in reducing clinical effects and disease transmission, but vaccination alone has never been effective in eradicating brucellosis from any animal population. Even when the prevalence of brucellosis is low, elimination of vaccination with reliance on test and removal programs can be associated with resurgence of human or livestock brucellosis. Efforts to reduce brucellosis vaccination in the United States in the early 1960s and early 1970s resulted in an increased number of $Brucella$-infected cattle herds (Dr Mike Gilsdorf, personal communication, 2009). Currently available brucellosis vaccines for cattle (strains RB51 and 19) are highly effective in reducing production losses caused by brucellosis and in reducing transmission but are less effective in preventing livestock from being infected with field strains of $Brucella$ spp or seroconverting after exposure. Vaccination is not effective in preventing seroconversion if cattle are exposed to infectious dosages of B $abortus$ field strains. Vaccinated cattle can test seropositive after exposure irregardless of infection status.

Experimental efficacy studies ensure that all animals receive a known infectious dose of a virulent $Brucella$ strain at the most susceptible time (midgestation). However, vaccine-induced protection under field conditions is most likely greater than that in experimental studies because exposure times and dosages under field conditions may not be optimal for infection.[24] Field efficacy may be influenced by factors (nutrition, environment, stress, or concurrent infections) that deleteriously affect immunity. It has been demonstrated that abortion and infection rates are directly related to the exposure dose of a virulent B $abortus$ strain,[27,28] and high challenge dosages can overwhelm vaccine-induced protection.[29] Because of the large number of variables that may influence vaccine-induced protection against brucellosis, assignment of a specific numeric value for $Brucella$ vaccine efficacy under field conditions would be unreliable. Rather, numeric estimates of protection should be viewed as being approximations and as reflecting differences in effects between paired vaccinated and nonvaccinated animals under controlled conditions. It should also be noted that abortion or infection rates in field or experimental studies may be influenced by known or unknown factors.

Strain 19

The *B abortus* strain 19 vaccine (S19) was the principal vaccine used for cattle vaccination in the United States until 1996. It was first isolated in 1923, experimentally evaluated in the 1930s, and introduced for field use in the United States in 1941. Derived from a virulent isolate of *B abortus*, S19 was naturally attenuated when the virulent culture was inadvertently left at room temperature for 1 year. As a smooth strain, S19 expresses the O side chain on its lipopolysaccharide. The O side chain of S19 induces serologic responses on brucellosis surveillance tests, which cannot be differentiated from antibody responses caused by infection with field strains of *B abortus*. The persistence of S19 until adulthood in an estimated 2 animals per 100,000 calfhood vaccinates can contribute to retained titers that interfere with serologic surveillance. Retained titers from S19 vaccination can be problematic in countries, such as the United States, where serologic surveillance is emphasized. Some countries in South America continue to use the original full dosage of S19 (2.5–12 $\times$ 10^{10} CFUs) for calfhood vaccination, whereas the United States and other countries switched to a reduced dosage (3–10 $\times$ 10^9 CFUs) in the 1980s in an effort to reduce the number of calfhood vaccinates having retained antibody titers.

Numerous studies over many years have demonstrated that calfhood vaccination with full and reduced dose of S19 protects cattle against brucellosis. In a large field trial in the United States in 1936, full-dose S19 vaccination of more than 18,000 calves in 260 *Brucella*-infected herds led to normal parturition in more than 96% of the calves when they reached adulthood.[30] Similar efficacy results were demonstrated in cattle vaccinated with reduced dosages of S19.[31] Retrospective data have also demonstrated that S19 calfhood vaccination in *Brucella*-infected herds reduces the number of seroreactors and facilitates the elimination of brucellosis from the herd.[32] Based on experimental data that used the full calfhood dose and evaluated protection in cattle up to 9 years of age, it was estimated that approximately 65% to 75% of all vaccinated animals were completely protected for their productive lifespan.[28,33] Similar data for the duration of immunity has not been reported for the reduced calfhood dosage of S19.

S19 has also been effectively used as an adult vaccine in *Brucella*-infected herds and has facilitated reductions in brucellosis prevalence.[34–36] Low dosages (0.3–3 $\times$ 10^9 CFUs) of S19 in adult cows reduce brucellosis seroprevalence and fetal losses under field conditions. A large adult vaccination study in cattle demonstrated a reduction in human infections.[34] Adult vaccination seems beneficial particularly for larger herds in which test and slaughter methods alone might not be effective, and a large and perhaps prohibitive portion of seroreactors might have to be removed.[36] Although beneficial for controlling or eradicating *B abortus* from cattle, adult vaccination with S19 can be associated with adverse effects. In 2 studies in which calfhood vaccination status was not clarified, 22% of pregnant cattle aborted after vaccination with 5.8 $\times$ 10^9 CFUs of S19[35] and 14.3% of cattle between 1 and 9 months of gestation aborted after vaccination with 1.2 $\times$ 10^7 CFUs of S19.[37] In a large field study involving more than 10,000 dairy cattle in herds that routinely used calfhood vaccination, less than 1% of cattle aborted after vaccination with a standard dosage of S19.[36] In the later study, significant reductions in milk production for 8 to 12 days after vaccination were noted.

Strain RB51

In 1996, the United States essentially eliminated the use of S19 and switched to the *B abortus* strain RB51 vaccine. The RB51 strain is rough because it has minimal expression of the lipopolysaccharide O side chain. Because of the lack of O-side-chain expression, RB51 does not induce antibody responses that are detected by conventional brucellosis serologic tests. Cattle that were calfhood vaccinated with S19 did not seroconvert as adults when boostered with calfhood dosages of RB51. Under experimental conditions, cattle vaccinated with 1 to 3.4×10^{10} CFUs of RB51 have reduced incidents of abortion or *Brucella* infection at necropsy when compared with nonvaccinated cattle.[38,39] Ongoing experiments suggest that high levels of immunity persist for 4 to 5 years of age in animals that are calfhood vaccinated with RB51 (Olsen, unpublished, 2009).

As with S19, adult vaccination with RB51 has been used to protect cattle against brucellosis. Under experimental conditions, parenteral vaccination of pregnant cattle with 1 to 3×10^9 CFUs of RB51 is safe and efficacious for the subsequent pregnancy.[40] Like S19, RB51 can induce abortions under field conditions.[41] Current data suggest that calfhood vaccinated cattle can be safely booster vaccinated with RB51 ($1–3 \times 10^9$ CFUs) as pregnant adults.[42,43]

Comparison of S19 with RB51

At present, the greatest controversy in regard to *B abortus* vaccination is whether calfhood vaccination with RB51 induces equivalent protection in cattle as compared with S19 vaccination. Although several experimental and field studies have demonstrated that RB51 is efficacious in protecting cattle against experimental infection, there are only limited data in which the experimental design included simultaneous comparisons of both vaccines. In a series of calfhood vaccination studies at the National Animal Disease Center involving relatively small numbers of cattle, a nonsignificant reduction in the abortion rates was observed in S19 vaccinates (0 of 19) when compared with RB51 vaccinates (1 of 29). Cattle vaccinated with S19 had slight reductions in the infection rates at necropsy (1 of 22, 5%) when compared with those vaccinated with RB51 (3 of 29, 10%).

The prevalence of brucellosis within the livestock population, the intensity of serologic surveillance, the regulatory pressure, and economics are factors that may influence vaccine selection. In the absence of intense serologic surveillance, retained titers from S19 vaccination would be unlikely to present significant regulatory problems. In contrast, in the late 1980s and early 1990s in the United States, most seropositive or suspect responses detected at market surveillance were found by epidemiologic investigation to have resulted from S19 vaccination. In the United States, switching to RB51 vaccination has been beneficial in reducing economic costs associated with reactor traceback efforts, and it has facilitated the identification of remaining *Brucella*-infected herds. In countries with a high prevalence of brucellosis and/or limited regulatory programs, S19 may be the vaccine of choice because it may be slightly more protective and many countries can produce commercial S19 vaccines. However, in the United States, where prevalence of brucellosis is low and serologic surveillance is high, the RB51 vaccine is preferred because of its lack of interference with serologic surveillance and comparable efficacy in protecting against brucellosis.

Other Vaccines

A heat-killed *B abortus* strain 45/20 vaccine was developed in the 1920s and introduced for field use. As a rough strain, it offers serologic advantages like RB51 but cannot be used as a live vaccine because of its reversion to a smooth form in vivo.[44] Because it requires 2 injections and is not as protective as S19, its use worldwide has been very limited.[45]

Several potential new vaccine strains, predominantly genetically engineered strains,[46-48] have been evaluated in laboratory animal models. In addition, new encapsulation methods that may increase immunogenicity have been evaluated. The lack of development of new vaccine candidates may be partly because of the lack of progression from laboratory animals to the host species of interest, the high cost of efficacy studies in large ruminants, and the limited economic return on new brucellosis vaccines. In general, candidates that have progressed into ruminant studies at this time have not demonstrated protection that exceeds currently available vaccines.

The use of laboratory animal models, such as mice, for B abortus research is inexpensive when compared with studies done in the natural host. Inherent deficiencies in laboratory animals as predictive models for natural hosts may also explain conflicting results between mice and large ruminant studies[46,49] and may also have negatively impaired development of new vaccines. As laboratory animal models are generally used as positive predictors of efficacy in the host species of interest, the possibility that protective cattle vaccines may have been discarded because of negative results in murine models cannot be eliminated.

OTHER RESERVOIR HOSTS

Regulatory programs have been very effective in reducing or eliminating the prevalence of targeted diseases in domestic livestock, but spillover of the disease from domestic livestock to wildlife has allowed the establishment of new reservoir hosts. The establishment of wildlife reservoirs of disease has complicated regulatory efforts by allowing transmission back to domestic livestock and has allowed the persistence of B abortus.[24] It is ironic that most experts agree that brucellosis in wildlife reservoirs originated from Brucella infections in domestic livestock. Numerous studies have documented spillover into hosts in whom the disease is not manifested and transmission does not occur (dead-end or spillover hosts). However, current problems in the UnitedStates are associated with wildlife species in which the disease is manifested and transmission does occur (maintenance hosts).

The United States currently has at least 2 wildlife species that function as maintenance hosts for B abortus: elk (Cervus elaphus nelsoni) and bison (Bison bison). Brucellosis in bison remains controversial because of its infection of a historically important free-ranging herd in arguably the most eminent park in the United States. Since the elimination of hands-on management of bison in Yellowstone National Park in 1967,[50] the herd has increased from 397 animals to peak populations of approximately 3000 to 5000 bisons. Wolves have been reintroduced into the environment, but predation does not have a significant effect on the bison population.[50] Seroprevalence of brucellosis in the Yellowstone National Park bison is approximately 50%,[51] and data suggest that B abortus can be isolated from approximately 46% of seropositive bisons.[52] Bulls have a high seroprevalence for brucellosis, and recent data have suggested that behavior may play a role in the transmission to males. Experimental studies have demonstrated that bisons can transmit B abortus to cohoused cattle,[53] although documentation of transmission under field conditions is lacking. Lack of documented transmission is most likely because of regulatory efforts to maintain spatial and temporal separation of free-ranging bison from cattle. The risk of interspecies transmission may also be prevented by the rapid removal of aborted fetuses from the landscape by numerous predators in the environment. At present, no cases of human brucellosis have been linked to brucellosis in bison.

In the Greater Yellowstone Area (GYA), the total population of elk (*C elaphus nelsoni*) is estimated at 120,000 animals.[54] Because of the loss of traditional winter-feeding ranges due to development and agriculture, beginning in 1909, the state of Wyoming and the US Fish and Wildlife Service established 23 feedgrounds, which provide hay during winter months. Seroprevalence of brucellosis averages approximately 35% in adult female elk on Wyoming feedgrounds compared with 2% to 3% in elk that over-winter off the feedgrounds.[55] In the neighboring state of Idaho, seroprevalence in areas of artificial feeding ranged from 12% to 80%, whereas hunter surveys suggested population seroprevalence of only 2% to 3%.[56] Epidemiologic data have suggested that the 10 *Brucella*-infected cattle herds identified in the GYA since 2002 have re-sulted from wildlife transmission, with elk implicated as the most likely source. Brucel-losis in elk has been epidemiologically linked to 2 zoonotic infections in which the only significant risk factor was contact with elk carcasses.[57]

Although feral swine are most commonly infected with *Brucella suis*, recent work has suggested that they may also serve as maintenance hosts for *B abortus*.[58] Field transmission of *B abortus* from feral swine to cattle has not been documented at present. However, Texas and other southeastern states report numerous cases of seropositive cattle, which are shown by bacterial culture to be infected with *B suis*.

OTHER BRUCELLA SPP IN CATTLE

Feral swine are rapidly expanding their ranges across the United States, with at least 44 of 50 states reporting populations.[59] Feral swine populations were estimated at 4 million animals in 1999 by one report,[60] whereas another report estimated in 2000 that Texas alone had 3 million.[61] In at least 14 states, brucellosis has been docu-mented to be present in feral swine populations,[62] with some populations demon-strating high seroprevalence.[63] Feral swine shed *B suis* for extended periods of time in urine and mucosal secretions. Numerous field cases have been documented in which cattle were infected with *B suis* from feral swine. Cattle infected with *B suis* have positive responses on brucellosis serologic tests, which cannot be differentiated from responses after *B abortus* infection. Differentiating *B suis* from *B abortus* requires bacteriologic isolation, which is not always successful.

In some areas of the world, *Brucella melitensis* has become endemic in cattle pop-ulations.[64] Although extremely rare in the United States, *B melitensis* was isolated from a cow in southern Texas in 1999.[65] Previously, *B melitensis* was last detected in sheep and goats in southern Texas in 1969. Limited data are currently available on vaccines to protect cattle against *B melitensis*. Currently, the World Organization for Animal Health, formerly known as the Office International des Epizooties, does not recom-mend the use of the *B melitensis* Rev.1 vaccine in cattle.[66] Data to support the use of other vaccines in protecting cattle against *B melitensis* are currently lacking.

New and phenotypically diverse strains of *Brucella* have been isolated from sea mammals (eg, dolphins, porpoises, seals, beluga whales).[67] Some isolates have caused zoonotic infections in people in England, Peru, and New Zealand. Under experimental conditions, cattle infected conjunctivally or intravenously with a seal *Brucella* isolate from Puget Sound, Washington, did seroconvert on brucellosis sero-logic tests. Abortion occurred in 2 of 3 animals after intravenous injection but not in cattle conjunctivally exposed.[68] The marine *Brucella* are intriguing, as current data suggest that lungworms (*Parafilaroides* and *Phocoena*) may play a role in natural trans-mission in seals and porpoises.[69] However, current knowledge suggests that marine strains of *Brucella* are of low risk for causing brucellosis in cattle.

HUMAN INFECTION

Although reproductive losses caused by *B abortus* can be expensive to cattle producers, the primary impetus for regulatory programs to control brucellosis in cattle is to prevent zoonotic infections in humans. Multiple studies have demonstrated that addressing brucellosis in animal reservoirs is the most cost-efficient mechanism for controlling human brucellosis.[20–23] Human infection with *B abortus* can occur from direct contact with infected animals or tissues or fluids associated with abortion. However, consumption of nonpasteurized dairy products from *Brucella*-infected animals is the most frequent route of human infection. Entry can occur across mucosal surfaces by aerosolization into respiratory tissues, by oral consumption, or by penetration through breaks in the epidermis. Inadvertent exposure to live vaccine strains, most commonly via needle sticks, has also been a frequent source of human infections, especially in the veterinarian profession.[70] *Brucella* spp are probably also the most common zoonotic agent for causing laboratory-associated infections. Human-to-human transmission through breast milk or coitus has been occasionally described for *B melitensis*[71] but does not appear to be of significance for *B abortus*.

Human infection with *B abortus* can cause chronic, debilitating clinical illness with nonpathognomonic symptoms.[72,73] Typically, infected humans have recurrent episodes of fever (undulant fever), splenomegaly, hepatomegaly, and asthenia and frequently have malodorous perspiration. Although generally targeted to lymphoreticular tissues, *Brucella* can localize in almost any tissue, including joints, brain, and cardiac muscle, with inflammatory responses leading to complications, such as osteoarthritis, meningitis, and myocarditis. Bone and joint involvement is the most common complication of human brucellosis,[73] whereas endocarditis is most frequently associated with fatalities.

Between the years of 1996 and 2005, the United States had 1057 cases of brucellosis reported to the Centers for Disease Control and Prevention (105.7 cases/year; www.cdc.gov/mmwr). This number is less when compared with the reported average of 218 human cases per year in 1967 to 1972 when brucellosis was widespread in domestic livestock. Before the initiation of the State/Federal Cooperative Brucellosis Control Program, the Centers for Disease Control and Prevention reported 6321 human cases of brucellosis in 1947.

SUMMARY

Brucellosis is a zoonotic disease that causes reproductive losses in cattle and has international trade implications. During the last 80 years, the United States has invested considerable financial resources in eliminating this disease. With the exception of the introduction of the *B abortus* RB51 strain in 1996, tools to control or eradicate brucellosis have not significantly changed for decades. Vaccination and serologic detection remain important for regulatory programs. Although brucellosis is associated with economic losses for producers, justification for the cost of regulatory programs is based on data that indicate that addressing the disease in animals is the most cost-effective mechanism to prevent human disease. As the United States nears completion of programs to eradicate brucellosis from domestic livestock, the persistence of *Brucella* spp within wildlife reservoirs will increase in importance. Although eradicating brucellosis in wildlife reservoirs will be difficult and costly, it is unlikely that the United States can be considered totally free of brucellosis in cattle, without resolution of the disease in free-ranging wildlife reservoirs.

REFERENCES

1. Ragan VE. The brucellosis eradication program in the United States. In: Kreeger TJ, editor. Brucellosis in elk and bison in the Greater Yellowstone Area. Cheyenne (WY): Wyoming Game and Fish Department; 2002. p. 7–16.
2. Olsen SC, Thoen CO, Cheville NF. Brucella. In: Gyles CL, Thoen CO, Prescott JF, et al, editors. Pathogenesis of bacterial infections of animals. Ames (IA): Blackwell Publishing; 2004. p. 309–19.
3. Herrera E, Palomares G, Diaz-Aparicio E. Milk production increase in a dairy farm under a six-year brucellosis control program. Ann N Y Acad Sci 2008;1149: 296–9.
4. Jubb KVF, Kennedy PC, Palmer NC. Female genital system. In: Maxie MG, editor. Pathology of domestic animals, 5th edition. vol. 3. New York: Saunders; 2007. p. 484–6.
5. Alton GG, Jones LM, Angus RD, et al. Techniques for the brucellosis laboratory. Paris: Institut National de la recherché agronomique; 1988. p. 13–62.
6. Whatmore AM, Perrett LL, MacMillan AP. Characterisation of the genetic diversity of Brucella by multilocus sequencing. BMC Microbiol 2007;20(7):34.
7. Vizcaino N, Cloeckaert A, Verger J, et al. DNA polymorphism in the genus Brucella. Microbes Infect 2000;2:1089–100.
8. Bricker BJ, Ewalt DR, Halling SM. Brucella "HOOF-Prints": strain typing by multi-locus analysis of variable number tandem repeats (VNTRs). BMC Microbiol 2003;3:15.
9. Enright FM. The pathogenesis and pathobiology of Brucella infection in domestic animals. In: Nielsen K, Duncan JR, editors. Animal brucellosis. Boca Raton (FL): CRC Press, Inc; 1990. p. 301–20.
10. Cheville NF, McCullough DR, Paulson LR. Brucellosis in the Greater Yellowstone Area. Washington, DC: National Research Council; 1998. p. 25.
11. Roop RM, Gee JM, Robertson GT, et al. Brucella stationary-phase gene expression and virulence. Annu Rev Microbiol 2003;57:57–76.
12. Keppie J, Williams AE, Witt K, et al. The role of erythritol in tissue localization of the brucellae. Br J Exp Pathol 1965;46:104–8.
13. Cutler SJ, Whatmore AM, Commander NJ. Brucellosis-new aspects of an old disease. J Appl Microbiol 2005;98:1270–81.
14. Jiménez de Bagüés MP, Terraza A, Gross A, et al. Different responses of macrophages to smooth and rough Brucella spp.: relationship to virulence. Infect Immun 2004;72:2429–33.
15. Bellaire BH, Roop RM, Cardelli JA. Opsonized virulent Brucella abortus replicates within nonacidic, endoplasmic reticulum-negative, LAMP-1-positive phagosomes in human monocytes. Infect Immun 2005;73:3702–12.
16. Olsen SC, Bellaire BH, Roop RM, et al. Brucella. In: Byles CL, Prescott JP, Songer JG, et al, editors. Pathogenesis of bacterial infections in animals. Ames (IA): Blackwell Publishing; 2010, in press. Chapter 22.
17. Rittig MG, Alvarez-Martinez MT, Porte F, et al. Intracellular survival of Brucella spp. in human monocytes involves conventional uptake but special phagosomes. Infect Immun 2001;69:3995–4006.
18. Celli J. Surviving inside a macrophage: the many ways of Brucella. Res Microbiol 2006;157:93–8.
19. Pappas G, Akritidis N, Bosilkoviski M, et al. Brucellosis. N Engl J Med 2005;352: 2325–36.
20. Roth F, Zinsstag J, Orkhon D, et al. Human health benefits from livestock vaccination for brucellosis: case study. Bull World Health Organ 2003;81:867–76.

21. Bernués A, Manrique E, Maza MT. Economic evaluation of bovine brucellosis and tuberculosis eradication programmes in a mountain area of Spain. Prev Vet Med 1997;30:137–49.
22. Jelastopulu E, Bikas C, Petropoulos C, et al. Incidence of human brucellosis in a rural area in Western Greece after the implementation of a vaccination programme against animal brucellosis. BMC Public Health 2008;8:241.
23. Minas A, Minas M, Stournara A, et al. The "effects" of Rev-1 vaccination of sheep and goats on human brucellosis in Greece. Prev Vet Med 2004;64:41–7.
24. Olsen SC, Stoffregen WS. Essential role of vaccines in brucellosis control and eradication programs for livestock. Expert Rev Vaccines 2005;4:915–28.
25. Nicoletti P, Winter AJ. The immune response to *Brucella abortus*—the cell-mediated response to infections. In: Nielsen K, Duncan JR, editors. Animal brucellosis. Boston: CRC Press; 1990. p. 83–96.
26. Huang LY, Krieg AM, Eller N, et al. Induction and regulation of Th1-inducing cytokines by bacterial DNA, lipopolysaccharide, and heat-inactivated bacteria. Infect Immun 1999;67:6257–63.
27. Alton GG, Jones LM, Garcia-Carillo C, et al. *Brucella abortus* 45/20 vaccines in goats: immunity experiment. Am J Vet Res 1972;33:1747–51.
28. Manthei CA. Summary of controlled research with strain 19. Proc Annu Meet U S Livest Sanit Assoc 1959;63:91–7.
29. Confer AW, Hall SM, Faulkner CB, et al. Effects of challenge dose on the clinical and immune responses of cattle vaccinated with reduced doses of *Brucella abortus* strain 19. Vet Microbiol 1985;10:561–75.
30. Wright AE. Report of the cooperative bovine brucellosis work in the United States. Proc Annu Meet U S Livest Sanit Assoc 1942;47:149–54.
31. Deyoe BL, Dorsey TA, Meredith KB, et al. Effect of reduced dosages of *Brucella abortus* strain 19 in cattle vaccinated as yearlings. Proc Annu Meet U S Anim Health Assoc 1979;83:92–104.
32. Jones LM, Berman DT. The role of living vaccines in prophylaxis. Dev Biol Stand 1976;31:328–34.
33. Manthei CA. Application of research to bovine brucellosis control and eradication programs. J Dairy Sci 1968;51:1115–20.
34. Al-Khalaf SA, Mohamad BT, Nicoletti P. Control of brucellosis in Kuwait by vaccination of cattle, sheep and goats with *Brucella abortus* strain 19 or *Brucella melitensis* strain Rev. 1. Trop Anim Health Prod 1992;24:45–9.
35. Nicoletti P. The effects of adult cattle vaccination with strain 19 on the incidence of brucellosis in dairy herds in Florida and Puerto Rico. Proc Annu Meet U S Anim Health Assoc 1979;83:75–80.
36. Nicoletti P. A preliminary report on the efficacy of adult cattle vaccination using strain 19 in selected dairy herds in Florida. Proc Annu Meet U S Anim Health Assoc 1976;80:91–100.
37. Corner LA, Alton GG. Persistence of *Brucella abortus* strain 19 infection in adult cattle vaccinated with reduced doses. Res Vet Sci 1981;31:342–4.
38. Cheville NF, Olsen SC, Jensen AE, et al. Effects of age at vaccination on efficacy of *Brucella abortus* strain RB51 to protect cattle against brucellosis. Am J Vet Res 1996;57:1153–6.
39. Poester FP, Goncalves VS, Paixao TA, et al. Efficacy of strain RB51 vaccine in heifers against experimental brucellosis. Vaccine 2006;24:5327–34.
40. Olsen SC. Responses of adult cattle to vaccination with a reduced dose of *Brucella abortus* strain RB51. Res Vet Sci 2000;69:135–40.

41. Van Metre DC, Kennedy GA, Olsen SC, et al. Brucellosis induced by RB51 vaccine in a pregnant heifer. J Am Vet Med Assoc 1999;215:1491–3.
42. Samartino LE, Fort M, Gregoret R, et al. Use of *Brucella abortus* vaccine strain RB51 in pregnant cows after calfhood vaccination with strain 19 in Argentina. Prev Vet Med 2000;45:193–9.
43. Leal-Hernandez M, Diaz-Aparicio E, Perez R, et al. Protection of *Brucella abortus* RB51 revaccinated cows, introduced in a herd with active brucellosis, with presence of atypical humoral response. Comp Immunol Microbiol Infect Dis 2005;28: 63–70.
44. McEwen AD. Experiments on contagious abortion. Immunization studies with vaccines of graded virulence. Vet Rec 1938;50:1097–2002.
45. Sutherland SS, Robertson AG, LeCras DV, et al. The effects of challenge with virulent *Brucella abortus* on beef cattle vaccinated as calves or adults with either *Brucella abortus* strain 19 or 45/20. Aust Vet J 1981;57:470–3.
46. Fiorentino MA, Campos E, Cravero S, et al. Protection levels in vaccinated heifers with experimental vaccines *Brucella abortus* M1-luc and INTA 2. Vet Microbiol 2008;132:302–11.
47. Vemulapalli R, He Y, Sriranganathan N, et al. *Brucella abortus* RB51: enhancing vaccine efficacy and developing multivalent vaccines. Vet Microbiol 2002;90:521–32.
48. Yang X, Becker T, Walters N, et al. Deletion of znuA virulence factor attenuates *Brucella abortus* and confers protection against wild-type challenge. Infect Immun 2006;74:3874–9.
49. Olsen SC, Boyle SM, Schurig GG, et al. Immune responses and protection against experimental challenge after vaccination of bison with *Brucella abortus* strain RB51 or RB51 overexpressing superoxide dismutase and glycosyltransferase genes. Clin Vaccine Immunol 2009;16:535–40.
50. Meyer ME, Meagher M. Brucellosis in free-ranging bison (*Bison bison*) in Yellowstone, Grand Teton, and Wood Buffalo National Parks: a review. J Wildl Dis 1995; 31:579–98.
51. Pac HI, Frey K. Some population characteristics of the northern Yellowstone bison herd during the winter of 1988–1989. Bozeman (MT): Montana Department of Fish, Wildlife, and Parks; 1991. p. 5–11.
52. Rhyan JC, Gidlewski T, Roffe TJ, et al. Pathology of brucellosis in bison from Yellowstone National Park. J Wildl Dis 2001;37:101–9.
53. Davis DS, Templeton JW, Ficht TA, et al. *Brucella abortus* in captive bison. I. Serology, bacteriology, pathogenesis, and transmission to cattle. J Wildl Dis 1990;26:360–71.
54. Toman TT, Lemke T, Kuck L, et al. Elk in the Greater Yellowstone Area: status and management. In: Thorne ET, Bryce MS, Nicoletti P, et al. Brucellosis, bison, elk and cattle in the Greater Yellowstone Area: defining the problem, exploring solutions. Cheyenne (WY): Wyoming Game and Fish Department; 1997. p. 56–64.
55. Claus D, Kilpatrick S, Dean R, et al. Brucellosis-feedground-habitat program: an integrated management approach to brucellosis in elk in Wyoming. In: Kreeger TJ, editor. Proceedings of brucellosis in elk and bison in the Greater Yellowstone Area. Cheyenne (WY): Wyoming Game and Fish Department; 2002. p. 80–96.
56. Etter RP, Drew ML. Brucellosis in elk in eastern Idaho. J Wildl Dis 2006;42:271–8.
57. Greater Yellowstone Interagency Brucellosis Committee. Interspecies transmission of *Brucella abortus*. Available at: www.gyibc.com/reference_Material; 1997. Accessed 2009.

58. Stoffregren WC, Olsen SC, Wheeler CJ, et al. Diagnostic characterization of a feral swine herd enzootically infected with *Brucella*. J Vet Diagn Invest 2007;19: 227–37.
59. Hutton T, DeLiberto T, Owen S, et al. Disease risk associated with increasing feral swine numbers and distribution in the United States. Midwest Assoc.of Fish and Wildlife Agencies. 2006. Available at: www.mich.gov/documents/mda/Hutton_pig_paper_218759_7. Accessed 2009.
60. Pimental D, Lach L, Zuniga R, et al. Environmental and economic costs of nonindigenous species in the United States. BioScience 1999;50:53–65.
61. Muller T, Conrathis FJ, Hahn EC. Pseudorabies virus infection (Aujeszky's disease) in wild swine. Infect Dis Rev 2000;2:27–34.
62. Zygmont SM, Nettles VF, Shotts EB, et al. Brucellosis in wild swine: a serologic and bacteriologic survey in the southeastern United States and Hawaii. J Am Vet Med Assoc 1982;181:1285–7.
63. Gresham CS, Gresham CA, Duffy MJ, et al. Increased prevalence of *B. suis* and pseudorabies virus antibodies in adults of an isolated feral swine population in costal South Carolina. J Wildl Dis 2003;38:653–6.
64. Samaha H, Al-Towaily M, Khoudair RM, et al. Multicenter study of brucellosis in Egypt. Emerg Infect Dis 2008;14:1916–8.
65. Kahler SC. *Brucella melitensis* infection discovered in cattle for first time, goats also infected. J Am Vet Med Assoc 2000;216:648.
66. Bovine brucellosis. In: Linnane S, Pearson JE, editors. Manual of diagnostic tests and vaccines for terrestrial animals. Paris: Office International des Epizooties; 2008. p. 624–59.
67. Dawson CE, Stubberfield EJ, Perrett LL, et al. Phenotypic and molecular characterization of *Brucella* isolates from marine mammals. BMC Microbiol 2008;8:224.
68. Rhyan JC, Gidlewski T, Ewalt DR, et al. Seroconversion and abortion in cattle experimentally infected with *Brucella* sp. isolated from a Pacific harbor seal (*Phoca vitulina richardsi*). J Vet Diagn Invest 2001;13:379–82.
69. Garner MM, Lambouurn DM, Jeffries SJ, et al. Evidence of *Brucella* infection in Parafilaroides lungworms in a Pacific harbor seal (*Phoca vitulina richardsi*). J Vet Diagn Invest 1997;9:298–303.
70. Berkelman RL. Human illness associated with use of veterinary vaccines. Clin Infect Dis 2003;37:407–14.
71. Tikare NV, Mantur BG, Bidari LH. Brucellar meningitis in an infant—evidence for human breast milk transmission. J Trop Pediatr 2008;54:272–4.
72. Franco MP, Mulder M, Gilman RH, et al. Human brucellosis. Lancet Infect Dis 2007;7:775–86.
73. Mantur BG, Amarnath SK, Shinde RS. Review of clinical and laboratory features of human brucellosis. Indian J Med Microbiol 2007;25:188–202.

Attaching-effacing *Escherichia coli* Infections in Cattle

Rodney A. Moxley, DVM, PhD*, David R. Smith, DVM, PhD

KEYWORDS

- *Escherichia coli* • Attaching-effacing *E coli* • Cattle
- Diarrheagenic pathogens

Escherichia coli was first recognized as a cause of diarrhea and septicemia in calves more than 115 years ago.[1] Intestinal infection with *E coli* manifested principally by diarrhea is commonly known as enteric colibacillosis, in contrast to septicemic and enterotoxemic colibacillosis, which are characterized by systemic infection and per-acute collapse.[2,3] Diarrheagenic *E coli* are now broadly placed into 6 classes based on virulence mechanisms.[4,5] One of these classes, enterotoxigenic *E coli* (ETEC), is the most common cause of diarrhea in beef and dairy calves in the first 4 days of life.[3,6] ETEC are characterized principally by the production of fimbriae and entero-toxins, with strains producing K99 (now called F5) fimbria and heat-stable entero-toxin-a (STa) as the main ones causing disease in calves.[3–6] Two other diarrheagenic classes, namely enterohemorrhagic *E coli* (EHEC) and enteropathogenic *E coli* (EPEC), are important causes of disease in human beings, but less well substantiated causes of diarrhea in calves.[3–6]

E coli strains that cause hemorrhagic colitis (HC) and hemolytic uremic syndrome (HUS) in humans, express high levels of Shiga toxin (Stx), cause attaching-effacing (A/E) lesions in intestinal epithelial cells, and possess a specific 60-MDa EHEC plasmid are known as EHEC.[7] Hence, using this original definition, the causation of human illness (HC or HUS) was an obligatory criterion for identification of an isolate as EHEC.[7] One feature EHEC and EPEC have in common is the causation of intestinal epithelial lesions known as attaching and effacing (A/E).[4,5,8] Attaching-effacing *E coli* (AEEC) is a designation for those *E coli* strains known to cause A/E lesions or at least carry the genes for this trait, and therefore include organisms that fall into either the EHEC or EPEC classes.[4,5,8] A distinction between EHEC and EPEC is that the former produce Stx, whereas the latter do not.[4,5] *E coli* strains that produce or carry genes for the production of Stx (also known as Verotoxin or Verocytotoxin [VT], and formerly

School of Veterinary Medicine & Biomedical Sciences, University of Nebraska-Lincoln, Fair Street & East Campus Loop, Lincoln, NE 68583-0905, USA
* Corresponding author.
E-mail address: rmoxley1@unl.edu (R.A. Moxley).

Vet Clin Food Anim 26 (2010) 29–56
doi:10.1016/j.cvfa.2009.10.011
0749-0720/10/$ – see front matter © 2010 Elsevier Inc. All rights reserved.

known as Shigalike toxin [SLT]) have been called Shiga toxin–producing *E coli* (STEC) or Verotoxin-producing *E coli* (VTEC).[4,5,9–13] Mainil and Daube[12] proposed that all *E coli* strains producing or carrying the genes for Stx but not A/E should be called STEC or VTEC, whereas those positive for both should be called EHEC. Unless stated otherwise, this nomenclature is adopted for use in this article. In addition, the term Stx is used instead of SLT or VT, and STEC instead of VTEC.

Cattle are a major reservoir of STEC and EHEC, including the prototype of this class, *E coli* O157:H7, which was the first *E coli* serotype recognized to cause HC and HUS in humans.[13–19] Worldwide, *E coli* O157:H7 is the EHEC serotype most often associated with causation of HUS.[20] EPEC and EHEC strains can belong to more than 1000 O:H serotypes[21]; there are more than 435 serotypes of STEC,[13,21,22] and more than 120 O serogroups of EHEC and STEC[12] have been recovered from cattle. Because cattle are carriers of many different serotypes of EHEC, much emphasis has been placed on the public health and food safety concerns associated with the fecal shedding of these organisms. However, much less emphasis has been given to their roles as diarrheagenic pathogens of cattle. Mainil and Daube[12] noted that certain subgroups are pathogens of cattle; in their review, they indicated that the most important ones causing diarrheal disease in calves were O5:H⁻, O26:H⁻, O26:H11, O111:H⁻, and O118:H6 . In contrast, in a more recent review article on the pathophysiology of calf diarrhea it was stated that the claim that AEEC are pathogens of calves is questionable.[6] The goal of the present article is to address the question of pathogenicity, with a review that focuses on the results of studies of natural and experimental infections with these organisms. The authors' conclusion is that there is overwhelming evidence that many different serogroups of AEEC are diarrheagenic pathogens of calves.

THE ATTACHING-EFFACING LESION

The first report of A/E lesions in any species was in 1969 by Staley and colleagues[23] in a study involving newborn gnotobiotic piglets inoculated with *E coli* O55:B5:H7. The purpose of the study was to demonstrate the "ultramicroscopic sequence of the attachment and penetration of *E coli* into ileal epithelial cells of the neonatal pig." The origin of the *E coli* strain was not stated, but O55:H7 is a classic EPEC of humans, and thought to be the evolutionary precursor of *E coli* O157:H7.[24] The ultrastructural lesions described in the article by Staley and colleagues[23] were bacterial attachment to enterocytes with degeneration and exfoliation of microvilli. These investigators also were particularly interested in bacterial uptake or phagocytosis by enterocytes of the newborn piglet, and this process was extensively described. The existence of different diarrheagenic classes, the importance of ETEC in the causation of porcine enteric colibacillosis, and the association of ETEC with the intestinal epithelium were not known at the time of this publication, nor was it known that pathogenic *E coli* strains might vary in their attachment mechanisms. Ten years later, Moon and colleagues[25] reported that different *E coli* strains vary in the mechanisms they use to associate with the intestinal epithelium. This study contrasted the rather loose adherence of ETEC mediated by pili with that of the *E coli* that tightly attach.[25] At this time, *E coli* that attach had already been described to occur in rabbits.[26] In their article, Moon and colleagues[25] showed a photomicrograph of bacteria attached to the surface of absorptive enterocytes in a typical A/E pattern in the colon of a calf. The investigators hypothesized that these organisms were *E coli*, and stated this could be evidence that a new enteropathogenic type of *E coli*, one that is nonenterotoxigenic and noninvasive, was emerging in cattle and other animal species.

In 1982, Rothbaum and colleagues[27] described the presence of "enterocyte-adherent *E coli*" in biopsies of the jejunum, rectum, or both in human infants with protracted diarrhea. The ultrastructural appearance of the association between bacteria and enterocyte was that of the A/E lesion, and the causative organisms were *E coli* O119:B14, a classic EPEC serotype.[27] In 1983, Moon and colleagues[8] coined the term "attaching and effacing" for the lesion characterized by intimate bacterial attachment and effacement of microvilli, as originally described by Staley and colleagues[23] and later reported to occur in rabbits and humans.[26,27] These investigators also coined the term "attaching-effacing *E coli* (AEEC)" for those *E coli* organisms that cause A/E lesions.[8]

EVIDENCE OF AEEC AS CATTLE PATHOGENS BASED ON STUDIES OF NATURAL AND EXPERIMENTAL DISEASE
Disease in Calves Caused by E coli O5, O26, O111, O118, and O145 Infection

A series of 3 articles describing a dysentery syndrome that occurred in 8- to 21-day-old calves at a research farm in England from the autumn of 1981 until the spring of 1983 were the first reports to confirm the presence of AEEC in cattle.[28–30] On this farm, the syndrome affected calves derived from a herd of Friesian cows that, when 3 days old, had been allocated to an individual pen. During the stated period, 12 of approximately 400 calves that had been allocated to the pen developed dysentery. Dysentery was first seen in calves at 8 to 21 days of age (mean 15 days), and characterized by the passage of copious bright red blood in the feces. Feces became liquid in all dysenteric calves concurrent with or 1 to 5 days before the onset of dysentery. Most calves had no signs of systemic illness at the onset of dysentery, nor pyrexia, and initially, normal appetite was maintained; however, signs of dehydration, dullness, anorexia, reluctance to move, weight loss, and death occurred in some cases. In addition, persistent grinding of the teeth, abdominal distention with pain on palpation, and a noticeable smell of necrotic tissue were recorded in some calves.

In the first attempt to identify the cause of the dysentery syndrome, Chanter and colleagues[28,29] administered intestinal contents and feces from affected calves, or microorganisms isolated from them, to 1-day-old gnotobiotic calves. Inoculated calves passed normal feces for 2 to 4 days after inoculation, and for the next 4 to 7 days (until euthanasia), they passed mucoid, liquid feces containing many small clots of fresh blood. At necropsy, the walls of the colon and rectum were thickened, and there was patchy reddening on the longitudinal folds of the mucosae of the cecum, colon, and rectum. Petechial hemorrhages were numerous and occasionally larger hemorrhages were seen, with clotted blood adherent to the mucosal surface. In some areas, there was an adherent layer of mucus stained with intestinal contents. The production of dysentery and colonic lesions was strongly associated with colonization by an atypical form of *E coli*, designated S102-9. On quantitative bacterial culture, the mucosae of the ileum, colon and rectum contained as many as 10^6, 10^{10}, and 10^9 *E coli*, respectively, and these numbers were approximately 4 times higher than those in the gut lumen. The calves were bacteremic, but bacterial counts in the blood were less than that typically seen with septicemia-inducing *E coli* strains. The majority of biochemical reactions of this organism were typical of *E coli*, but it produced urease, and was anaerogenic and nonmotile; its serotype was O5:K⁻:H⁻. Colonies on MacConkey agar had a characteristic red center and a clear outer zone; the surrounding medium did not exhibit a red precipitate. Strain S102-9 was identified as *E coli*, in particular by its ability to produce acid in MacConkey broth at 44°C and indole at 44°C.

In a separate report from the same study, the etiology was also addressed, but this report focused more on the pathologic changes of the dysentery syndrome.[29] Lesions in calves with the naturally and experimentally produced syndrome were limited to the intestinal tract, although gross lesions in the large intestines of gnotobiotic and farm calves varied.[29] Ceca appeared normal on gross examination except in one farm calf in which it was hyperemic and had undergone intussusception into the colon. Colonic lesions varied from mild patchy reddening with petechial hemorrhages, adherent mucus, and blood clots. No gross lesions were seen in the rectum in any of the calves with the exception of hyperemia of superficial extremities of the longitudinal folds. In the ileum in 4 of 5 farm calves and a gnotobiotic calf, villi were atrophic, fused, and covered by cuboidal or flattened enterocytes. Bacteria were seen in association with irregularly arranged and exfoliated enterocytes in one gnotobiote. There was an increase in the numbers of neutrophils in the lamina propria of the villi of one farm calf, and in the gnotobiote with adherent bacteria. In all calves, cecal lesions were mild; foci of adherent bacteria were associated with clumps of irregularly arranged and exfoliated enterocytes, and increased numbers of neutrophils were seen in the lamina propria. Neutrophils were seen rarely in the crypts, or on the luminal surface.

In all calves, lesions were most severe in the colon and rectum, where there was hyperemia of mucosal capillaries with occasional petechial hemorrhages on the luminal surface. Bacteria appeared to be adherent to the mucosal surface between the mouths of the crypts and sometimes into the crypts for approximately 10% of their length. Adherent bacteria could be seen in sections stained with hematoxylin and eosin, but were more clearly visible in sections stained with Giemsa or in semithin sections of tissue embedded in epoxy resin and stained with toluidine blue. The epithelial surfaces containing adherent bacteria were irregular, due to enterocyte degeneration and exfoliation. The mucosa was often edematous and infiltrated with neutrophils, which also had entered some crypt lumens and exuded onto the luminal surface. The mucosal surface also contained mucus, exfoliated enterocytes, and erythrocytes.

Typical A/E lesions were seen in the colon in farm and gnotobiotic calves by scanning and transmission electron microscopy. Under scanning electron microscopy, the distribution of bacilli on the surfaces of enterocytes was sometimes restricted to intercryptal regions, but in some cases covered the entire surface. Microvilli of infected enterocytes were absent, or were abnormal in orientation or length, either shortened or elongated. Exfoliated enterocytes bearing these changes were also seen on infected surfaces. Bacteria were noted by transmission electron microscopy to be closely associated with the enterocyte cell membrane. At sites of bacterial adherence the microvilli were effaced, and other microvilli not containing adherent bacteria were frequently distorted and disorientated. At the points of bacterial attachment, the enterocyte cytoplasm typically was cup-shaped or arranged as a pedestal.

In histologic sections stained by an immunoperoxidase technique, several enteropathogens in a gnotobiotic calf inoculated with feces were detected, namely rotavirus, coronavirus, E coli S102-9, and Campylobacter spp. In contrast, the 2 gnotobiotic calves inoculated only with E coli (S102-9), confirmed that S102-9 was detectable in sections using the immunoperoxidase method; these calves were not tested for other enteric pathogens. In 3 of the 5 dysenteric farm calves, the mucosal surface of the large intestine contained surface-attached bacteria that stained positively with antiserum to E coli (S102-9). In the other 2 farm calves with dysentery, typical lesions were seen in the large intestine, but bacteria adherent to the mucosal surface did not stain positive with antisera to S102-9.

In a second study, the dysentery syndrome was experimentally induced in 5 4-day-old colostrum-fed calves after inoculation with S102-9.[30] The clinical, microbiological, and pathologic features were essentially the same as those described in the first 2 reports.[28,29] However, in this study immunity and age resistance were investigated; dysentery was not seen following a second challenge in calves that had recovered, nor was it seen in an age-matched calf at 24 days of age, nor in a 51-day-old calf. S102-9 did not produce heat-stable enterotoxin, but did produce a toxin cytopathic for Vero and HeLa cells (ie, Stx). In addition, the investigators also conducted a survey of field cases of calf diarrhea in southern England during the winters of 1981 to 1982 and 1982 to 1983.[30] Of 659 lactose-fermenting bacterial isolates, including 373 from calves with diarrhea, 4 had an atypical colony morphology on MacConkey agar indistinguishable from that of *E coli* S102-9, were anaerogenic and produced urease. Based on other tests, these isolates were identified as *E coli*. The 4 isolates originated from different farms and 3 were isolated from calves with diarrhea. Coronavirus was isolated from one of these calves and *Salmonella typhimurium* from another; the third isolate from a normal calf was designated 6/193, and the fourth from a calf with diarrhea in which other enteropathogens were not detected was designated 37/1. Preliminary serotyping of 37/1 and 6/193 revealed they were O5. Therefore, *E coli* phenotypically indistinguishable from S102-9 was detected in diarrheic calves from other farms in southern England; however, because only 4 of 659 isolates were identical to S102-9, this organism was concluded not to be an important cause of enteric disease in the survey. It was noted that one isolate with these properties had previously been associated with diarrhea in a calf in France.[29,31]

An *E coli* phenotypically very similar to S102-9 was isolated in the United States from a 2-day-old beef calf in Minnesota with nondysenteric diarrhea.[32] The clinical case isolate, 84-5406, was a urease-positive O5:K4:H− *E coli* that produced Stx, but did not produce enterotoxins and was noninvasive; its colony morphology on MacConkey agar was unremarkable. Isolate 84-5406 was sensitive to ampicillin, cephalothin, chloramphenicol, furazolidone, gentamycin, kanamycin, polymyxin B, spectinomycin, sulfasoxazole, and trimethoprim-sulfamethoxazole, and was resistant to penicillin and tetracycline. The calf from which this organism was isolated was co-infected with rotavirus and coronavirus, and had evidence of villous atrophy in the small intestine and diffuse colonization of the colonic epithelium by bacteria typical of AEEC. A conventional colostrum-deprived lamb was inoculated with a pure culture of 84-5406, and this animal developed bloody diarrhea and died within 5 days after inoculation. Histologically, the colon of the lamb was found to be diffusely colonized with bacteria, and the inoculum strain was isolated from this tissue. Three 1-day-old gnotobiotic calves subsequently were inoculated with 84-5406; the calves were checked at 12-hour intervals post inoculation (PI) for anorexia, depression, fever, diarrhea, and the presence of mucus or blood in the feces. The calves developed a mild fever (0.5°C elevation) at 36 hours PI, which peaked (0.9°C increase) at 48 hours PI and fluctuated slightly thereafter for 1 to 3 more days until it returned to normal. The calves became depressed when the temperatures reached 40.0°C, but none became anorectic. Two of the calves developed diarrhea by 36 hours PI. The diarrheic feces were loose, dark green, and mucoid, and by 60 hours PI the feces of one diarrheic calf contained frank blood. The diarrhea in the calf that did not become dysenteric lasted only 24 hours.

At necropsy, hyperemia of the longitudinal folds of the rectum was noted in both the 84-5406 and control calves, and microscopic lesions were limited to the intestines of the former.[32] Bacterial colonization was seen multifocally in the ileum, and diffusely in the large intestine. Bacteria were noted to be closely attached to the surfaces of enterocytes, and many cells with attached bacteria had become necrotic and sloughed into the intestinal lumen. Loss of enterocytes from the surfaces of villi had resulted in villous atrophy in the ileum (**Fig. 1**). Bacterial colonization and enterocyte sloughing in the cecum, colon, and rectum were diffuse (**Fig. 2**), and associated with minimal acute multifocal inflammatory reaction characterized by edema and neutrophilic infiltration in the lamina propria. Bacteria colonizing the intestines were noted to have stained positive with anti-O5 serum when observed by immunofluorescence microscopy. In contrast, the epithelium of the colon and rectum of gnotobiotic calves inoculated with sterile broth is smooth with intact enterocyte junctions and densely packed microvilli (**Figs. 3** and **4**). Under scanning electron microscopy, the colon and rectum in gnotobiotic calves inoculated with 84-5406 were noted to have diffuse AEEC bacterial colonization, causing epithelial sloughing and irregularity of the mucosal surface (**Fig. 5**). On higher magnification, microvillous effacement at sites of intimate bacterial attachment, that is, classic A/E lesions were seen both by scanning (**Fig. 6**) and transmission electron microscopy (**Fig. 7**). Extensive AEEC infection of individual enterocytes resulted in death and sloughing of these cells; this is shown by transmission electron microscopy in a calf infected with 84-5406 (**Fig. 8**). A diagnostic case of natural disease in a calf infected with an unidentified serotype of AEEC is shown histologically in **Fig. 9**. In the diagnostic case shown in **Fig. 9**, bacterial colonization was extensive and had caused death and exfoliation of colonic mucosal epithelial cells. Persistence of bacterial colonization and epithelial sloughing resulted in AEEC bacteria brought into close proximity to the underlying basement membrane.

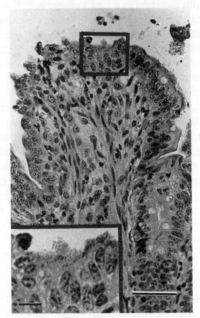

Fig. 1. Light micrograph of ileum from gnotobiotic calf inoculated with *E coli* O5:H⁻ strain 84-5406. There is multifocal enterocyte necrosis and detachment associated with microcolonies of bacteria (*inset*) attached to apical cell membranes. Loss of enterocytes has resulted in villous atrophy (as evidenced by a villus:crypt ratio of 1 in this affected villus). Bar = 100 μm. Inset shows detail of bacterial microcolonies (bar = 5 μm). (*From* Moxley RA, Francis DH. Natural and experimental infection with an attaching and effacing strain of *Escherichia coli* in calves. Infect Immun 1986;53(2):339–46; with permission. Copyright © 1986 American Society for Microbiology.)

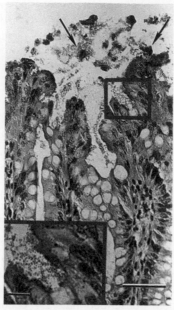

Fig. 2. Light micrograph of rectum from gnotobiotic calf inoculated with *E coli* O5:H⁻ strain 84-5406. Bacterial colonization is diffuse and extensive, with diffuse enterocyte necrosis and detachment (*arrows*). Colonization is mainly on the mucosal surface in intercryptal regions (denoted in scanning electron micrographs as ridges) and crypt openings; bacterial colonization deep into the crypts is not seen. Bar = 100 μm. Inset shows detail of bacterial microcolonies (bar = 5 μm). (*From* Moxley RA, Francis DH. Natural and experimental infection with an attaching and effacing strain of *Escherichia coli* in calves. Infect Immun 1986;53(2):339–46; with permission. Copyright © 1986 American Society for Microbiology.)

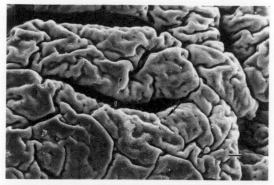

Fig. 3. Scanning electron photomicrograph of colon of a gnotobiotic calf that was sham-inoculated with sterile trypticase soy broth when 24 hours old and euthanized 7 days later. The mucosal surface is smooth and completely devoid of microbial flora. The mucosal surface is arranged in ridges (r) separated by furrows (f), into which crypts (not seen at this magnification) open. Small circular holes on the mucosal surface (*arrow*) demarcate pits created by goblet cells that have discharged their mucus. Hexagonal outlines of enterocytes (*arrowhead*) are evident at this magnification (original negative magnification ×500; bar = 20 μm).

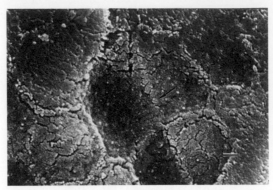

Fig. 4. Higher magnification scanning electron photomicrograph of colon of sham-inoculated gnotobiotic calf. Microvilli are seen as a dense mat on the surfaces of enterocytes. Outlines of enterocytes (*arrow*) appear as slight ridges (original negative magnification ×5000; bar = 1 μm).

Loss of epithelium had resulted in enteric mucosal atrophy and hemorrhage. Subsequent to the reports of S102-9 and 84-5406, other studies of natural and experimental AEEC infections in calves were reported in different countries.

Pospischil and colleagues[33] described naturally occurring AEEC infections in a retrospective study of the intestines of 3 calves in West Germany. The calves had diarrhea and catarrhal enteritis, and 2 were on a combined experimental rotavirus and ETEC study. Two of the calves were 7 days old and one was 23 days old. At necropsy, all 3 had catarrhal enteritis or gastroenteritis, and other complicating lesions. Histologically, there was diffuse atrophy and focal fusion affecting villi in the mid- and distal jejunum, and ileum. A/E bacteria were detected in the ileum, cecum and colon of all 3 calves, but were not seen in the proximal jejunum, mid-jejunum, or distal jejunum. Jejunal, ileal, and colonic epithelium of one calf contained numerous *Cryptosporidium*. A heavy layer of bacteria was seen in the cecum and colon, and on

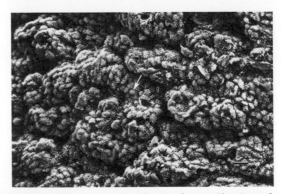

Fig. 5. Scanning electron photomicrograph of colon from calf 7 days after oral inoculation with strain 84-5406. The mucosal surface is roughened due to rounding and detachment of enterocytes, and diffuse bacterial attachment to the apical surfaces of these cells. Microvilli are visible; an individual enterocyte that has undergone rounding and is in the process of detachment is denoted by an arrow. Ridges (r) have atrophied due to cell loss, and in this figure are approximately one-half the width of that of the control calf. Furrows (f) demarcate boundaries of ridges, as in the control (original negative magnification ×500; bar = 20 μm).

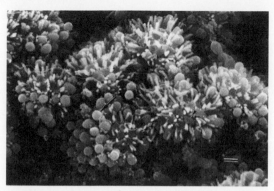

Fig. 6. Higher magnification scanning electron photomicrograph of colon shown in previous figure. Strain 84-5406 bacteria (*arrow*) cover the apical cell membranes of enterocytes. Cuplike or pedestal-like distortions of the apical cell membranes (*arrowhead*) are present at sites were bacteria were detached during tissue processing. Microvilli between attached bacterial cells are prominent and elongated. Enterocytes are swollen and are in the process of detachment from the mucosal surface (original negative magnification ×5000; bar = 1 μm). (*From* Moxley RA, Francis DH. Natural and experimental infection with an attaching and effacing strain of *Escherichia coli* in calves. Infect Immun 1986;53(2):339–46; with permission. Copyright © 1986 American Society for Microbiology.)

transmission electron microscopy, typical A/E lesions were seen. One *E coli* isolate from the colon of one calf, identified as O23:K⁻:NM, produced Stx.

Schoonderwoerd and colleagues[34] reported 2 natural cases of AEEC infection of 5-week-old veal calves with a Stx-producing *E coli* O111:NM isolate, and experimental reproduction of disease with the isolate in a colostrum-deprived calf. Natural infection was characterized by pseudomembranous ileitis, and mucohemorrhagic colitis and proctitis. The calves also had evidence of systemic infection with increased fluid

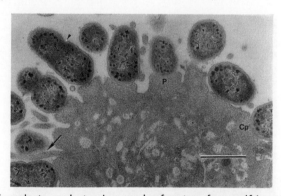

Fig. 7. Transmission electron photomicrograph of rectum from calf inoculated with strain 84-5406. The attachment of bacteria to this enterocyte results primarily in pedestal-like cell membrane evagination (P), with occasional cuplike invagination (Cp). Microvilli between sites of bacterial attachment are elongated (*arrow*). Some bacteria are in the process of binary fission (*arrowhead*). The cytoplasm lacks a discernible terminal web and contains numerous vacuoles (original negative magnification ×15,000; bar = 1 μm). (*From* Moxley RA, Francis DH. Natural and experimental infection with an attaching and effacing strain of *Escherichia coli* in calves. Infect Immun 1986;53(2):339–46; with permission. Copyright © 1986 American Society for Microbiology.)

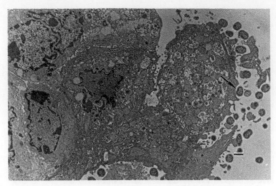

Fig. 8. Transmission electron photomicrograph of rectum from calf inoculated with strain 84-5406. An enterocyte containing many attached bacteria is necrotic, and in the process of sloughing from the mucosal surface. An individual attached bacterial cell is denoted by an arrow. Bacteria reside on pedestals, but bacterial release into the intestinal lumen is evident, some with bacteria still attached to fragmented remains of enterocytes (original negative magnification ×3000; bar = 1 μm).

and fibrin strands in some joints, a mild diffuse fibrinous peritonitis, swelling and hemorrhage in the kidneys, and enlargement of the mesenteric lymph nodes. Histologically, in the ileum there was villous atrophy in association with bacterial adherence, epithelial sloughing, fibrinosuppurative inflammation, and hemorrhage. Similar lesions were seen in the colon. Adherent bacteria in the ileum and colon stained positive with *E coli* O111 antiserum by immunohistochemistry. Cultures of the ileum and colon of both calves yielded a heavy growth of *E coli* O111:NM, which on further testing was shown to produce high levels of Stx. The *E coli* isolates were urease negative and unremarkable with regard to colony morphology. The isolates were resistant to

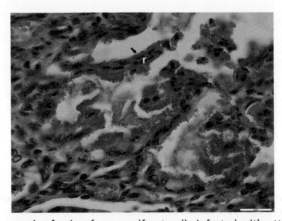

Fig. 9. Light micrograph of colon from a calf naturally infected with attaching-effacing *E coli*. AEEC had in this case had colonized both the small and large intestines. Bacterial proliferation has resulted in the formation of dense mats of organisms in intimate contact with the epithelium. Bacterial colonization extends to the depths of some crypts. Enterocytes with adherent bacteria have undergone atrophy. Sloughing of infected enterocytes has further resulted in atrophy of the ridges (r), with bacteria coming in close proximity to the basement membrane (*arrow*). Bar = 20 μm.

ampicillin, carbenicillin, sulfasoxazole, tetracycline, trimethoprim-sulfamethoxazole, and spectinomycin, and sensitive to chloramphenicol, gentamicin, neomycin, kanamycin, and nitrofurantoin. A 4-day-old colostrum-deprived Holstein bull calf that was negative for pathogens was inoculated orally with the *E coli* O111:NM isolate. The rectal temperature increased to 40°C on day 4 PI, and remained elevated until the next day when the calf was euthanized; the calf did not develop diarrhea during the 5-day PI period. At necropsy, the mesenteric lymph nodes were moderately enlarged, and the contents of the cecum and proximal colon were watery. Histologically, villous atrophy was seen in the duodenum, jejunum, and ileum. Bacterial adherence was detected only in the large intestine, more so in the colon than the cecum, and was associated with sloughing of mucosal epithelial cells and acute purulent inflammation. Adherent bacteria stained positive with anti-O111 serum by immunohistochemistry, and typical A/E lesions were detected in the large intestine by scanning and transmission electron microscopy. No evidence of bacterial invasion into the intestinal epithelium was detected.

Mainil and colleagues[35] tested 429 *E coli* isolates from calves younger than 1 month for the production of HeLa cell cytotoxins. The isolates came from calves that had enteric disease or systemic disease thought to have been caused by *E coli*. HeLa cell cytotoxic activity that was neutralizable with monoclonal antibodies to Stx1 or Stx2 were concluded to be due to those respective toxins; 4 isolates produced Stx1 and 1 produced Stx2. Four of the 5 isolates were typeable, and 1 each was found to be O26ab, O26, O22, and O111. Calves were experimentally inoculated with 2 of these isolates. The calves, when younger than 1 day, were allowed to suckle the dam, and then removed. Nine were inoculated when 5 to 10 days old; 6 calves were inoculated with isolate 1625 (O26:K⁻:H11, Stx1+), and the other 3 calves were inoculated with the nontypeable isolate, 211 (Rough:K?:H11, Stx2+). Isolate 1625 had been shown to cause A/E lesions in 4 of 6 inoculated rabbit loops, whereas isolate 211 did not induce A/E lesions in any of 6 inoculated rabbit loops. None of the calves inoculated with either isolate developed gross lesions in their alimentary tracts, and none developed diarrhea. Six of the calves were euthanized and necropsied, one from each strain inoculation group at 5, 7, and 9 days PI. The geometric mean viable *E coli* counts in the intestines for all calves combined were calculated. Bacterial counts in the intestines were 7×10^3 per 5-cm segment from the ileum, and 2×10^5 per 5-cm segment from the spiral colon. No microscopic lesions were seen in the intestinal tracts of any of the 3 calves inoculated with isolate 211, nor were they seen in the calf that was necropsied on day 9 after inoculation with strain 1625. However, spiral and pelvic colons from the 2 calves inoculated with isolate 1625 and examined at 5 or 7 days PI had a few focal lesions characteristic of those produced by AEEC. Lesions in the calves were qualitatively similar to those described in the calf from which strain 1625 was isolated originally, but were fewer in number and smaller in diameter. Presence of AEEC was confirmed by electron microscopy. Mainil and colleagues[35] concluded that increased Stx production and AEEC activity occur together in some *E coli* isolates from calves in the United States. However, the prevalence of such isolates in the collection studied was low. The bacteria apparently did not colonize well, and the A/E lesions induced in this study were not extensive enough to cause diarrhea. The AEEC lesions in the calf naturally infected with isolate 1625 were more numerous than those in the experimentally infected calves. Mainil and colleagues[35] noted that the isolate, which had been stored frozen for nearly 20 years before the study, might have lost virulence during storage, or the calves may have been immune or genetically resistant to the isolate.

Janke and colleagues[36,37] described natural cases of AEEC infections of calves presented to 2 veterinary diagnostic laboratories in South Dakota and Minnesota. Sixty cases of AEEC infection were detected from 59 farms in 7 states (South Dakota, Minnesota, Iowa, Nebraska, North Dakota, Wisconsin, and Michigan). Eighty-seven percent were dairy calves; 82% were Holstein or Holstein crossbreds. Diarrhea was the predominant clinical sign in calves with AEEC infection, with blood seen in the feces in 48% of the cases. However, 73% of the calves were infected concurrently with other enteric pathogens (cryptosporidia, rotavirus, coronavirus, ETEC, bovine viral diarrhea virus, and other coccidia). In 27% of the cases, AEEC was the only enteric pathogen identified. The age range of the calves was 2 days to 4 months, and the average age, excluding the 4-month-old animal, was 11.8 days. Eighty-eight percent of the calves were 2 to 21 days old; over half (51.7%) were 7 to 14 days old, and 36.6% were 2 to 6 or 15 to 21 days old (18.3% in each group). In 23.3% of the cases, extraintestinal lesions, such as pneumonia, arthritis, septicemia, and peritonitis, were detected. STEC were recovered from 31 of 46 calves; serotyping studies were conducted on 17 Stx-producing isolates. The predominant serotype was O111:NM; of 17 isolates, 9 (52.9%) were O111, 3 (17.6%) were O5:NM, 1 (5.9%) was O26:NM, and 4 (23.5%) were nontypeable. Fifteen of 60 calves (25%) at necropsy had grossly evident congestion and hemorrhage of the intestinal mucosa, and lesions were most pronounced in the large intestine. In 14 of 60 calves (23.3%), the feces were bloody. In the most severe cases, there was diffuse hyperemia and focal hemorrhage of the colonic mucosa, and the contents of the colon were blood-tinged with clots, necrotic debris, and mucus. In 2 calves, the cecum was hemorrhagic. Under light microscopy, A/E bacterial adherence to the intestinal mucosa was detected in the large intestine only in 34 of 60 calves (56.7%); in the small intestine only in 7 of 60 (11.7%); and in both locations in 19 of 60 (31.7%). Hence, A/E bacterial attachment was seen in the large intestine in 53 of 60 calves (88.3%). The investigators postulated that the reason for the preponderance of dairy calves in the study was because most were immunodeficient due to inadequate colostral intake.

Dorn and colleagues[38] characterized STEC isolates obtained during 1983 to 1989 from calves with diarrhea submitted as cases to diagnostic laboratories in South Dakota and Minnesota; an unspecified proportion of these isolates originated from previously published studies.[32,36,37] Thirty-six STEC isolates, each from a different calf, were identified for the study. These isolates came predominantly from calves designated as dairy or dairy-crossbred; only 4 of the isolates were from beef or beef-crossbred calves. One calf was 3 months old and all others of known age were less than 3 weeks old. Thirty-two of the 36 calves had bacteria colonizing the intestines and diarrhea, 3 had colonization with no observed diarrhea, and 1 had diarrhea but colonization was obscured by postmortem autolysis. Thirteen of the calves were observed by histopathology to have lesions of the colon. Twelve of the calves were observed to have bloody diarrhea. All 36 isolates fermented sorbitol within 24 hours. Twenty-one isolates were serogroup O111; 4 were O5, 2 were O26, 2 were O45, 1 was O69, 2 were O103, and 4 were nontypeable. The 4 O5:NM and 2 other isolates did not ferment raffinose. All but one isolate, 84-5406 (O5:NM),[32] hybridized with a probe for the 60-MDa EHEC plasmid. Thirty-two isolates hybridized with the stx_1 probe, 3 hybridized with both the stx_1 and stx_2 probes, and 1 (isolate 84-5406) hybridized with neither probe. The verotoxigenic activity of isolate 84-5406 was partially neutralized by monoclonal antibodies against Stx1.

At least 2 studies have provided evidence that non-Stx-producing AEEC are pathogens of calves and typically infect both the small and large intestines. Pearson and colleagues[39] reported the detection of AEEC in the small and large intestines of a 3-week-old calf with yellow, watery diarrhea. The calf had no evidence of blood in the intestines or feces, and no pathogens other than the AEEC were isolated. AEEC were detected by transmission electron microscopy of specimens obtained surgically under general anesthesia. Histologically, AEEC were detected in the proximal jejunum, lower jejunum, ileum, cecum, and colon. The bacteria stained positively by an immunohisto-chemical procedure using antiserum raised against an *E coli* recovered from the calf; however, they did not stain using antiserum to S102-9, the O5:NM Stx1-producing AEEC previously reported.[28–30] Affected areas of small intestine colonized with the AEEC had sloughing of enterocytes with villous atrophy, villous fusion, and inflammation of the mucosa characterized by infiltration with neutrophils and plasma cells. Lesions in the small intestine were most severe in the ileum. AEEC bacterial adherence and epithelial sloughing were also seen in the cecum and colon. By electron microscopy, typical A/E lesions and pedestal formation were seen in affected areas in the small and large intestines. The serotype of *E coli* isolated from this calf was not reported; however, it was a non-Stx-producer. Fischer and colleagues[40] detected a non-Stx-producing AEEC O26:NM isolate (7996-90) as the sole pathogen isolated from a 14-day-old Simmental calf with diarrhea. The isolate did not produce enterotoxins, Stx, or ETEC fimbriae, and was genotypically negative for the EPEC adherence factor (bundle forming pili), but it induced localized adherence in HEp-2 cells. In addition, it induced A/E lesions in Caco-2 (human colonic carcinoma cells), rabbit intestinal loops, and large intestines of gnotobiotic piglets.[40] The lack of Stx production, coupled with localized adherence on HEp-2 cells and induction of A/E lesions, were taken as conclusive evidence that the isolate was an EPEC.

Wray and colleagues[41] inoculated colostrum-fed and colostrum-deprived neonatal calves 1 of 2 *E coli* isolates that produced either Stx1 or Stx2. The Stx1+ isolate A56 was O26:K60:H11, and the Stx2+ isolate A52 was O8:K85:H9. Five calves at the time of inoculation were 1 day old, and the remaining 4 were 2, 4, 16, or 17 days old. Only calves that were colostrum-deprived and 1 day old when inoculated developed A/E lesions or diarrhea. Both A56 and A52 induced A/E lesions in the small and large intestines in respective calves. Three of 4 colostrum-deprived calves developed anorexia, a slight elevation in rectal temperature (<1°C), and diarrhea with blood and mucus in their feces. At necropsy, they had hyperemia of the mucosa of the ileum and colon and enlargement of the mesenteric lymph nodes. Histologically, both A56 and A52 induced villous atrophy in the ileum secondary to bacterial colonization and epithelial cell sloughing. Typical A/E lesions were seen in the ileum and colon by transmission electron microscopy with both strains. The investigators noted that this was the first report of a Stx2+ *E coli* being associated with disease in calves. However, what was perhaps more important was the demonstration of an apparently protective effect of age and colostrum in AEEC infections.

Stordeur and colleagues[42] isolated an *E coli* O118:H6 strain (340S89) from a 2-week-old Friesian calf that died of diarrhea. The strain was gene probe positive for intimin and Stx1, and caused A/E lesions in rabbits. In an attempt to reproduce disease with the strain, 4 naturally born calves that were isolated immediately after birth, and then were washed, disinfected, and fed colostrum were used. The colostrum was demonstrated to lack agglutinating antibodies against strain 340S89. At 6 hours of age, 3 of the calves were inoculated orally with strain 340S89, and at 44 or 64 hours PI they were euthanized. One calf that was not inoculated was used as a control. The 3 calves inoculated with 340S89 developed mild hyperthermia and nonbloody diarrhea at 24 hours PI; the control calf did not develop diarrhea or other clinical signs of disease. Strain 340S89 was re-isolated from the feces of the 3 inoculated calves, but not from the control calf. The 3 inoculated calves developed A/E lesions in the large intestine or both the small and large intestines, and a neutrophilic-lymphocytic enterocolitis.

Sandhu and Gyles[43] compared the pathologic effects of STEC that vary in their association with bovine and human disease. The pathogenicity of STEC serotypes associated with both dysentery in calves and HUS in humans (O5:H⁻, O26:H11, O111:H⁻, O113:H21) were compared with that of STEC O157:H7, which is associated with HUS in humans but less well documented disease in calves. The STEC were administered into ligated loops in the ileum and colon of 4 2- to 6-day-old calves. Strains of all serotypes tested except O113:H21, that is, O5:H⁻, O26:H11, O111:H⁻, O113:H21, and O157:H7, adhered focally to enterocytes and caused A/E lesions in both the ileum and colon. Acute neutrophilic inflammation was seen in inoculated loops, and these lesions were generally more severe in the ileum than the colon. Although the investigators did not discuss it, these results suggest that many different AEEC regardless of serotype are generally capable of causing A/E lesions in either the small or large intestine if present in high enough dosage, for example, enough to over-come immunity, and for long enough to make contact with mucosal enterocytes (eg, conditions present in a ligated gut loop).

Disease in Older Cattle Caused by AEEC Infection

There are at least 3 reports in the literature of older calves or adult cattle having entero-colitis and dysentery in association with AEEC infection. Janke and colleagues[36,37] described a case in a 4-month-old dairy calf in the Midwestern United States. However, the most remarkable cases were reports of fatal disease in a 19-month-old cow in Japan,[44] and another in an 8-month-old heifer in the United Kingdom.[45]

Wada and colleagues[44] reported that a 19-month-old Holstein cow manifested mu-cohemorrhagic diarrhea, anorexia, and depression after being out on a public pasture for approximately 2.5 weeks. This cow was shedding coccidial oocysts (300 per gram of feces) and was given sulfadimethoxine and Ringer solution intravenously; however, the aforementioned clinical signs continued, and the animal was euthanized. At necropsy, a large amount of bloody contents with mucus was present in the colon, and the mucosa contained petechial hemorrhages. The mesenteric lymph nodes were enlarged. Histologically, the mucosal epithelium in the colon was irregular and numerous gram-negative bacteria were notably adhered to the surfaces of entero-cytes. The lamina propria was hyperemic or hemorrhagic and contained a neutrophilic infiltrate. The intestinal crypts were dilated with mucus and the colonic lumen con-tained necrotic enterocytes, mucus, and erythrocytes. A small number of coccidia were detected in the mucosa. No lesions were seen in other parts of the alimentary tract. By immunohistochemistry, the adherent bacteria stained positive for *E coli* O15 antigen. AEEC and A/E lesions were found in the colonic tissue by transmission and scanning electron microscopy. The O15 *E coli* was not detected by culture of the rectal contents, and other tests for enteric pathogens on tissues, namely, BVD virus and *Salmonella*, were negative. *E coli* O15 is a classic EPEC serotype that causes disease naturally in rabbits (eg, strain RDEC-1) and experimentally in pigs.[8]

Pearson and colleagues[45] reported that a group of 40, 8- to 12-month old heifers in the United Kingdom developed diarrhea, and 6 developed dysentery within 1 month after being turned out to pasture in May. One 8-month-old heifer became severely ill within 5 days after the onset of diarrhea, and did not respond to antibiotic therapy. This animal collapsed, passing liquid and bloody feces, with pale mucous membranes and a hematocrit of 9.6%. The rest of the heifers responded to potentiated sulfon-amide and oral fluid therapy, and recovered. The heifer that collapsed was euthanized and immediately necropsied. A blood clot was present in the lumen of the distal portion of the small intestine, which extended anteriorly for approximately 2 meters from the ileo-ceco-colic junction. The cecum and colon had liquid contents with small blood clots. No ulcers or sites of origin of hemorrhage in the gastrointestinal tract were visible at necropsy. *E coli* O26:K60, a known pathogenic serotype, was isolated from a sample of feces of one of the heifers, although not from the animal that was necropsied. By polymerase chain reaction (PCR), the isolate was positive for stx_1, stx_2, β-intimin, enterohemolysin, and other EHEC virulence factors. Histologically, the necropsied heifer had neutrophilic enteritis with atrophy and fusion of villi, and presence of hemosiderin-laden macrophages in the mucosa of the duodenum and ileum. The colonic mucosa contained an inflammatory infiltrate; the mucosal epithelium was irregular but intact, and colonized with bacteria on the surface. The attached bacteria stained positive for O26 antigen by immunohistochemistry. Tissue from this area excised from paraffin blocks was found to have AEEC and A/E lesions by transmission electron microscopy.

Disease in Calves Caused by E coli O157:H7 and O157:NM Infection

Diarrhea and enteritis have been associated with naturally occurring *E coli* O157:H7 infections in 1- to 3-week-old calves in Argentina, England, and South Korea.[46–48] In 1977 Ørskov and colleagues[46] isolated 3 *E coli* O157:H7 strains from the feces of a calf with enteric colibacillosis in Argentina. The exact age of this animal apparently was not determined, but was stated to be between 1 and 3 weeks. All 3 isolates were later shown to produce Stx. Ørskov and colleagues stated that although this study included only 1 diseased animal, the predominance of this serotype in the calf with diarrhea may suggest an association with disease. Further, they noted that the isolation of *E coli* O157:H7 from this calf was support for the hypothesis that cattle are a reservoir of the organism for humans. Numerous other studies later demonstrated this to be the case, as reported in many different primary research articles and summarized in review articles.[4,5,10–19]

A second report of natural association with *E coli* O157:H7 and disease in a neonatal calf was that by Daniel and colleagues[47] in the United Kingdom. These investigators isolated *E coli* O157:H7 "in pure profuse growth" from the intestine of a 6-day-old suckling calf that had developed dysentery while at pasture and died. The calf had been treated with potentiated sulfonamide boluses and oral fluid therapy. At necropsy, the calf had necrotizing enteritis, hyperemia of the mucosa of the cecum and colon, and blood-tinged fluid and cellular debris in the intestines. The calf also had a thickened umbilicus, hemorrhage from the mesenteric blood vessels along their junction with the small intestine, and enlarged mesenteric lymph nodes. The investigators noted the "calf had received an adequate intake of colostrum." Unfortunately, the intestines were not examined histologically due to advanced postmortem autolysis. The *E coli* O157:H7 isolate from the necropsied calf produced Stx2. One month later, on a return visit to the farm, rectal swabs were taken from 47 cows and 47 calves, and subsequently, Stx2+ *E coli* O157:H7 was isolated from 7 of these calves. Three of the 7 calves were 2 months old and shared a pen. The other 4 calves were 5 to 7 months old, and 2 of these shared a pen. Further testing revealed that the original isolate and 4 others were of the Stx2c subtype, and had identical pulsed field gel electrophoresis profiles.

Dean-Nystrom and colleagues[49–51] demonstrated by experimental inoculation that *E coli* O157:H7 can cause A/E lesions, enterocolitis and diarrhea in both colostrum-deprived and colostrum-fed neonatal calves, and A/E lesions without diarrhea in 3- to 4-month-old weaned calves. In addition, they demonstrated that intimin expression by the infecting organism is necessary for the formation of A/E lesions and subsequent colonization.[50] Dean-Nystrom and colleagues[49] reported, "EHEC O157:H7 pathogenicity in cattle appears to be age related, even within the neonatal period." The virulence of EHEC O157:H7 bacteria was greater in calves inoculated when less than 12 hours old than in those 30 to 36 hours old. All calves inoculated when less than 12 hours old were colostrum-deprived, whereas calves inoculated when 30 to 36 hours old were either colostrum-fed or colostrum-deprived. Both calves less than 12 hours old and those 30 to 36 hours old at the time of inoculation developed diarrhea and A/E lesions in the small and large intestines by 18 hours PI; however, the virulence was greater in the younger calves as evidenced by the greater extent of A/E lesions in these animals. Some calves inoculated when less than 12 hours old were allowed to survive until 3 days PI, and by this time the severity of diarrhea and inflammation, and the frequency and extent of A/E lesions had increased compared with those euthanized at 18 hours PI. The colostrum was shown to contain antibodies against O157 lipopolysaccharide and Stx1, but not Stx2. Both colostrum-fed and colostrum-deprived calves inoculated with strain 3081, which is gene probe positive for stx_1 and stx_2 (as well as the intimin gene eae and CVD419, the EHEC plasmid), developed A/E lesions. Two of 3 colostrum-deprived calves compared with 1 of 4 colostrum-fed calves developed diarrhea. Calves with the most severe lesions had necrotizing, fibrinosuppurative enterocolitis associated with A/E lesions and enterocyte sloughing. Lesions were severe enough in one calf to cause severe dehydration and death by day 2 PI; this calf had been inoculated when less than 12 hours old. Collectively, A/E lesions in different calves were found in the jejunum, ileum, colon, and rectum.

Dean-Nystrom and colleagues[51] inoculated 3- to 4-month-old weaned calves with E coli O157:H7 and found that the rectum was the major site of colonization. A/E lesions were seen in the rectum and cecum of calves with the highest levels of E coli O157:H7. These investigators hypothesized that E coli O157:H7 causes A/E lesions in older calves like those in neonatal calves, but these were not detected in earlier studies because intestinal levels of this organism at necropsy were too low (ie, <10^6 colony-forming units [CFU]/g of tissue) for focally distributed microscopic lesions to be detected. Because fasted ruminants were known to shed higher numbers of E coli and other enteric pathogens than well-fed animals,[52] Dean-Nystrom and colleagues[51] fasted 4-month-old weaned calves for 48 hours before inoculation with EHEC O157:H7 strain 86-24 to increase intestinal levels of EHEC O157:H7 at necropsy. Fasted calves were inoculated via stomach tube with 10^{10} CFU of E coli O157:H7 (9 calves) or nonpathogenic E coli strain (3 calves), necropsied at 4 days PI, and examined histologically. Nine of 9 calves inoculated with E coli O157:H7 and 2 of 3 calves inoculated with nonpathogenic E coli developed watery diarrhea by 18 hours and 3 days after inoculation, respectively. However, 5 calves infected with E coli O157:H7 and both of the diarrheic control calves had coccidia (based on histology). The occurrence of diarrhea in calves inoculated with E coli O157:H7 2 days earlier than in control calves may have been evidence that this organism contributes to diarrhea in some weaned calves. At 4 days PI, higher numbers of inoculated bacteria were recovered from the intestines of weaned calves inoculated with E coli O157:H7 than from the control calves. Multifocal A/E lesions were found in the rectum of 3 calves inoculated with E coli O157:H7 and also in the cecum of 2 of these calves. These lesions were similar to those in neonatal calves; however, the extent of intestinal damage in the rectum and cecum in weaned calves infected with E coli O157:H7 was less than that in similarly infected neonatal calves. No A/E bacteria were found in the spiral colon or ileum of any of the E coli O157:H7 infected calves or in any site in control calves. The A/E bacteria were identified as E coli O157:H7 by immunoperoxidase staining with anti-E coli O157:H7 serum. The calves that had A/E bacteria had higher numbers of

E coli O157:H7 bacteria in the rectum and cecum than did calves in which no lesions were found. A/E bacteria were found in the 3 calves that had greater than 10^6 CFU of *E coli* O157:H7 per gram of rectal tissue, but not in those with lower counts. Two of the 3 calves with rectal lesions that had greater than 10^5 CFU of *E coli* O157:H7 per gram of cecal tissue also had A/E bacteria in the cecum. Coccidia were seen in the intestinal mucosa of 2 of the 3 calves that had A/E bacteria. These studies clearly demonstrated that weaned calves, like neonatal calves, are colonized by *E coli* O157:H7 (ie, have higher intestinal levels of inoculated bacteria at 4 days PI than do calves inoculated with a nonpathogenic control *E coli* strain) and are susceptible to intestinal damage induced by *E coli* O157:H7. High bacterial counts and A/E lesions were found only in the rectum and cecum and only in some of the calves inoculated with *E coli* O157:H7. Dean-Nystrom and colleagues[50] hypothesized that the rectum and cecum may be the principal sites of *E coli* O157:H7 colonization during the carrier-shedder state in cattle.

Escherichia coli O157:H7 Infection as a Cause of Subclinical Disease in Cattle

Naylor and colleagues[53] identified lymphoid-follicle dense mucosa at the terminal rectum as the principal site of colonization of EHEC O157:H7 in cattle, and later demonstrated the presence of A/E lesions at this location and the requirement for bacterial gene products that mediate these effects at that location.[54] In the first study,[53] colonization of the terminal rectum was detected in a 12-month-old steer that had been naturally infected, and also in experimentally infected 8- to 14-week-old calves. In the second study,[54] A/E lesions were demonstrated in 3- and 5-month-old experimentally infected calves, and the same 12-month-old naturally infected steer as the one reported previously.[53] The identification of the terminal rectum as the principal site for EHEC O157:H7 bacterial colonization and A/E lesion formation may explain why, with few exceptions,[51,55–57] these lesions were not detected in intestinal tissue in studies involving 5-day-old gnotobiotic[58] or conventional neonates and young (2–8-week-old) calves,[59–61] or cattle older than this infected with EHEC O157:H7.[60] In only one other study[51] had rectal tissue from an older (in this case 3–4-month-old) inoculated animal been examined, and in only one study had tissue from the rectum from adult cattle been shown to be susceptible to *E coli* O157:H7-induced A/E lesions; and this was in explants, not live animals.[55] Hence, the studies by Naylor and colleagues[53,54] were the first to show A/E lesions in a live, naturally infected adult (12-month-old) bovine, and first to show they were limited to the terminal rectum.

Although the terminal rectum was shown to be the principal site of *E coli* O157:H7 in cattle, in the same study Naylor and colleagues[53] found that the rumen, small intestine and proximal colon, and cecum, the last immediately distal to the ileocecal valve, are minor sites of colonization. In 2 of 54 animals studied, colonization was detected in these other sites. These findings are consistent with the results of previous experimental inoculation studies.[60,61] Other studies have demonstrated that small intestinal (ileal) tissue of conventional calves older than neonates is susceptible to A/E lesions with *E coli* O157:H7 when inoculated into ligated loops. The age of the calves in most of these studies ranged from 28 to 38 days[57,62,63]; however, as noted previously, ligated ileal loops of conventional neonatal (2- to 6-day-old) calves[44] also support these lesions. Ileal explants from an adult cow similarly were susceptible to A/E lesions.[56]

Because the ligated loop and explant models involved inoculation of a small area of tissue with a relatively great inoculum level, the development of A/E lesions in these tissues, which sometimes are not considered a major colonization site in vivo (eg, small intestine), suggest bacterial dosage may potentially be a significant factor affecting whether A/E lesions develop in the intact host. Vlisidou and colleagues[57] reported an interesting observation in that the neuroendocrine hormone norepinephrine augmented *E coli* O157:H7-induced enteritis and adherence in the bovine calf ligated ileal loop model, and these effects were dependent on the ability of *E coli* O157:H7 to induce A/E lesions. Epinephrine and norepinephrine cross-talk with a bacterial quorum-sensing system regulating expression of genes that encode for numerous protein virulence factors involved in colonization, for example, the type III secreted proteins and flagellum.[64] Quorum-sensing is a mechanism that the bacteria use to sense the density of their species in an environment and colonize an area like the mucosal surface. Quorum-sensing is an intriguing area of research currently under investigation with regard to mechanisms by which EHEC O157:H7 and other AEEC colonize and cause disease.

Other studies have demonstrated that inflammation, innate immune responses, and systemic and mucosal antibody responses occur in response to *E coli* O157:H7 colonization and infection of the intestinal mucosa in cattle of various ages, including adults, and these findings are now taken as evidence that this organism is a pathogen of the bovine host. Bretschneider and colleagues[65-67] demonstrated that adult cattle (mean age, 16 months) orally inoculated with *E coli* O157:H7 and shedding this organism in their feces developed antigen-specific IgA and IgG rectal mucosal and IgG serum antibodies to O157 lipopolysaccharide, and to type III secreted proteins known to be involved in A/E lesion formation, namely EspA, EspB, and the translocated intimin receptor (Tir). Collectively, Dean-Nystrom and colleagues,[50] Cornick and colleagues,[68] Naylor and colleagues,[54] and Vlisidou and colleagues,[63] through the use of bacterial constructs containing deletions in genes encoding intimin (*eae*) and type III secreted proteins, namely Tir (*tir*), demonstrated that the A/E attachment mechanism mediated by these gene products plays a critical role in colonization of the bovine intestine, including the terminal rectum. Bretschneider and colleagues[66] reported that *E coli* O157:H7 strains that expressed reduced amounts of H7 flagellin protein including those that were completely nonflagellated did not effectively colonize the intestines of inoculated adult cattle. The results of a study by Dobbin and colleagues[69] suggested that a regulator of flagellar gene expression, and not the flagella itself, played a significant role in colonization. However, Mahajan and colleagues[70] demonstrated that H7 flagella facilitate attachment of *E coli* O157:H7 to bovine rectal epithelial cells in vitro. These investigators hypothesized that the H7 flagellum does indeed play a significant role in colonization, first through its role in providing motility, and second by "browsing" the epithelial surface, then tethering the bacterium to accessible receptors, for example, mucin or other glycoconjugates. Colonization is then thought to progress into a secondary phase involving a decrease in expression of the flagella, and an increase in expression of type III secreted proteins with A/E lesion formation. Naylor and colleagues[71] and Nart and colleagues[72] demonstrated that cattle develop humoral and mucosal antibody responses, respectively, against O157, H7, and other antigens in response to colonization. Antibodies of the IgG and IgA class were both found in the serum and rectal mucosa. Bretschneider and colleagues,[65] and Naylor and colleagues[71] both found that circulating antibodies of the IgA class decrease in titer following repeated bacterial challenge, suggesting that the circulating antibodies are consumed, perhaps by translocation into the gut lumen, in response to infection. Bretschneider and colleagues[65] found that IgA antibodies to type III secreted proteins and not those to O157 lipopolysaccharide (LPS) decreased after the second challenge. Both studies also demonstrated that cattle shed less bacteria in the feces on subsequent challenges. Hence, antibodies directed against proteins that mediate colonization are used for protection against subsequent challenge. Nart and colleagues[73] reported that *E coli* O157:H7 infection of cattle induced a quantifiable neutrophilic inflammatory response in the lamina propria of the rectum when bacterial numbers reached 10^5 CFU/cm^2. These animals also developed IgA antibody responses to whole *E coli* O157:H7 cells. The investigators concluded that, based on the identification of a pathologic change and the production of a local immune response in the terminal rectum, *E coli* O157:H7 should not be considered a commensal organism in cattle.[73]

Proposed Role of Shiga Toxin in the Bovine Host

Mainil and Daube[12] reported in a major review article that more than 85% of EHEC isolated from cattle are positive for stx_1 only (as opposed to stx_2, both stx_1 and stx_2, or no *stx*), and this group of AEEC in particular are diarrheagenic pathogens of calves. An important question is the role of Stx, if any, in EHEC colonization of the bovine intestine. Stx is a potent cytotoxin that plays a key role in the induction of vascular lesions and other pathogenetic events that characterize HC and HUS in humans. However, unlike human beings, cattle lack the receptor for Stx in their blood vessels, and this has been proposed as a major reason why cattle do not usually develop severe hemorrhagic colitis and have never been found to develop HUS following EHEC infection.[74] Cattle do, however, have receptors for Stx in some cells, and this may potentially contribute to disease. Hoey and colleagues[75] reported the finding of Stx receptors in crypt epithelial cells in the intestine, but the toxin does not traffic to the endoplasmic reticulum; it ends up in lysosomes, which probably prevents toxicity. Stamm and colleagues[76] identified novel mesenchymal, nonepithelial Stx target cells in the crypt area of the bovine colonic mucosa. These investigators reported that bovine crypt epithelial cells are resistant to the effects of Stx1, but some intestinal mucosal mesenchymal cells, preliminarily characterized as mucosal macrophages, are Stx1-responsive and may participate in the interaction of STEC with the bovine intestinal mucosa. Menge and colleagues[77] found that intraepithelial lymphocytes in cattle have receptors for Stx, and reported that Stx1 reduces the proliferative responses of these cells to mitogenic stimuli, and reduces expression of CXCL8 (interleukin-8) by these cells. Hoffman and colleagues[78] found that the development of a cellular immune response against STEC antigens is significantly delayed in calves following inoculation with Stx2-producing *E coli* O157:H7. Fecal shedding of Stx2+ O157 was significantly higher than that of Stx-nonproducing *E coli* O157:H7. This shedding occurred despite the development of antibodies against O157 LPS. Hoffman and colleagues[78] hypothesized that Stxs cause immunosuppression by interfering with antigen-specific cell-mediated immune responses, which promote STEC colonization in the bovine host.

EVIDENCE OF AEEC AS CATTLE PATHOGENS BASED ON EPIDEMIOLOGIC STUDIES
Escherichia coli O5, O26, O111, O118, and O145 Infection of Calves

Several serogroups of AEEC and STEC have been isolated from diarrheic calves in different countries. In the United Kingdom, Sherwood and colleagues[79] reported that 13 of 306 (3%) of diarrheic calves had *E coli* in their feces that produced detectable Stx, and they belonged to the O4, O8, O19, O26, O111, O149, O168, and O nontypeable groups. Serogroup O111 was isolated from 3 calves, O26 was isolated from 2 calves, and the others were isolates from one each. Two calves were concurrently infected with *Cryptosporidium* spp, and one with rotavirus and coronavirus. The isolates were not tested for the intimin gene; hence, it was not reported whether these were AEEC. Wieler and colleagues[80] reported that out of 174 *E coli* strains isolated from diarrheic calves in Germany and Belgium, that were positive for *stx* genes, 122 strains (70.1%) were also positive for *eae*. One hundred 7 of these *eae*-positive strains (87.7%) harbored stx_1 genes, 13 strains (10.7%) had stx_2 genes, and 2 strains (1.6%) had both *stx* genes. The strains displayed 17 different O types, the majority (97 strains [79.5%]) belonging to O5 (5 strains), O26 (21 strains), O111 (13 strains) O118 (36 strains), O145 (9 strains), and O157 (13 strains).

Orden and colleagues[81] screened fecal samples from 221, 1- to 30-day-old diarrheic dairy calves in Spain. A total of 861 culture isolates from these samples were identified as *E coli*. *E coli* isolates were tested for Stx first by Vero cell assay and then for *stx* genes by PCR; if an isolate was positive by either method it was called STEC. All isolates that were positive for Stx by Vero cell assay were found to be *stx*+ by PCR. Isolates also were tested by PCR for *eae* and *espB*. STEC (in this study this term included all Stx+ that were either *eae*+ or *eae*−) and *eae*+ non-STEC were detected in 20 (9.0%) and 18 (8.1%) of the diarrheic calves tested, respectively. Of the STEC, 69.8% were positive for stx_1, 20.9% were positive for stx_2, and 9.3% were positive for stx_1 and stx_2. STEC isolates in a high percentage (76.7%) of diarrheic dairy calves belonged to the O4, O26, O39, O91, O113, O128, and O145 serogroups. Data from calves was grouped according to age as follows: 1 to 7 days, 8 to 14 days, 15 to 21 days, and 22 to 30 days; and odds ratios (OR) with 95% confidence intervals for infection with STEC and *eae*-positive non-STEC were calculated. The odds of STEC infection in 22- to 30-day-old diarrheic calves was significantly higher in comparison with the 1- to 7-day-old (OR = 14.09), 8- to 14-day-old (OR = 8.18), and 15- to 21 day-old (OR = 5.73) calves. The odds of infection with *eae*-positive non-STEC in the 22- to 30-day-old calves was greater in comparison with the 1- to 7-day-old calves (OR = 5.74).

China and colleagues[82] conducted a large-scale epidemiologic study in Belgium that addressed whether AEEC are pathogens of calves. A total of 695 calves were included in the study: 295, 2- to 10-week-old calves that had died of diarrheal disease; 311, 4- to 6-week-old healthy calves from 5 different farms without a serious diarrheal problem; and 89 newborn to 3-month-old calves from 7 farms with severe diarrhea problems. In the case of animals that died, intestinal contents instead of feces was cultured, and they were sampled only once (ie, post mortem). In the case of healthy calves on farms without a diarrhea problem, fecal samples were collected only once. Fecal samples were collected twice per week for 12 weeks from calves with or without diarrhea on farms that had a history of recurrent diarrheal disease. Farms with a history of recurrent diarrhea had these signs despite vaccination for ETEC, rotavirus, coronavirus, and antibiotic therapy. Both colony hybridization with gene probes and PCR were used to assay for *eaeA*, *espB*, stx_1, and stx_2. Strains were called AEEC if they had a positive result for *eaeA*; EPEC if they were *eaeA*+ but negative for *stx*; VTEC (STEC) if they were *stx*+, but negative for *eaeA*; and EHEC if they were *eaeA*+ and *stx*+. AEEC strains were identified in 91% of calves on farms with recurrent diarrhea problems, and in 66% of the calves, there was a correlation between the presence of AEEC and diarrhea. Feces from 1- to 12-week-old calves were positive for AEEC; 90% of these samples came from 2- to 8-week-old calves, and the mean age of the calves with AEEC was 5 weeks. The number of Stx positive bacteria was significantly higher in calves that died of diarrhea than in healthy or sick calves, and this finding was interpreted as evidence that Stx played an underlying role in the pathogenesis of disease. China and colleagues[82] stated that AEEC are clearly present in large numbers in farms with recurrent problems of diarrhea with variation from farm to farm. The proportion of calves with diarrhea and AEEC (66%) was significantly higher than the proportion of healthy calves with AEEC (25% in farms with diarrhea and 24% in farms without diarrhea).

Lee and colleagues[83] investigated the rates of occurrence of EHEC O26 and O111 in calves with or without diarrhea on farms in South Korea. These investigators conducted an observational study involving a total of 442 diarrheic and nondiarrheic young beef and dairy calves (<16 weeks old) from 115 different farms. EHEC O26 and O111 were detected in 14.4% and 12.5% of the diarrheic calves, respectively, compared with 7.6% and 5.9% of the nondiarrheic calves. The authors of this article (R.A.M., D.R.S.) analyzed the data from this study using multivariate logistic regression to evaluate the effect of calf age and clinical signs of diarrhea on the probability to recover EHEC O26 and O111 from these calves. There were significant (P<.05) interactions between the age of the calf and presence of diarrhea on the probability for recovering EHEC O26 or O111 from the feces. Of 163 calves 3 weeks old or less, 18 of 110 (16%) calves with diarrhea, and 1 of 53 (2%) calves without diarrhea shed EHEC O26. Of the 279 older calves, 19 of 147 (13%) calves with diarrhea shed EHEC O26, and 13 of 132 (10%) calves without diarrhea shed EHEC O26. Among calves 3 weeks old or less, the odds for calves with diarrhea to be shedding EHEC O26 was 10.2 times greater than the odds for nondiarrheic calves; yet, among calves older than 3 weeks the odds for calves with diarrhea to be shedding EHEC O26 was only 1.4 times greater. Of 239 calves 4 weeks old or less, 21 of 157 (13%) calves with diarrhea, and 2 of 82 (2%) calves without diarrhea shed EHEC O111. Of the 203 older calves, 11 of 100 (11%) calves with diarrhea shed EHEC O111, and 9 of 103 (9%) calves without diarrhea shed EHEC O111. Among calves 4 weeks old or less, the odds for calves with diarrhea to shed EHEC O111 was 6.2 times greater than the odds for nondiarrheic calves; yet, among calves older than 4 weeks the odds for calves with diarrhea to shed EHEC O111 was only 1.3 times greater. These interactions between age and diarrhea on recovery of EHEC O26 and O111 suggest that neonatal calves were more likely to exhibit clinical signs with these infections than older calves.

Pearce and colleagues[84] conducted a study in northern Scotland that investigated the shedding of *E coli* O26, O103, O111, O145, and O157 in a cohort of beef calves from birth over a 5-month period. *E coli* O26 was shed by 94% of the calves, and more than 90% of the O26 isolates were positive for *stx₁*, *eae*, and enterohemolysin (*ehl*) genes. *E coli* O103 was shed by 51% of the calves. Forty-eight percent of the O103 isolates were positive for *eae* and *ehl*; none were positive for *stx₁*. No O111 was detected, and shedding of O145 and O157 was rare. All but one O157 isolate was positive for *stx₂*, *eae*, and *ehl*. No association between fecal shedding of *E coli* O26 and O103 and diarrhea in the calves was found. A major finding was that the pattern of shedding of O26 and O103 in calves was very different. *E coli* O26 was shed by a higher proportion of dams at calving than at the end of the study; this suggested higher O26 exposure to newborn calves from the dam; in addition the *stx₁*, *eae*, and *ehl* genes were more common in O26 than O103 and the investigators hypothesized that the products of these genes might play an important role in colonization in the calf gut. With regard to why no relationship between shedding and diarrhea was detected, Pearce and colleagues suggested that the dams may have transferred protective antibodies in the colostrum to their calves, thereby preventing diarrhea; however, this was not tested. The investigators also commented that because calves were sampled weekly, they may have missed diarrheic episodes lasting less than 7 days.

Blanco and colleagues[22] characterized the virulence factors and O groups of 514 STEC isolates from diarrheic and healthy cattle in Spain. The isolates belonged to

164 different seropathotypes (associations between serotypes and virulence genes); however, only 12 accounted for 43% of the isolates. Seropathotype O157:H7 stx_2 eae ehxA (46 isolates) was the most common, followed by O157:H7 stx_1 stx_2 ehxA (34 isolates), O113:H21 stx_2 (25 isolates), O22:H8 stx_1 stx_2 ehxA (15 isolates), O26:H11 stx_1 eae ehxA (14 isolates), and O77:H41 stx_2 ehxA (14 isolates). STEC isolates belonged to 66 O serogroups and 113 O:H serotypes, including 23 new serotypes. Sixty-seven percent belonged to 1 of 15 serogroups, namely, O2, O4, O8, O20, O22, O26, O77, O91, O105, O113, O116, O157, O171, O174, and OX177. Fifty-two percent belonged to only 10 serotypes, namely, O4:H4, O20:H19, O22:H8, O26:H11, O77:H41, O105:H18, O113:H21, O157:H7, O171:H2, and ONT:H19. The eae (intimin) genes were subtyped and a new variant, namely, eae-ξ, was discovered. With this discovery, at least 15 different intimin types and subtypes have now been identified (α1, α2, β1, β2, γ1, γ2/θ, δ/κ, ϵ, ζ, η, ι, λ, μ, ν, and ξ). The extensive number of combinations serotypes, coupled with variations of virulence factors (seropathotypes) highlights the increasingly complex diversity of STEC infections in cattle. In this study, the overall prevalence rates of STEC colonization were estimated to be 37% in calves and 27% in cows. Isolates that were positive for stx_2 and those positive for both stx_1 and stx_2 were present in similar proportions in calves and cows. In contrast, isolates that were positive for eae and stx_1 were more commonly recovered from calves than cows. Although they did not report an analysis of data comparing the diarrheic versus healthy calves in this study, these investigators cited their previous surveys in which they found a significantly higher percentage of Stx1-producing E coli in diarrheic calves, which suggested a pathogenic role in neonatal calf diarrhea.

Aidar-Ugrinovich and colleagues[85] conducted a study that investigated the occurrence, serotypes, and virulence markers of STEC and EPEC strains in diarrheic and nondiarrheic calves in Brazil. A total of 546 fecal samples from 264 diarrheic calves and 282 healthy calves on beef farms in São Paulo were screened by PCR. STEC and EPEC were isolated in 10% and 2.7% of the 546 animals, respectively. E coli O157:H7 was not detected in any of the calves. The most frequent serotypes among STEC strains detected were O7:H10, O22:H16, O111:H⁻, O119:H⁻, and O174:H21; the most prevalent EPEC strains detected were O26:H11, O123:H11, and O177:H11. Several serotypes detected in this study constituted ones not previously reported among STEC, namely, O7:H7, O7:H10, O48:H7, O111:H19, O123:H2, O132:H51, O173:H⁻, and O175:H49. In this study, the investigators found no differences in carriage of STEC and EPEC in diarrheic and healthy cattle; however, they stated that "a significantly higher number of Stx1-producing E coli were found in diarrheic calves, suggesting a pathogenic role in neonatal calf diarrhea."

Escherichia coli O157:H7 and O157:NM Infection of Calves

Kang and colleagues[48] conducted an observational study similar to a previous one by this group involving EHEC O26 and EHEC O111[83] to investigate the rates of occurrence of EHEC O157:H7/NM in diarrheic and nondiarrheic calves younger than 20 weeks on farms in South Korea. A total of 498 diarrheic and nondiarrheic calves on 115 farms were included. EHEC O157:H7/NM was detected in 24 of 244 (10%) of the diarrheic calves, respectively, compared with 7 of 254 (3%) of the nondiarrheic calves. The authors of this article (R.A.M., D.R.S.) analyzed the data from this study using multivariate logistic regression to evaluate the effect of calf age and clinical signs of diarrhea on the probability to recover EHEC O157:H7/NM from these calves. Analysis revealed a significant ($P = .001$) interaction between the age of the calf and presence of diarrhea on the probability for recovering EHEC O157:H7/NM from the feces. Of 194 calves 4 weeks of age or less, 17 of 125 (14%) calves with diarrhea, and 1 of 69

(1.4%) calves without diarrhea shed EHEC O157:H7/NM. Of the 304 older calves, 7 of 119 (6%) calves with diarrhea shed EHEC O157:H7/NM, and 6 of 185 (3%) calves without diarrhea shed EHEC O157:H7/NM. Among calves 4 weeks old or less, the odds for calves with diarrhea to be shedding EHEC O157:H7/NM was 10.7 times greater than the odds for nondiarrheic calves; yet, among calves older than 4 weeks the odds for calves with diarrhea to be shedding EHEC O157:H7/NM was only 1.9 times greater. The interaction between age and diarrhea on recovery of EHEC O157:H7/NM was nearly identical to those observed with EHEC O26 and O111, and suggests that neonatal calves were more likely to exhibit clinical signs with EHEC O157:H7/NM infection than older calves.

SUMMARY

A review of the literature provides overwhelming evidence that AEEC are pathogens of cattle, mainly calves between the ages of 1 and 5 weeks. AEEC predominantly infect the large intestine and may cause diarrhea, with roughly one-fourth of the cases manifested clinically as dysentery, and pathologically as colitis or enterocolitis. AEEC infections are usually seen in conjunction with other enteric pathogens, for example, *Cryptosporidium* spp, other coccidia, rotavirus, and coronavirus, and these organisms significantly increase the severity of the clinical illness. In neonatal calves and in some cases, older animals, the infections can be fatal, but mainly when superimposed on another enteric infection. Most cases of clinical illness are caused by serogroups O5, O26, O111, O118, and O145, but other serogroups may be involved, which varies in different parts of the world. *E coli* O157:H7 and O157:NM are pathogens of the neonate, but epidemiologic evidence suggests they may be associated with diarrheal disease in older calves. By definition, AEEC cause attaching-effacing lesions, which are ultrastructural, and characterized by effacement of microvilli and intimate attachment of the bacterium to the apical cell membrane of the enterocyte. The causation of A/E lesions requires products of bacterial genes that induce microvillous effacement and intimate attachment. These genes are located on the locus of enterocyte effacement on the bacterial chromosome and their products include, but are not limited to, type III secreted proteins and the outer membrane protein, intimin. Most clinically apparent AEEC infections in calves are caused by strains that, by definition, produce intimin but also typically produce Shiga toxin (Stx), and especially Stx1. Although cattle do not have vascular receptors for Stx, they do have receptors on intraepithelial lymphocytes and cells that have preliminarily been identified as mucosal macrophages in the intestine. By acting on these cells, Stx is thought to cause immunosuppressive effects, especially affecting cell-mediated immune responses, and these may interfere with the ability of the host to clear the infection or develop fully protective immunity on recovery. AEEC pathologically are most likely to cause clinically evident disease when bacterial colonization is extensive enough to cause significant sloughing of enterocytes. Enterocyte loss and inflammation may be severe enough to result in diarrhea and dysentery.

REFERENCES

1. Gay CC, Besser TE. *Escherichia coli* septicaemia in calves. In: Gyles CL, editor. *Escherichia coli* in domestic animals and humans. Wallingford (CT): CAB International; 1994. p. 75–90.
2. Gay CC. *Escherichia coli* and neonatal disease of calves. Bacteriol Rev 1965;29: 75–101.

3. Butler DG, Clarke RC. Diarrhoea and dysentery in calves. In: Gyles CL, editor. *Escherichia coli* in domestic animals and humans. Wallingford (CT): CAB International; 1994. p. 91–116.
4. Nataro JP, Kaper JB. Diarrheagenic *Escherichia coli*. Clin Microbiol Rev 1998; 11(1):142–201.
5. Kaper JB, Nataro JP, Mobley HLT. Pathogenic *Escherichia coli*. Nat Rev Microbiol 2004;2(2):123–40.
6. Foster DM, Smith GW. Pathophysiology of diarrhea in calves. Vet Clin North Am Food Anim Pract 2009;25(1):13–36.
7. Levine MM. *Escherichia coli* that cause diarrhea: enterotoxigenic, enteropathogenic, enteroinvasive, enterohemorrhagic, and enteroadherent. J Infect Dis 1987;155(3):377–89.
8. Moon HW, Whipp SC, Argenzio RA, et al. Attaching and effacing activities of rabbit and human enteropathogenic *Escherichia coli* in pig and rabbit intestines. Infect Immun 1983;41(3):1340–51.
9. O'Brien AD, Holmes RK. Shiga and Shiga-like toxins. Microbiol Rev 1987;51(2): 206–20.
10. O'Brien AD, Kaper JB. Shiga toxin-producing *Escherichia coli*: yesterday, today, and tomorrow. In: Kaper JB, O'Brien AD, editors. *Escherichia coli* O157:H7 and other Shiga toxin-producing *E coli* strains. Washington, DC: ASM Press; 1998. p. 1–11.
11. Paton JC, Paton AW. Pathogenesis and diagnosis of Shiga toxin-producing *Escherichia coli* infection. Clin Microbiol Rev 1998;11(3):450–79.
12. Mainil JG, Daube G. Verotoxigenic *Escherichia coli* from animals, humans and foods: who's who? J Appl Microbiol 2005;98(6):1332–44.
13. Gyles CL. Shiga toxin-producing *Escherichia coli*: an overview. J Anim Sci 2007; 85(Suppl 13):E45–62.
14. Riley LW, Remis RS, Helgerson SD, et al. Hemorrhagic colitis associated with a rare *Escherichia coli* serotype. N Engl J Med 1983;308:681–5.
15. Armstrong GL, Hollingsworth J, Morris JG. Emerging food-borne pathogens: *Escherichia coli* O157:H7 as a model of entry of a new pathogen into the food supply of the developed world. Epidemiol Rev 1996;18(1):29–51.
16. Stevens MP, van Diemen PM, Dziva F, et al. Options for the control of enterohaemorrhagic *Escherichia coli* in ruminants. Microbiology 2002;148(Pt 12):3767–78.
17. Moxley RA. *Escherichia coli* O157:H7: an update on intestinal colonization and virulence mechanisms. Anim Health Res Rev 2004;5(1):15–33.
18. Hussein HS, Sakuma T. Prevalence of Shiga toxin-producing *Escherichia coli* in dairy cattle and their products. J Dairy Sci 2005;88(2):450–65.
19. Hussein HS. Prevalence and pathogenicity of Shiga toxin-producing *Escherichia coli* in beef cattle and their products. J Anim Sci 2007;85(Suppl 13):E63–72.
20. Tarr PI, Gordon CA, Chandler WL. Shiga-toxin-producing *Escherichia coli* and haemolytic uraemic syndrome. Lancet 2005;365(9464):1073–86.
21. Bardiau M, Labrozzo S, Mainil JG. Putative adhesins of enteropathogenic and enterohemorrhagic *Escherichia coli* of serogroup O26 isolated from humans and cattle. J Clin Microbiol 2009;47(7):2090–6.
22. Blanco M, Blanco JE, Mora A, et al. Serotypes, virulence genes, and intimin types of Shiga toxin (verotoxin)-producing *Escherichia coli* isolates from cattle in Spain and identification of a new intimin variant gene (eae-ξ). J Clin Microbiol 2004; 42(2):645–51.
23. Staley TE, Jones EW, Corley LD. Attachment and penetration of *Escherichia coli* into intestinal epithelium of the ileum in newborn pigs. Am J Pathol 1969;56(3): 371–92.

24. Feng P, Lampel KA, Karch H, et al. Genotypic and phenotypic changes in the emergence of *Escherichia coli* O157:H7. J Infect Dis 1998;177(6):1750–3.
25. Moon HW, Isaacson RE, Pohlenz J. Mechanisms of association of enteropathogenic *Escherichia coli* with intestinal epithelium. Am J Clin Nutr 1979;32(1):119–27.
26. Takeuchi A, Inman LR, O'Hanley PD, et al. Scanning and transmission electron microscopic study of *Escherichia coli* O15 (RDEC-1) enteric infection in rabbits. Infect Immun 1978;19(2):686–94.
27. Rothbaum R, McAdams AJ, Giannella R, et al. A clinicopathologic study of enterocyte-adherent *Escherichia coli*: a cause of protracted diarrhea in infants. Gastroenterology 1982;83(2):441–54.
28. Chanter N, Morgan JH, Bridger JC, et al. Dysentery in gnotobiotic calves caused by atypical *Escherichia coli*. Vet Rec 1984;114(3):71.
29. Hall GA, Reynolds DJ, Chanter N, et al. Dysentery caused by *Escherichia coli* (S102-9) in calves: natural and experimental disease. Vet Pathol 1985;22:156–63.
30. Chanter N, Hall GA, Bland AP, et al. Dysentery in calves caused by an atypical strain of *Escherichia coli* (S102-9). Vet Microbiol 1986;12(3):241–53.
31. De Rycke J, Boivin R, Le Roux P. Demonstration of strains of *Escherichia coli* with septicemic characteristics in the feces of calves with mucoid enteritis. Ann Rech Vet 1982;13(4):385–97.
32. Moxley RA, Francis DH. Natural and experimental infection with an attaching and effacing strain of *Escherichia coli* in calves. Infect Immun 1986;53(2):339–46.
33. Pospischil A, Mainil JG, Baljer G, et al. Attaching and effacing bacteria in the intestines of calves and cats with diarrhea. Vet Pathol 1987;24(4):330–4.
34. Schoonderwoerd M, Clarke RC, van Dreumel AA, et al. Colitis in calves: natural and experimental infection with a verotoxin-producing strain of *Escherichia coli* O111:NM. Can J Vet Res 1988;52(4):484–7.
35. Mainil JG, Duchesnes CJ, Whipp SC, et al. Shiga-like toxin production and attaching effacing activity of *Escherichia coli* associated with calf diarrhea. Am J Vet Res 1987;48(5):743–8.
36. Janke BH, Francis DH, Collins JE, et al. Attaching and effacing *Escherichia coli* infections in calves, pigs, lambs, and dogs. J Vet Diagn Invest 1989;1(1):6–11.
37. Janke BH, Francis DH, Collins JE, et al. Attaching and effacing *Escherichia coli* infection as a cause of diarrhea in young calves. J Am Vet Med Assoc 1990; 196(6):897–901.
38. Dorn CR, Francis DH, Angrick EJ, et al. Characteristics of Vero cytotoxin producing *Escherichia coli* associated with intestinal colonization and diarrhea in calves. Vet Microbiol 1993;36(1–2):149–59.
39. Pearson GR, Watson CA, Hall GA, et al. Natural infection with an attaching and effacing *Escherichia coli* in the small and large intestines of a calf with diarrhoea. Vet Rec 1989;124(12):297–9.
40. Fischer J, Maddox C, Moxley R, et al. Pathogenicity of a bovine attaching effacing *Escherichia coli* isolate lacking Shiga-like toxins. Am J Vet Res 1994;55(7):991–9.
41. Wray C, McLaren M, Pearson GR. Occurrence of 'attaching and effacing' lesions in the small intestine of calves experimentally infected with bovine isolates of verocytotoxic *E coli*. Vet Rec 1989;125(14):365–8.
42. Stordeur P, China B, Charlier G, et al. Clinical signs, reproduction of attaching/ effacing lesions, and enterocyte invasion after oral inoculation of an O118 enterohaemorrhagic *Escherichia coli* in neonatal calves. Microbes Infect 2000;2(1): 17–24.
43. Sandhu KS, Gyles CL. Pathogenic Shiga toxin-producing *Escherichia coli* in the intestine of calves. Can J Vet Res 2002;66(2):65–72.

44. Wada Y, Nakazawa M, Kubo M. Natural infection with attaching and effacing *Escherichia coli* (O15) in an adult cow. J Vet Med Sci 1994;56(1):151–2.

45. Pearson GR, Bazeley KJ, Jones JR, et al. Attaching and effacing lesions in the large intestine of an eight-month-old heifer associated with *Escherichia coli* O26 infection in a group of animals with dysentery. Vet Rec 1999;145(13):370–3.

46. Ørskov F, Ørskov I, Villar JA. Cattle as a reservoir of verotoxin-producing *Escherichia coli* O157:H7. Lancet 1987;2(8553):276.

47. Daniel R, Matthews L, Willshaw G. Isolation of *E coli* O157 from a calf with dysentery. Vet Rec 1998;143(2):56.

48. Kang SJ, Ryu SJ, Chae JS, et al. Occurrence and characteristics of enterohemorrhagic *Escherichia coli* O157 in calves associated with diarrhoea. Vet Rec 2004; 98(3–4):323–8.

49. Dean-Nystrom EA, Bosworth BT, Cray WC Jr, et al. Pathogenicity of *Escherichia coli* O157:H7 in the intestines of neonatal calves. Infect Immun 1997;65(5):1842–8.

50. Dean-Nystrom EA, Bosworth BT, Moon HW, et al. *Escherichia coli* O157:H7 requires intimin for enteropathogenicity in calves. Infect Immun 1998;66(9): 4560–3.

51. Dean-Nystrom EA, Bosworth BT, Moon HW. Pathogenesis of *Escherichia coli* O157:H7 in weaned calves. Adv Exp Med Biol 1999;473:173–7.

52. Rasmussen MA, Cray WC Jr, Casey TA, et al. Rumen contents as a reservoir of enterohemorrhagic *Escherichia coli*. FEMS Microbiol Lett 1993;114(1):79–84.

53. Naylor SW, Low JC, Besser TE, et al. Lymphoid follicle-dense mucosa at the terminal rectum is the principal site of colonization of enterohemorrhagic *Escherichia coli* O157:H7 in the bovine host. Infect Immun 2003;71(3):1505–12.

54. Naylor SW, Roe AJ, Nart P, et al. *Escherichia coli* O157:H7 forms attaching and effacing lesions at the terminal rectum and colonization requires the *LEE4* operon. Microbiology 2005;151(Pt 8):2773–81.

55. Baehler AA, Moxley RA. *Escherichia coli* O157:H7 induces attaching-effacing lesions in large intestinal mucosal explants from adult cattle. FEMS Microbiol Lett 2000;185(2):239–42.

56. Phillips AD, Navabpour S, Hicks S, et al. Enterohaemorrhagic *Escherichia coli* O157:H7 target Peyer's patches in humans and cause attaching/effacing lesions in both human and bovine intestine. Gut 2000;47(3):377–81.

57. Vlisidou I, Lyte M, van Diemen PM, et al. The neuroendocrine stress hormone norepinephrine augments *Escherichia coli* O157:H7-induced enteritis and adherence in a bovine ligated ileal loop model of infection. Infect Immun 2004;72(9): 5446–51.

58. Woodward MJ, Gavier-Widen D, McLaren IM, et al. Infection of gnotobiotic calves with *Escherichia coli* O157:H7 strain A84. Vet Rec 1999;144(17):466–70.

59. Wray C, McLaren IM, Randall LP, et al. Natural and experimental infection of normal cattle with *Escherichia coli* O157. Vet Rec 2000;147(3):65–8.

60. Cray WC, Moon HW. Experimental infection of calves and adult cattle with *Escherichia coli* O157:H7. Appl Environ Microbiol 1995;61(4):1586–90.

61. Brown CA, Harmon BG, Zhao T, et al. Experimental *Escherichia coli* O157:H7 carriage in calves. Appl Environ Microbiol 1997;63(1):27–32.

62. Stevens MP, Marchès O, Campbell J, et al. Intimin, Tir, and Shiga toxin 1 do not influence enteropathogenic responses to Shiga toxin-producing *Escherichia coli* in bovine ligated intestinal loops. Infect Immun 2002;70(2):945–52.

63. Vlisidou I, Dziva F, La Ragione RM, et al. Role of intimin-Tir interactions and the Tir-cytoskeleton coupling protein in the colonization of calves and lambs by *Escherichia coli* O157:H7. Infect Immun 2006;74(1):758–64.

64. Pacheco AR, Sperandio V. Inter-kingdom signaling: chemical language between bacteria and host. Curr Opin Microbiol 2009;12(2):192–8.
65. Bretschneider G, Berberov EM, Moxley RA. Isotype-specific antibody responses against *Escherichia coli* O157:H7 locus of enterocyte effacement proteins in adult beef cattle following experimental infection. Vet Immunol Immunopathol 2007; 118(3–4):229–38.
66. Bretschneider G, Berberov EM, Moxley RA. Reduced intestinal colonization of adult beef cattle by *Escherichia coli* O157:H7 *tir* deletion and nalidixic-acid-resistant mutants lacking flagellar expression. Vet Microbiol 2007;125(3–4):381–6.
67. Bretschneider G, Berberov EM, Moxley RA. Enteric mucosal antibodies to *Escherichia coli* O157:H7 in adult cattle. Vet Rec 2008;163(7):218–9.
68. Cornick NA, Booher SL, Moon HW. Intimin facilitates colonization by *Escherichia coli* O157:H7 in adult ruminants. Infect Immun 2002;70(5):2704–7.
69. Dobbin HS, Hovde CJ, Williams CJ, et al. The *Escherichia coli* O157 flagellar regulatory gene *flhC* and not the flagellin gene *fliC* impacts colonization of cattle. Infect Immun 2006;74(5):2894–905.
70. Mahajan A, Currie CG, Mackie S, et al. An investigation of the expression and adhesion function of H7 flagella in the interaction of *Escherichia coli* O157:H7 with bovine intestinal epithelium. Cell Microbiol 2009;11:121–37.
71. Naylor SW, Flockhart A, Nart P, et al. Shedding of *Escherichia coli* O157:H7 in calves is reduced by prior colonization with the homologous strain. Appl Environ Microbiol 2007;73(11):3765–7.
72. Nart P, Holden N, McAteer SP, et al. Mucosal antibody responses of colonized cattle to *Escherichia coli* O157-secreted proteins, flagellin, outer membrane proteins and lipopolysaccharide. FEMS Immunol Med Microbiol 2008;52(1): 59–68.
73. Nart P, Naylor SW, Huntley JF, et al. Responses of cattle to gastrointestinal colonization with *Escherichia coli* O157. Infect Immun 2008;76(11):5366–72.
74. Pruimboom-Brees IM, Morgan TW, Ackermann MR, et al. Cattle lack vascular receptors for *Escherichia coli* O157:H7 Shiga toxins. Proc Natl Acad Sci U S A 2000;97(19):10325–9.
75. Hoey DE, Sharp L, Currie C, et al. Verotoxin 1 binding to intestinal crypt epithelial cells results in localization to lysosomes and abrogation of toxicity. Cell Microbiol 2003;5(2):85–97.
76. Stamm I, Mohr M, Bridger PS, et al. Epithelial and mesenchymal cells in the bovine colonic mucosa differ in their responsiveness to *Escherichia coli* Shiga toxin 1. Infect Immun 2008;76(11):5381–91.
77. Menge C, Blessenohl M, Eisenberg T, et al. Bovine ileal intraepithelial lymphocytes represent target cells for Shiga toxin 1 from *Escherichia coli*. Infect Immun 2004;72(4):1896–905.
78. Hoffman MA, Menge C, Casey TA, et al. Bovine immune response to Shigatoxigenic *Escherichia coli* O157:H7. Clin Vaccine Immunol 2006;13(12): 1322–7.
79. Sherwood D, Snodgrass DR, O'Brien AD. Shiga-like toxin production from *Escherichia coli* associated with calf diarrhea. Vet Rec 1985;116(8):217–8.
80. Wieler LH, Vieler E, Erpenstein C, et al. Shiga toxin-producing *Escherichia coli* strains from bovines: association of adhesion with carriage of *eae* and other genes. J Clin Microbiol 1996;34(12):2980–4.
81. Orden JA, Ruiz-Santa-Quiteria JA, Cid D, et al. Verotoxin-producing *Escherichia coli* (VTEC) and *eae*-positive non-VTEC in 1-30-days-old diarrhoeic dairy calves. Vet Microbiol 1998;63(2–4):239–48.

82. China B, Pirson V, Mainil J. Prevalence and molecular typing of attaching and effacing *Escherichia coli* among calf populations in Belgium. Vet Microbiol 1998;63(2–4):249–59.
83. Lee JH, Hur J, Stein BD. Occurrence and characteristics of enterohemorrhagic *Escherichia coli* O26 and O111 in calves associated with diarrhea. Vet J 2008; 176(2):205–9.
84. Pearce MC, Jenkins C, Vali L, et al. Temporal shedding patterns and virulence factors of *Escherichia coli* serogroups O26, O103, O111, O145, and O157 in a cohort of beef calves and their dams. Appl Environ Microbiol 2004;70(3): 1708–16.
85. Aidar-Ugrinovich L, Blanco J, Blanco M, et al. Serotypes, virulence genes, and intimin types of Shiga toxin-producing *Escherichia coli* (STEC) and enteropathogenic *E coli* (EPEC) isolated from calves in São Paulo, Brazil. Int J Food Microbiol 2007;115(3):297–306.

Bovine Pasteurellosis and Other Bacterial Infections of the Respiratory Tract

Dee Griffin, DVM, MS

KEYWORDS

- BRD • Pasteurellosis • Pneumonia • Bovine
- Management • Feedlot • Treatment • Vaccination

VCNA EMERGING REEMERGING AND PERSISTENT INFECTIOUS DISEASES OF CATTLE

The commonly discussed bacterial pathogens associated with the bovine respiratory disease (BRD) complex are *Pasteurella multocida*, *Mannheimia haemolytica* (formerly *Pasteurella hemolytica*), *Histophilus somni* (formerly *Hemophilus somnus*), and *Mycoplasma bovis* (formerly *Mycoplasma agalactiae* subspecies bovis). All 4 of these pathogens receive attention as primary pathogens. Generally considered commensal bacteria, all but *Mycoplasma bovis* are found mainly in the upper respiratory tract. All are opportunist, generally relying on respiratory viral damage and stress-based immune suppression to become deadly BRD pathogens.[1]

Pasteurella Multocida

Pasteurella multocida has 5 capsular serogroups (A, B, D, E, and F) and somatic serotypes 1 to 16.[2–4] The most commonly isolated *Pasteurella multocida* in bovine respiratory disease is A:3 followed by a much smaller isolation rate for D:3.[5] *Pasteurella multocida* is more commonly identified in respiratory disease affecting younger cattle in syndromes including enzootic neonatal calf pneumonia and in shipping fever of weaned calves.[6] The involvement of more than just *Pasteurella multocida* in the development of pneumonia is accepted. Multiple factors including immune moderating stresses such as adverse climate and other environmental conditions, adverse nutritional conditions such as damaged feedstuffs and abrupt ration changes, animal handling and transportation, and the interaction of other cattle health diseases such as concomitant infections with the other previously listed BRD bacterial pathogens, gastrointestinal bacterial pathogens, and parasites.[1,7–10]

Department of Veterinary and Biomedical Sciences, Great Plains Veterinary Educational Center, University of Nebraska – Lincoln, PO Box 148, Clay Center, NE 68933-0148, USA
E-mail address: dgriffin@gpvec.unl.edu

Vet Clin Food Anim 26 (2010) 57–71
doi:10.1016/j.cvfa.2009.10.010
0749-0720/10/$ – see front matter © 2010 Elsevier Inc. All rights reserved.

vetfood.theclinics.com

Pasteurella multocida is readily isolated from nasal secretions and deep pharyngeal collections in young calves and weaning and feeder cattle.[2,7] The reported isolation rates in clinically normal cattle are between 20% and 60%.[2] High bacterial recovery rates in clinically normal animals suggest *Pasteurella multocida* is a commensal organism, and recovery in cattle suffering from clinically respiratory disease may not be a true association with a causal relationship. *Pasteurella multocida* isolation from nasal secretion of calves suffering from clinical respiratory disease is about twice as high as the isolation rate in clinically normal calves.[2,5] Although *Pasteurella multocida* can be highly infectious, the bacterium is not considered to be highly contagious.[2,5,11]

Most respiratory disease cases reported from cattle producers are based on a simple set of observations that are generally applied to cattle considered at a high risk for developing BRD. Most commonly targeted herds of cattle are stressed or newly received cattle. The observations most commonly targeted are signs that include depression (D), appetite loss (A), respiratory character change (R), and temperate elevation (T), collectively referred to as DART. These clinical signs are not pathognomonic for bacterial pneumonia but they have been used for decades in the treatment management of BRD.[12] The common and consistent uses of the DART signs as a diagnostic proxy for BRD make case treatment records a useful means of examining incidence rates, and various management, environmental, and nutritional causal relationships. BRD mortality in groups of cattle is poorly related to the BRD case treatment records.[13–16] The poor correlation between morbidity based on the DART signs and BRD mortality makes it difficult to design interventions directed at specific potential pathogens such as *Pasteurella multocida* vaccine development. It is difficult to use antimicrobial minimum inhibitory concentration laboratory results from fatal BRD cases in the management of clinical cases based on the DART signs.[9,17–20]

Enzootic calf pneumonia (ECP) is the most common respiratory disease in cattle ascribed to *Pasteurella multocida*. ECP is most often discussed as a disease of calves, whereas shipping fever, also known as the BRD complex or syndrome, is discussed as a disease of older weanling, stocker, or feeder cattle.[5] Differences between ECP and the BRD complex are arbitrary based on the age and common management stresses such as marketing and transportation. ECP is most frequently described as a dairy-calf disease and generally not considered important in suckling beef calves as the preweaning incidence of respiratory disease is believed to be low; however, this may be an incorrect assumption. Treatment of suckling beef calves is problematic because it involves capturing a calf for treatment that is being guarded by a protective mother. The possibility of injury to the calf while trying to capture it for treatment, or injury to the person by the calf's mother while trying to treat the calf, is considerable. Therefore, observations based on case treatment records, as commonly performed with other forms of BRD, are difficult and it is impossible to estimate BRD in suckling calves across the beef industry. In beef-cow calf operations BRD in sucking calves is sometimes referred to as "summer pneumonia." *Pasteurella multocida* is commonly isolated from specimens collected from live and dead calves.[2,5] Generally, these complaints arise when the calves are 2 to 4 months of age. Ear infections in newly weaned beef calves, often assumed to be caused by *Mycoplasma bovis*, frequently yield *Pasteurella multocida* as the only isolate.

Colostral failure of passive transfer (FTP) is a well-documented condition associated with many calfhood diseases. The ramification of FTP beyond calfhood to the incidence of diseases more commonly observed at weaning has also been reported.[9] However, the link between FTP and BRD associated with *Pasteurella multocida* has not been established.[2,21] Passively acquired antibodies to *Pasteurella multocida* are reported to be undetectable in calves more than 2 months of age.[2] The short half-life of the *Pasteurella multocida* passively acquired antibodies makes it difficult to understand how FTP could be associated with *Pasteurella multocida* BRD in calves more than 2 months of age, as described by dairy-calf ranch operators and beef-cow calf production units. BRD diagnosis in these situations is generally based on DART signs and, therefore, only circumstantially related to BRD and cannot be definitively correlated to *Pasteurella multocida*.

Isolation of *Pasteurella multocida* as a principle bacterium recovered from pneumonic lungs at necropsy is considered more indicative of a causal relationship.[22–24] Diagnostic microbiologists more frequently report *Pasteurella multocida* in fatal cases of BRD from feedlots. This is contrary to decades of reports implicating *Mannheimia haemolytica* as the principle bacterial pathogen associated with fatal BRD in feedlots. Increased reporting of *Pasteurella multocida* as a principle bacterial isolate from fatal cases of BRD has led to questions concerning pathogenic drifts of the bacterium.[2,9,25,26]

Historical cattle-feeding industry data indicate change in the weight and age of cattle entering feedyards. The most prominent observations are the increase in genetic size of cattle and the need to introduce these larger breeds to the food chain before they reach full maturity, and the increased cost of grazing compared with confinement feeding. The result has been an increasing number of cattle entering the feeding industry as weaned calves. This shift in the age for feeder cattle could account for the change in frequency of isolation of *Pasteurella multocida* compared with the frequency of isolation of *Mannheimia haemolytica* in fatal cases of BRD in feedlots.[27–30]

Mannheimia Haemolytica

Mannheimia haemolytica is generally considered the most important bacterial pathogen in BRD of cattle post weaning. *Mannheimia haemolytica* has 12 capsular serotypes (A1, A2, A5, A6, A7, A8, A9, A12, A13, A14, A16, and A17).[25,26,31,32] The most common serotypes isolated from BRD lungs at necropsy are primarily A1 followed by A6.[26] *Mannheimia haemolytica* is a commensal bacterium that can generally be found in the tonsillar tissue draining the retropharyngeal lymph node.[26,32] Isolation of the bacterium from nasal swabs taken from healthy, nonstressed cattle is not typically rewarding. However, the isolation rate and organism numbers increase as cattle are stressed.[26] Weaning, comingling of cattle from different sources, marketing, and transportation are the common stresses responsible for weakening the immune system, which is a common link to developing *Mannheimia haemolytica* BRD.[1,8] Production management stresses such as dehorning and castration added to the stresses already mentioned are often associated with high BRD morbidity and mortality. In these situations, the frequency of *Mannheimia haemolytica* isolation from the lungs of fatal BRD cases increases.[1,8,16,27] Upper respiratory viral infections with agents such as bovine herpes virus 1(BHV-1), bovine virus diarrhea virus (BVDV) type 1 or type 2, bovine respiratory syncytial virus (BRSV), and parainfluenza virus 3 (PI-3) are considered key elements in the pathogenesis of life-threatening BRD associated with *Mannheimia haemolytica, Pasteurella multocida,* and *Histophilus somni*.[9,12,31,33,34] The cellular damage caused by viral replication in the upper respiratory has a profound adverse effect on the innate bacterial clearance mechanism.[6,26,35] In addition, viral-induced immune suppression including diminished T lymphocyte, B lymphocyte, monocyte, and macrophage activity has been established.[2,6,27,36–38]

The virulence factors possessed by *Mannheimia haemolytica* are impressive. Those factors that play a role in bacterium attachment and colonization include adhesion protein, capsular polysaccharide, fimbriae, sialoglycoprotease, and neuraminidase. The capsular polysaccharide of the organism negatively affects the phagocytic ability of the neutrophils and the sialoglycoprotease affects the effectiveness of opsonizing antibodies.[6,27,35] Iron-regulated outer membrane proteins are virulence factors that allow *Mannheimia haemolytica* to replicate in a low-iron host-regulated environment.[6,27] Lipid A of the lipopolysaccharide (LPS) cell wall component is a critical virulence factor related to the macrophage activation associated with endotoxin. Lipid A is associated with the release of tumor necrosis factor, vascular damage, and the observed inflammatory signs of high fevers and hypotensive shock.[6,27,36] Although LPS is important in the pathogenesis, its value in a vaccination immune response is questionable as antibody titers to LPS do not correlate with protection in experimental *Mannheimia haemolytica* challenge.[27] Lipoproteins identified among the virulence factors hold some promise as a potential component of a *Mannheimia haemolytica* vaccine.[27,37,39] The lipoprotein PlpE has been found to be immunogenic, and when combined with available *Mannheimia haemolytica* vaccines enhanced protection.

Leukotoxin (LKT) is the most widely held important *Mannheimia haemolytica* virulence factor associated with lung damage that allows the bacterium to evade destruction by the host's phagocytic cells.[27] As the amount of LKT increases during an infection, the severity of the cellular effect increases from apoptosis to necrosis.[27,36] The necrotizing damage and cellular infiltrate found in cattle that die from *Mannheimia haemolytica* pneumonia is impressive. The vascular damage and inflammatory mediators are responsible for the massive fibrin response commonly observed at necropsy.[6,26,27]

Although *Mannheimia haemolytica* is highly infectious, similar to *Pasteurella multocida* the bacterium is generally not considered highly contagious.[27] This is contrary to development of BRD and a serologic response in noninoculated calves when experimentally comingled with inoculated calves. Observations in feedlots continue to point to severe cases of BRD and seem to be confined to sets of cattle. The disease does not move in an epidemic fashion within a feedyard.[11] The common observations in severely affected groups of cattle are their dubious production, health, and marketing management backgrounds.[6,8,13,17,34,40]

Histophilus Somni

Histophilus somni (formerly *Haemophilus somnus*) in calves and feeder cattle is, like the other BRD bacteria discussed earlier, a commensal gram-negative bacterium residing in the nasopharyngeal region but may preferentially colonize the lower respiratory tract.[6,11,31,41] The isolation rate in clinically normal cattle entering feedyards is reported in as few as 15% to more than 50% of newly received cattle.[31,41] The isolation rate in feeder cattle showing clinical BRD signs is reported to be higher than in clinically normal cattle.[42] The isolation rate is reported to be inversely related to the geometric mean *Histophilus somni* antibody titer for groups of newly received cattle.[11,42] This isolation rate suggests immunization sufficiently spaced before weaning, comingling, marketing, or transportation stresses might be a key management consideration for minimizing histophilosis.[42,43] The major outer membrane protein and lipooligosaccharide virulence factors are similar to *Mannheimia haemolytica*, but in addition, histamine release and an exopolysaccharide produced play a role in the pathogenesis.[42,44] The usefulness of *Histophilus somni* bacterins is discussed later.

The bacterium has been associated with several disease manifestations, including fibrinopurulent bronchopneumonia as a singular etiologic pathogen or as a pathogen component of the BRD complex; abscessing laryngitis; thromboembolic meningoencephalitis; polyarthritis-polyserositis; fibrinous pericarditis; and sudden death associated with cardiovascular left ventricular papillary muscle necrosis related to septicemia.[43,45] Generally, the respiratory form is considered the predecessor by weeks to months of the other body system maladies. Clinically, the pneumonia caused by *Histophilus somni* is indistinguishable from pneumonia caused by the other BRD bacterial pathogens.[6] Massive fibrin deposition is the most commonly associated observation on gross examination of affected lungs, but similar observations are reported for *Pasteurella multocida* and *Mannheimia haemolytica*. *Histophilus somni*, *Pasteurella multocida,* and *Mannheimia haemolytica* are commonly isolated together from the same diseased lung sample.[42] When these similarities are considered, along with the commensal nature of the organism, a definitive diagnosis of histophilosis can be precarious. Often a BRD-related diagnosis depends on isolating high numbers of the bacterium, but this likelihood can be marginal for samples taken from cattle that have been treated with an antibiotic before an isolation attempt.[42] The other body system maladies attributed to *Histophilus somni* are less complicated or confused with other potential pathogens. For these conditions, clinical signs or gross and histologic lesions that include vascular inflammation, thrombosis, infarction, and impressive polymorphonuclear leucocytic infiltration are frequently sufficient for an acceptable diagnosis.[26,42,46]

Mycoplasma Bovis

The role of *Mycoplasma bovis* in BRD of young calves is better understood than it is in stocker and feeder cattle.[6,11,23,26,47–50] Although the role of *Mycoplasma bovis* can be heavily debated, data defining its relationship in the BRD complex are not so clear as they are for the 3 bacterial BRD pathogens mentioned earlier. *Mycoplasma bovis* can play a role in enzootic pneumonia with or without associated otitis media, shipping fever, and chronic pneumonia complicated with arthritis or tenosynovitis.[47–49]

Mycoplasma bovis, a facultative anaerobe, has a trilayered membrane instead of a cell wall. The use of nasal swabs has not been so productive in studying the movement of this bacterium as the bacterium is more often found in the deeper respiratory system.[47,50]

Serology using enzyme-linked immunosorbent assay is the practical method used to identify movement of the organism. Strain typing requires molecular techniques such as arbitrarily primed polymerase chain reaction.[47] These techniques have been used mostly to help understand the epidemiology of the movement of the organism. The incidence within herds varies from absent to more than 90%.[49,51] The prevalence increases as cattle are stressed and comingled. Movement within herds includes dam to offspring transmission. Matched strains between dam and offspring have been identified. The bacterium found in mammary glands is apparently ingested, and aerosolized milk during suckling is the potential route for inoculation of the respiratory tract.[47] This mechanism may also be responsible for otitis media development. After entering the respiratory system, *Mycoplasma bovis* can move between the respiratory cells to enter the blood stream.[47] A bacteremia can be identified within a day of infection and persist for more than a week.[47] The organism can be isolated from other body system tissues after the bacteremia ends.[6,47] This is likely the mechanism for the arthritis most often associated with the respiratory form of *Mycoplasmosis*.[6,47,48]

Mycoplasma bovis can survive in the environment for days to weeks if protected from ultraviolet radiation.[47] Serology has identified movement of the bacterium within herds and this is most likely by animal to animal. When naïve cattle are mixed with cattle infected with *Mycoplasma bovis* the bacterium can be found in some of the naïve cattle within a day and in most of the naïve cattle within a week.[6,48] Once established in the respiratory tract, *Mycoplasma bovis* may persist for the life of the animal.[47,52] Experimentally infected cattle often stay asymptomatic or develop only mild clinical disease. Severe clinical disease has been reproduced using stress models similar to those used to study the other bacteria most commonly associated with BRD.[6,47] Pneumonia and arthritis are most typically seen 8 to 10 days post inoculation.[47,48] Virulence of *Mycoplasma bovis* is associated with 5 variable surface lipoproteins (Vsp); VspA, VspB, VspC, VspF, and VspO.[47] A synergistic effect seems to exist between *Mycoplasma bovis* and *Mannheimia haemolytica,* as a more severe disease is created when more calves infected with *Mycoplasma* are challenged with *Mannheimia* than when calves not infected with *Mycoplasma* are challenged.[6,47,48] The other associated causes of BRD, including stress, comingling, viral infection, and other respiratory bacterial pathogens, all play an important role.[6] The same components associated with BRD cause doubt that *Mycoplasma bovis* has a primary role in many BRD cases.[47,48,53-55]

Treatment of *Mycoplasma bovis* infections has not proven rewarding. The absence of a cell wall in *Mycoplasma* eliminates the consideration of β-lactam antibiotics. The systems and techniques used to evaluate the antibiotic sensitivity of *Mycoplasma bovis* have repeatedly found several antibiotics that should be effective. Consistent finding of *Mycoplasma bovis* in the lungs of treated cattle, including lungs from packing plants collected for clinically normal cattle, suggest that the antibiotics used and the animal's immune system were not sufficient for the animal to rid itself of the infection.[47,48,51,52]

The lung lesions range from mild collapse consolidated anterior-ventral areas to chronic caseonecrotic bronchopneumonia. The latter appears as nodules of caseous necrosis surrounded by collapsed consolidated lung. The centers are not typically liquefied unless the lesion is contaminated with other bacteria. Bronchiectasis may be visible.[47,48]

Culture techniques are difficult. Handing specimen samples properly is critical for a diagnostic laboratory to isolate the bacterium. Samples must be refrigerated and delivery should be expedited so the sample arrives within 24 hours. Transport media such as Stuarts or Eaton's are frequently suggested. If nasal swabs are attempted, Dacron-tipped plastic swabs are less apt to interfere with isolation than cotton-tipped wooden swabs.[47]

PATHOLOGY RELATED TO BACTERIAL BRD PATHOGENS

Of the respiratory pathology associated with the principle BRD bacterial pathogens (*Pasteurella multocida, Mannheimia haemolytica, Histophilus somni,* and *Mycoplasma bovis*), only *Mycoplasma bovis* offers grossly visible differences.[17,23,46,56] It is not uncommon to isolate all 4 of these potential pathogens in the same fatal BRD case.[26] *Pasteurella multocida, Mannheimia haemolytica,* and *Histophilus somni* can all produce similar bronchopneumonic inflammatory responses in the anterior-ventral lung lobes.[5,26,27,42,45-47] The vascular damage and severe inflammatory response commonly lead to fibrin deposition and necrosis of lung parenchyma.[26,27,42,45]

Instead of trying to associate gross visible observations with a particular bacterial pathogen at necropsy, the client would be better served if the practitioner determined the duration of the damage.[46] The duration presented at necropsy can vary from areas in the lung that are weeks to months old to areas that are hours to days old. By understanding the duration presented at necropsy and the sequence of events represented in the animal's background and treatment history, the practitioner can better guide the proper selection and use of available treatment.[53,57]

Lung lesion scoring at packing plants provides an opportunity to extend the information available beyond treatment histories and necropsy examinations. Lung lesion scoring observation in packing plants makes it obvious that not all cattle with lung lesions have been previously treated during the animal's stay in the feedlot.[58,59] Two possibilities could account for this observation: either the animal did not present sufficient DART signs in the judgment of the cattle's caretaker to warrant the animal being pulled for BRD treatment, or the BRD lung lesion occurred before the animal entered the feeding operation.[10,28] The lung lesion rate is variable but is generally associated with the background history of the cattle being observed. Cattle that have management histories that indicate that accepted cattle health practice was properly implemented, and minimal health detrimental events such as comingling and prolonged marketing and transport stress, generally have had much fewer (< 15% affected rate) and less severe (< 5% of the anterior lobes involved) lung lesions observable at the packing plant. The loss of gain performance associated with BRD in cattle with this level of involvement is low, usually less than 0.1 pounds (lbs) average daily gain (ADG) for affected cattle. On the other extreme are those groups of cattle that come from many smaller herds with questionable cattle health management practices. These groups are inevitable because the average beef herd size in the United States is approximately 40 cows, with an average estimated calving rate less than 80%. The typical feedlot pen finishes 100 to 200 feeder cattle. Therefore each pen would at least have single gender cattle from 10 herds. The marketing and transportation stress combined with the lack of health management preparation often leads to entire pens becoming sick with BRD based on the DART signs. It is not uncommon to find lung lesions in more than 50% of cattle that lack a proper health management history and for the lesions to involve 15% or more of the lung. The loss of gain performance associated with BRD in cattle with this level of involvement can be high, more than 1 pound ADG in severely affected cattle, but usually the ADG loss is approximately a third of a pound ADG for affected cattle.[10] This loss equates to 60 pounds lowered weight gain in a 200-day finish feeding period. At $0.90 per pound this is $56 loss in saleable weight. In addition to loss of gain there is also a negative effect on the United States Department of Agriculture (USDA) carcass quality grade. If the carcass quality grade is pushed into the next lower category and the price difference is $10 per hundredweight of carcass the average affected 750 pound carcass would be valued $75 less than carcasses from nonaffected cattle.

VACCINATION AS A BRD MANAGEMENT TOOL

Most BRD occurs in younger cattle with no history of health management following times of weaning or marketing stress.[1,10] Rapid induction of a cell-mediated immune response through the use of a modified live virus (MLV) vaccine is the primary BRD preventive focus when cattle like these arrive at a feedlot or backgrounding facility. MLV vaccines have uniformly shown value in experimental viral challenge models.[60–67] BHV-I infectious bovine rhinotracheitis (IBR) MLV vaccine seems to be the most accepted BRD complex management tool of newly received cattle.[10] Most cattle meeting this classification also receive a BVD MLV and a BRSV MLV vaccine.[6,10,13] Consulting cattle veterinarians seem not to have strong opinions about the necessity of including a PI-3 MLV vaccine, but do seem to have strong negative opinions about the usefulness of a killed virus or bacterial vaccine in newly received highly stressed cattle, citing the length of time required for an immune response to be too long to be of benefit.[10,13,18,28,33]

The most value recognized from BRD vaccinations occurs when they are administered before the marketing and transportation stresses so common to severe respiratory disease in groups of cattle.[13,17,33,34,53] BRD bacterins have a poor efficacy history. A neutral to negative effect has been commonly reported.[10,13,17] Vaccine usefulness for the common bacterial BRD pathogens *Pasteurella multocida*, *Mannheimia haemolytica*, *Histophilus somni*, and *Mycoplasma bovis* should be considered individually; however, the interactions among these potential pathogens in BRD make vaccine evaluation difficult.[47,52,55]

Numerous studies have demonstrated the relationship of high *Pasteurella multocida* antibody titers in calves and feeder cattle to improved gain performance.[2,5,11] This finding corresponds to the contentions of the importance of antibodies in resistance to pasteurellosis infection.[2,22] Live and killed vaccines are currently available. Live streptomycin-dependent *Pasteurella multocida* vaccine has shown improved health, including reduced lung damage scores, and gain performance when compared with nonvaccinated cattle in field efficacy and experimental challenge models. Killed *Pasteurella multocida* vaccines have not shown a significant reduction in morbidity, mortality, or lung lesions.[17]

The importance of LKT in *Mannheimia haemolytica* and the ability to remove most of the other components of the bacterial cell that had potential negative effects led to development of *Mannheimia haemolytica* LKT cell free vaccines.[27] Field efficacy results of these vaccines in highly stressed cattle are marginal for moderating morbidity and mortality, but better for reduction in lung damage scores collected at packing plants.[27] The relationship between lung damage scores and gain performance has been documented.[27] The value of these vaccines in immune management preconditioning programs has gained in acceptance. Given the wide variation in, or the lack of, documented usefulness, it becomes important for the veterinary practitioner to seek out creditable controlled field trial data before selecting or recommending a *Mannheimia haemolytica* vaccine.

A modified live *Mannheimia haemolytica* is available and a limited amount of data document the value of its use in newly received highly stressed feeder cattle. The conundrum is the widely accepted practice of metaphylactic use of antibiotics. This practice would seem to limit, if not eliminate, the value of a live bacterial vaccine. The recognition of other antigen fractions such as lipoproteins and sialoglycoprotease as potential adjuncts to improve vaccine performance, and novel routes of administration such as mucosal delivery, continues to be explored.

Histophilus somni bacterins have not proven effective as an arrival management tool of newly received feeder cattle.[10,13,17,45] Antibodies seem to play an important role in *Histophilus somni* protection.[42] The usefulness of available bacterins for positively affecting BRD morbidity or mortality tend to be slightly positive or neutral when used in preconditioning vaccination regimens and tend to be neutral to negative when used at feedlot arrival.[13,34,45] Negative observations of vaccination at feedlot arrival are hypothesized to be related to either an IgE anaphylaxic-like response from whole cell bacterins or an interaction between *Histophilus somni* when the animal is concurrently infected with BRSV.[42,44] The use of *Histophilus somni* bacterins at the initial feedlot processing potentially affects those conditions associated with the bacterium later in the feeding period after the immune system has had time to properly process the vaccine antigen.[17,34] Data to support this hypothesis are marginal. Failure of arrival bacterin use to control later feeding stage histophilosis condition may be caused by the walling-off, carrier-state phenomena related to isolated pockets of

the organism in different body systems following the initial BRD episode.[6,42] Specula-
tion around these types of observations and the observed ability of *Histophilus somni*
to survive macrophage phagocytosis led to the belief that the bacterium is a facultative
intracellular organism that would require a more meaningful cellular immune response
than would be considered typical for a bacterin.[42] This hypothesis is not completely
synchronous with the strength of the inverse relationship between *Histophilus somni*
titers at feedlot arrival and histophilosis.

Evaluation of *Mycoplasma bovis* vaccination data is not rewarding.[10,13,17] There are
no controlled, replicated, field trial data to support the selection and use of any available *Mycoplasma bovis* single antigen vaccine licensed by the USDA Animal and Plant
Health Inspection Service Veterinary Services. Available vaccines produce acceptable
antibody titers but this bacterium demonstrates variable expression of its surface
proteins, which limits the usefulness of humoral antibody protection.[47,52,55]

BRD BACTERIAL PATHOGEN TREATMENT MANAGEMENT

Innovations in new vaccines and medications in recent decades have not affected the
negative influence of BRD on production losses and costs,[10,13,17–19] although BRD
risks have changed in the same period. The cattle received at feedyards have changed
from predominately long yearlings and older cattle weighing on average more than 750
pounds to weaned calves and short yearlings weighing on average less than 650
pounds that have a higher risk of BRD. In recent years the term "ultra high risk" has
surfaced to describe groups of light-weight, highly stressed cattle that have acquisition source histories indicating a likelihood of 100% BRD morbidity.

Several decades ago sulfas, penicillin, oxytetracycline, tylosin, erythromycin, and
neomycin were the antibiotics cattle producers and veterinarians used to treat the
bacterial component of BRD. Although discussion of antibiotic resistance is common,
animal diagnostic laboratory data in recent decades show only fluctuations in BRD
bacterial sensitivity patterns with no long-term resistance documented.[68] Generally
the BRD bacterial pathogens are not highly contagious and with minor biosecurity
practices resistant pathogens leave the feedyard when the cattle are sold. Resistant
pathogens still in the cattle's are killed when renderers process the tissues in which
they reside at 275°C.

An educational film entitled "Pull 'em Deep" was produced several decades ago to
help train cattle caretakers in beef feedlots to deal with BRD. The point of the film was
simple: treatment outcomes will be better if the treatment is started early, before the
lung damage is so severe that recovery is doubtful. To some extent, it is simple math-
ematics: if a bacterium divides once an hour, in 24 hours 1 bug becomes 16 million
bacteria; if a sick animal is missed in the early stages of the disease, then that 1
day's growth of a BRD bacterial pathogen could be the difference between life and
death for the animal.

In recent decades, the pharmaceutical industry and the US Food and Drug Administration (FDA) have provided effective antibiotic choices. However, antibiotics do not
fix destroyed lung tissue so the principles taught in the "Pull' em Deep" film are not
only still important but the information these feedyards that handle cattle at higher
risk of BRD receive makes intercepting the disease process during the early stages
critical for protecting the animal's health and well-being. Cattle are prey animals
that have millions of years of genetic selection to help them avoid looking sick and
thereby avoid predation.

With this aim, the metaphylactic approach to BRD management was developed and
evaluated.[69–74] The metaphylaxis concept in BRD management attempts to identify

groups of newly received feeder cattle that are in the incubation or early subclinical phase of BRD and to provide an appropriately selected antibiotic to address the bacterial BRD component. Evaluation of the cattle's description and prior background is the accepted method of assessment. The cattle's description includes their weight, age, and need for dehorning or castration. The background information includes available health management history, degree of comingling, and elapsed BRD incubation time at arrival at the feedyard. BRD metaphylaxis has repeatedly been shown to decrease BRD morbidity and mortality without compromising the ability to treat cattle that are subsequently identified with clinical BRD. Antibiotic metaphylaxis has not changed the importance of identifying cattle early in the clinical stages of BRD. Caretakers are taught DART, that is to evaluate the animal's depression (D), appetite (A), respiration (R), and if these are not within normal limits to pull the animal out of the group for closer evaluation that includes evaluation of its rectal temperature (T). Cattle meeting the BRD DART criteria are started on antibiotic therapy. Treatment regimens should include antibiotic pharmacodynamic and pharmacokinetic evaluation.[6,68,75–79]

The American Veterinary Medical Association Animal Medicinal Drug Use Clarification Act provides the mechanism for veterinarians to adjust regimens to address the animal's health and well-being. The responsibility for avoiding violative residues is paramount and the likelihood of a residue occurring will increase if the label directions approved by the FDA are not followed, if the prescribing veterinarian is not diligent in adjusting the withdrawal time, or if the cattle caretaker/manager does not follow the veterinarian's prescribed adjusted withdrawal time. Beyond adjusting the withdrawal time as recommended by the Food Animal Residue Avoidance Databank (FARAD), the urine can be tested for the presence of antibiotics in cattle that do not return to normal growth performance following treatment. The PHAST (Pre-Harvest Antibiotic Screen Test), which uses *Bacillus megaterium* spores, and the PremiTest (DSM Innovation Center, Geleen, The Netherlands), which uses *Bacillus stearothermophilus*, are examples of tests that have sensitivity levels for detecting antibiotics in urine, an indirect measure of a potential antibiotic residue that might be found in the kidney.

BOTTOM-LINE BRD RISK MANAGEMENT AND EVALUATION

The goal should be to preserve and strength animals' innate and acquired resistance. Proper preparation of the animals' immune system helps them defend themselves from pathogen challenges. Proper animal handling also plays an important role in lessening the effect of stress on the immune defense system. These techniques are key to keeping cattle healthy. Failure to manage these important production management health interfaces can have serious consequences (**Fig. 1**).

"Source, source, and source" are important keys to managing or minimizing production losses related to the BRD complex. The first source is related to the cattle's production management background. Calves born to healthy mothers are more likely to stay healthy than calves born to nutritionally and immunologically mismanaged mothers. The second source is the production and health management history common to the cattle in question from birth to marketing from the farm of origin. The third source is related to comingling and handling stress during the marketing and transportation from farm of origin to the next phase in production.

When evaluating cattle source, it is more common for proper production management practices to be followed in larger herds in which cattle are the principle source of income. Only slightly more than 50% of the beef calves marketed in the United States come from herds of more than 100 beef cows, which means that approximately half the calves marketed each year in the United States come from herds that provide

Interaction of Resistance vs. Challenge & Stress

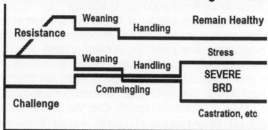

Fig. 1. The interaction between the animal's resistance to BRD pathogens and the loss of resistance caused by stress-induced increases in cortisol level during weaning and handling through marketing, transportation, and feedyard adaptation overcomes the animal's ability to fight off infections. If resistance to disease can be improved through preweaning health and production management the animal is more likely to remain healthy.

less than $10,000 to the family income. These part-time beef-cattle producers and the marketing channels used to gather and move their calves to the next level of production are important. The hobby nature of these groups of cattle producers leads to inconsistency of health management practices, and their marketed calves can present serious health management challenges. Some areas of the United States have common histories in which this is a concern. A small herd size does not mean the calves are high-risk purchases. The USDA Cooperative Extension Service and cattle producers associations have developed production and health management guidelines for preparing calves to enter market channels. These guidelines include proper selection and use of health management products. To achieve a price more representative of the improved value of well-managed cattle, the cattle are commonly marketed as collected groups. Although this procedure does not address comingling, the health preparation before marketing decreases BRD associated loses and costs.

REFERENCES

1. Aich P, Potter AA, Griebel PJ. Modern approaches to understanding stress and disease susceptibility: a review with special emphasis on respiratory disease. Int J Gen Med 2009;2:19–32.
2. Dabo SM, Taylor JD, Confer AW. *Pasteurella multocida* and bovine respiratory disease. Anim Health Res Rev 2008;8(2):129–50.
3. Dabo SM, Confer AW, Quijano-Blas RA. Molecular and immunological characterization of *Pasteurella multocida* serotype A:3 OmpA: evidence of its role in *P. multocida* interaction with extracellular matrix molecules. Microb Pathog 2003;35: 147–57.
4. Boyce JD, Adler B. The capsule is a virulence determinant in the pathogenesis of *Pasteurella multocida* M104 (B:2). Infect Immun 2000;68(6):3463–8.
5. Harper M, Boyce J, Adler B. *Pasteurella multocida* pathogenesis: 125 years after Pasteur. FEMS Microbiol Lett 2006;265:1–10.
6. Apley M. Bovine respiratory disease pathogenesis, clinical signs, and treatment in lightweight calves. Vet Clin North Am Food Anim Pract 2006;22(2):399–411.
7. Hunt ML, Adler B, Townsend KM. The molecular biology of *Pasteurella multocida*. Vet Microbiol 2000;72:3–25.

8. Carrol JA, Forsberg NE. Influence of stress and nutrition on cattle immunity. Vet Clin North Am Food Anim Pract 2007;23(1):105–49.

9. Chiase NK, Greene LW, Purdy CW, et al. Effect of transport stress on respiratory disease, serum antioxidant status, and serum concentrations of lipid peroxidation biomarkers in beef cattle. Am J Vet Res 2004;65(6):860–4.

10. Duff GC, Galyean ML. Board-invited review: recent advances in management of highly stressed newly received feeder cattle. J Anim Sci 2007;85:823–40.

11. Booker CW, Guichon PT, Jim GK, et al. Seroepidemiology of undifferentiated fever in feedlot calves in western Canada. Can Vet J 1999;40:40–8.

12. Aubry P, Warnick LD, Guard CL, et al. Health and performance of young dairy calves vaccinated with a modified-live Mannheimia haemolytica and Pasteurella multocida vaccine. J Am Vet Med Assoc 2001;219(12):1739–42.

13. Irsik M. Preparation prevents poor performance. Proceedings maintaining quality in the market place, Beef Short Course, KSU; 2005.

14. Seeger JT, Grotelueschen DM, Stokka GL. Comparison of feedlot health, nutritional performance, carcass characteristics and economic value of unweaned beef calves with an unknown health history and weaned beef calves receiving various herd-of-origin health protocols. Bovine Practitioner 2008;42(1):27–39.

15. Richeson JT, Beck PA, Gadberry MS, et al. Effects of on-arrival versus delayed modified live virus vaccination on health, performance, and serum infectious bovine rhinotracheitis titers of newly received beef calves. J Anim Sci 2008;86:999–1005.

16. Richeson JT, Kegley EB, Gadberry MS, et al. Effects of on-arrival versus delayed modified live virus vaccination on health, performance, bovine virus diarrhea virus type I titers, and stress and immune measures of newly received beef calves. J Anim Sci 2008;86:999–1005.

17. Smith RA. Feedlot diseases and their control. Proceedings: WBC Congress. Quebec (Canada); 2004.

18. McIntosh WMA, Schulz S, Dean W, et al. Feedlot veterinarians' moral and instrumental beliefs regarding antimicrobial use in feedlot cattle. J Community Appl Soc Psychol 2009;19:51–67.

19. Irsik M, Langemeier M, Schroeder T, et al. Estimating the effects of animal health on performance of feedlot cattle. Bovine Practitioner 2006;40(2):65–74.

20. King ME, Salman MD, Wittum TE, et al. Effect of certified health programs on the sale of beef calves marketed through a livestock videotape auction service from 1995 through 2005. J Am Vet Med Assoc 2006;229(9):1389–400.

21. Kirkpatrick JG, Step DL, Payton ME, et al. Effect of age at the time of vaccination on antibody titers and feedlot performance in beef calves. J Am Vet Med Assoc 2008;233(1):136–42.

22. Prado ME, Prado TM, Payton M, et al. Maternally and naturally acquired antibodies to Mannheimia haemolytica and Pasteurella multocida in beef calves. Vet Immunol Immunopathol 2006;111:301–7.

23. Binder A, Amtsberg G, Dose S, et al. [Examination of cattle with respiratory diseases for Mycoplasma and bacterial bronchopneumonia agents]. Zentralbl Veterinarmed B 1990;37(6):430–5 [in German].

24. Fuller TE, Kennedy MJ, Lowery DE. Identification of Pasteurella multocida virulence genes in septicemic mouse model using signature-tagged mutagenesis. Microb Pathog 2000;29:25–38.

25. Loneragan GH, Gould DH, Mason GL, et al. Involvement of microbial respiratory pathogens in acute interstitial pneumonia in feedlot cattle. Am J Vet Res 2001;62(10):1519–24.

26. Booker CW, Abutarbush SM, Morley PS, et al. Microbiological and histopathological findings in cases of fatal bovine respiratory disease of feedlot cattle in western Canada. Can Vet J 2008;49:473–81.
27. Rice JA, Casrrasco-Medina L, Hodgins DC, et al. Mannheimia haemolytica and bovine respiratory disease. Anim Health Res Rev 2008;8(2):117–28.
28. Snowder GD, Van Vleck LD, Cundiff LV, et al. Bovine respiratory disease in feedlot cattle: environmental, genetic and economic factors. J Anim Sci 2006;84: 1999–2008.
29. Macartney JE, Bateman KG, Ribble CS. Comparison of prices paid for feeder calves sold at conventional auctions versus special auctions of vaccinated or conditioned calves in Ontario. J Am Vet Med Assoc 2003;223(5):670–6.
30. Macartney JE, Bateman KG, Ribble CS. Health performance of feeder calves sold at conventional auctions versus special auctions of vaccinated or conditioned calves in Ontario. J Am Vet Med Assoc 2003;223(5):67783.
31. DeRosa DC, Mechor GD, Staats JJ, et al. Comparison of *Pasteurella* spp. Simultaneously isolated from nasal and transtracheal swabs from cattle with clinical signs of bovine respiratory disease. J Clin Microbiol 2000;38(1):327–32.
32. Katsuda K, Kamiyama M, Kohmoto M, et al. Serotyping of *Mannheimia haemolytica* isolates from bovine pneumonia: 1987–2006. Vet J 2008;178:146–8.
33. Speer NC, Young C, Roeber D. The importance of preventing bovine respiratory disease: a beef industry review. Bovine Practitioner 2001;36(2):189–96.
34. Thomson DU, White BJ. Backgrounding beef cattle. Vet Clin North Am Food Anim Pract 2006;22(2):373–9.
35. Swain SD, Siemsen DW, Hanson AJ, et al. Activation-induced mobilization of secretory vesicles in bovine neutrophils. Am J Vet Res 2001;62(11):1776–81.
36. McClenahan D, Fagliari J, Evanson O, et al. Role of inflammatory mediators in priming, activation, and deformability of bovine neutrophils. Am J Vet Res 2000;61(5):492–8.
37. Shewen PE, Carraso-Medina L, McBey BA, et al. Challenges in mucosal vaccination of cattle. Vet Immunol Immunopathol 2009;128:192–8.
38. Srikumaran S, Kelling CL, Ambagala A. Immune evasion by pathogens of bovine respiratory disease complex. Anim Health Res Rev 2008;8(2):215–29.
39. Cho YS, Lee HS, Lim Sk, et al. Safety and efficacy testing of a novel multivalent bovine respiratory vaccine composed of five bacterins and two immunogens. J Vet Med Sci 2008;70(9):959–64.
40. Epperson B. Lifetime effects of respiratory and liver disease in cattle. Range Beef Cow Symposium XVI, Greeley, CO, December 14–16, 1999.
41. Angen O, Thomsen J, Larsen LE, et al. Respiratory disease in calves: Microbiological investigations on trans-tracheally aspirated bronchoalveolar fluid and acute phase protein response. Vet Micro 2009;137(1–2):165–71.
42. Corbeil LB. Histophilus somni host-parasite relationships. Anim Health Res Rev 2008;8(2):151–60.
43. Kahn CM, Line S. Histophilosis. Merck vet manual. 9th edition; 2005. p. 606–7.
44. Berghaus LJ, Corbeil LB, Berghaus RD, et al. Effects of dual vaccination for bovine respiratory syncytial virus and *Haemophilus somnus* on immune responses. Vaccine 2006;24:6018–27.
45. Orr JP. *Haemophilus somnus* infection: a retrospective analysis of cattle necropsied at the Western College of Veterinary Medicine from 1970–1990. Can Vet J 1992;33:719–22.
46. Daoust PY. Morphologic study of bacterial pneumonia of feedlot cattle: determination of age of lesions. Can Vet J 1989;30:155–60.

47. Caswell JL, Archambault M. *Mycoplasma bovis* pneumonia in cattle. Anim Health Res Rev 2008;8(2):161–86.
48. Maunsell FP, Donovan GA. *Mycoplasma bovis* infections in young calves. Vet Clin North Am Food Anim Pract 2009;25(1):139–77.
49. Byrne WJ, McCormick J, Brice N, et al. Isolation of *Mycoplasma bovis* from bovine clinical samples in the republic of Ireland. Vet Rec 2001;148(11):331–3.
50. Khodakaram-Tafti A, Lopez A. Immunohistopathological findings in the lungs of calves naturally infected with *Mycoplasma bovis*. J Vet Med A Physiol Pathol Clin Med 2004;51:10–4.
51. Rosenbusch RF, Kinyon JM, Apley M, et al. In vitro antimicrobial inhibition profiles of *Mycoplasma bovis* isolates recovered from various regions of the United States from 2002 to 2003. J Vet Diagn Invest 2005;17:436–41.
52. Martin SW, Nagy E, Armstrong D, et al. The associations of viral and mycoplasmal antibody titers with respiratory disease and weight gain in feedlot calves. Can Vet J 1999;40:560–70.
53. Woolums AR, Loneragan GH, Hawkins LL, et al. Baseline management practices and animal health data reported by US feedlots responding to a survey regarding acute interstitial pneumonia. Bovine Practitioner 2005;39(2):116–24.
54. Shahriar FM, Clark EG, Janzen E, et al. Coinfection with bovine viral diarrhea virus and *Mycoplasma bovis* in feedlot cattle. Can Vet J 2002;43:863–8.
55. VandenBush TJ, Rosenbusch RF. Characterization of the immune response to *Mycoplasma bovis* lung infection. Vet Immunol Immunopathol 2003;94: 23–33.
56. Lubbers BV, Apley MD, Coetzee JF, et al. Use of computed tomography to evaluate pathologic changes in the lungs of calves with experimentally induced respiratory tract disease. Am J Vet Res 2007;68(11):1259–64.
57. Woolums AR, Loneragan GH, Hawkins LL, et al. A survey of the relationship between management practices and risk of acute interstitial pneumonia at US feedlots. Bovine Practitioner 2005;39(2):125–33.
58. Thompson PN, Stone A, Schultheiss WA. Use of treatment records and lung lesions scoring to estimate the effect of respiratory disease on growth during early and late finishing periods in South Africa feedlot cattle. J Anim Sci 2006; 84:488–98.
59. Daniel JA, Held JE, Brake DG, et al. Evaluation of the prevalence and onset of lung lesions and their impact on growth of lambs. Am J Vet Res 2006;67(5): 890–4.
60. Potter A, Gerdts V, Van Drunen Little-van den Hurk SD. Veterinary vaccines: alternatives to antibiotics? Anim Health Res Rev 2008;9(2):187–99.
61. White BJ, McReynolds S, Goehl D, et al. Effect of vaccination and weaning timing on backgrounding morbidity in preconditioned beef feeder calves. Bovine Practitioner 2008;42(2):111–6.
62. Wildman BK, Perrett T, Abutarbush SM, et al. A comparison of 2 vaccination programs in feedlot calves at ultra-high risk of developing undifferentiated fever / bovine respiratory disease. Can Vet J 2008;49:463–72.
63. Makoschey B, Munoz-Bielsa J, Oliviero L, et al. Field efficacy of combination vaccines against bovine respiratory pathogens in calves. Acta Vet Hung 2008; 56(4):485–93.
64. Frank GH, Briggs RE, Duff GC, et al. Effects of vaccination before transit and administration of florfenicol at time of arrival in feedlot on the health of transported calves and detection of *Mannheimia haemolyticia* in nasal secretions. Am J Vet Res 2002;63(2):251–6.

65. Confer AW, Ayalew S, Montelongo M, et al. Immunity of cattle following vaccination with *Mannheimia haemolytica* chimeric PlpE-LKT (SAC89) protein. Vaccine 2009;27:1771–6.
66. Confer AW, Montelongo M. Onset of serum antibodies to Pasteurella (Mannheimia) haemolytica following vaccination with five commercial vaccines. Bovine Practitioner 2001;35:141–8.
67. Perrett T, Wildman BK, Abutarbush SM, et al. A comparison of two *Mannheimia haemolytica* immunization programs in feedlot calves at high risk of developing undifferentiated fever/bovine respiratory disease. Bovine Practitioner 2008; 42(1):64–75.
68. Call DR, Davis MA, Sawant AA. Antimicrobial resistance in beef and dairy cattle production. Anim Health Res Rev 2008;9(2):159–67.
69. Guthrie CA, Rogers KC, Christmas RA, et al. Efficacy of metaphylactic tilmicosin for controlling bovine respiratory disease in high-risk northern feeder calves. Bovine Practitioner 2004;38(1):46–53.
70. McCary DG, Corbin MJ, Carter B, et al. A comparison of 3-, 5-, 7-, and 10-day post-metaphylaxis evaluation periods on health and performance following on arrival treatment with tilmicosin in feeder cattle – summary of two studies. Bovine Practitioner 2008;42(2):117–27.
71. Step DL, Engelken T, Romano C, et al. Evaluation of three antimicrobial regimens used as metaphylaxis in stocker calves at high risk of developing bovine respiratory disease. Vet Ther 2007;8(2):136–47.
72. Bryant TC, Nichols JR, Adams JR, et al. Effect of tilmicosin alone or in combination with *Mannheimia haemolytica* toxoid administered at initial feedlot processing on morbidity and mortality of high-risk calves. Bovine Practitioner 2008; 42(1):50–4.
73. Robb EJ, Hibbard B, Follis SL, et al. Duration of efficacy of ceftiofur crystalline free acid compared to tilmicosin when administered at various times before intratracheal *Mannheimia haemolytica* challenge in calves. Bovine Practitioner 2004; 38(2):177.
74. Carter BL, McClary DG, Mechor GD, et al. Comparison of 3-, 5-, and 7-day post-treatment evaluation periods for measuring therapeutic response to tilmicosin treatment of bovine respiratory disease. Bovine Practitioner 2006;40(2):97–101.
75. Brumbaugh GW, Herman JD, Clancy JS, et al. Effect of tilmicosin on chemotatic, phagocytic, and bactericidal activities of bovine and porcine alveolar macrophages. Am J Vet Res 2002;63(1):36–41.
76. Kehrenberg C, Salmon SA, Watts JL, et al. Tetracycline resistance genes in isolates of *Pasteurella multocida*, *Mannheimia haemolytica*, *Mannheimia glucosida* and *Mannheimia varigena* from bovine and swine respiratory disease: intergeneric spread of the tet(H) plasmid pMHT1. J Antimicrob Chemother 2001; 48:631–40.
77. Perrett T, Wildman BK, Fuch MT, et al. A comparison of florfenicol and tulathromycin for treatment of undifferentiated fever in feedlot calves. Vet Ther 2008;9(2): 128–40.
78. Post KW, Cole NA, Raleigh RH. In vitro antimicrobial susceptibility of *Pasteurella haemolytica* and *Pasteurella multocida* recovered from cattle with bovine respiratory disease complex. J Vet Diagn Invest 1991;2:124–6.
79. Thomas A, Nicolas DI, Mainil AL. Antibiotic susceptibilities of recent isolates of *Mycoplasma bovis* in Belgium. Vet Rec 2003;153(14):428–31.

Moraxella bovoculi and Infectious Bovine Keratoconjunctivitis: Cause or Coincidence?

John A. Angelos, DVM, PhD

KEYWORDS

• Moraxella bovoculi • Moraxella bovis
• Infectious bovine keratoconjunctivitis • Pinkeye • Cattle

Infectious bovine keratoconjunctivitis (IBK, or pinkeye) is the most common ocular disease of cattle and occurs in cattle populations throughout the world. All cattle breeds are considered susceptible, although a lower incidence of IBK has been reported in Brahman cattle and cattle with more periocular pigmentation.[1,2] Cattle with IBK exhibit corneal ulcers, corneal edema, photophobia, blepharospasm, and lacrimation. Although many corneal ulcers associated with IBK heal with varying degrees of corneal scarring, corneas may rupture, leading to permanent blindness.

Moraxella bovis has been accepted as the sole causative agent of IBK, and is currently the only agent for which Koch's postulates have been established for IBK.[3] Recently, however, a coccoid Moraxella was described that was also associated with IBK: M bovoculi.[4] This article describes known pathogenic and clinical features associated with M bovoculi that can help practitioners prevent IBK associated with M bovoculi.

In the long list of IBK-related studies published over many years, other bacteria isolated from the eyes of IBK-affected cattle were reported that did not fit the morphologic description of M bovis (ie, gram-negative rod or diplobacillus). These other organisms had been variously referred to as hemolytic gram-negative cocci or micrococci. In a 1917 translation of a 1911 manuscript, a gram-negative micrococcus isolated from cattle with IBK was described, however, it did not cause IBK after inoculation into the eyes of cattle.[5] In 1966, hemolytic gram-negative cocci were isolated from calves with severe keratitis and corneal ulceration.[6] Neisseria spp were subsequently reported in 24 of 25 outbreaks of IBK; however, M bovis was isolated in only two of the outbreaks.[7] In 1970, Neisseria (Branhamella) catarrhalis was reported to be isolated from nearly 45% of IBK cases, whereas M bovis was found in only 28% of IBK cases.[8] M bovis and organisms identified as Neisseria spp that were likely

Department of Medicine and Epidemiology, School of Veterinary Medicine, University of California, 2108 Tupper Hall, Davis, CA 95616, USA
E-mail address: jaangelos@ucdavis.edu

Vet Clin Food Anim 26 (2010) 73–78
doi:10.1016/j.cvfa.2009.10.002
0749-0720/10/$ – see front matter © 2010 Elsevier Inc. All rights reserved.

coccoid forms of Moraxella species have also been cultured from the eyes of normal cattle.[9,10] When the eyes of experimental calves were irradiated and then infected with N ovis (later renamed M ovis), however, lesions typical of IBK did not develop.[11] Based on these experimental observations, a definitive role for gram-negative cocci in the pathogenesis of IBK is questionable.

During a drug efficacy trial that was conducted in northern California during summer 2002, IBK-affected eyes of dairy and beef calves were cultured, and in most calves, hemolytic gram-negative cocci but not M bovis were isolated.[12] In a few cases, both M bovis and hemolytic gram-negative cocci were isolated. The hemolytic gram-negative cocci were subsequently characterized; biochemical and molecular data supported that these isolates were distinct from M bovis and M ovis and warranted their classification as a novel species that was named M bovoculi.[4] M bovoculi has probably circulated in cattle populations for many years, and could even have been present in the earliest reports of hemolytic gram-negative cocci or Neisseria spp. Hemolytic gram-negative cocci isolated from cases of IBK that have been historically designated as M ovis, M ovis–like, B ovis, or B ovis–like may also have been M bovoculi. Depending on the spectrum of biochemical tests that are performed on M ovis and M bovoculi, these species may appear identical (**Table 1**).

An exact role for M bovoculi in the pathogenesis of IBK is currently uncertain because no published studies have definitively linked corneal injury to M bovoculi infection. However, anecdotal evidence exists of autogenous vaccination with M bovoculi bacterins being successful in preventing IBK. These observations suggest a role for M bovoculi in IBK pathogenesis.

Biochemical testing and molecular methods now allow coccoid Moraxellae isolated from the eyes of cattle to be more easily differentiated. In the original characterization of M bovoculi, a phenylalanine deaminase test could differentiate M bovoculi (positive reaction) from M ovis and M bovis (negative reactions)[4] (**Fig. 1**).

Subsequently, the authors identified phenylalanine deaminase–negative M bovoculi. To differentiate these organisms from M ovis and M bovis, a rapid molecular method was developed that involves polymerase chain reaction (PCR) amplification of the interspacer region between the 16S rRNA and 23S rRNA genes followed by restriction digestion of the amplicon.[13] In this test, oligonucleotide primers for the interspacer region are used to amplify genomic DNA; the resulting ~ 600 bp amplicon is then subjected to restriction endonuclease digestion with AfaI. The amplicon generated for M bovoculi is cleaved into ~ 450 bp and ~ 150 bp fragments, whereas the amplicon generated for M bovis and M ovis are not cut with AfaI. Using this method, M bovoculi can be readily distinguished from M bovis and M ovis.

For M bovis, pathogenicity is linked to the expression of a cytotoxin that is known to be an RTX (Repeats in the structural ToXin) toxin.[14] Other significant food animal pathogens that encode RTX toxins include Mannheimia haemolytica, the cause of bovine shipping fever, and Actinobacillus pleuropneumoniae, the cause of swine pleuropneumonia. The M bovis cytotoxin is contained in an operon composed of 4 genes (mbxCABD) that encode proteins for cytotoxin activation (mbxC gene product), cytotoxin (mbxA gene product), and secretion (mbxB and mbxD gene products). In addition, a closely linked gene involved in secretion (tolC) flanks the mbxD gene.[15]

When M bovoculi was examined for the presence of similar RTX genes, a complete RTX operon (designated the mbvCABD operon) was identified.[16] A high degree of nucleotide and deduced amino acid sequence similarity exists between the M bovoculi and M bovis RTX operon genes. Along with mbvCABD, a closely linked tolC gene is also present flanking mbvD. These results suggest a possible role for M bovoculi in the pathogenesis of IBK.

Table 1
Phenotypic and biochemical characteristics of *Moraxella bovoculi*, *ovis*, and *bovis*

Characteristic	*Moraxella bovoculi*	*Moraxella ovis*[a]	*Moraxella bovis*[a]
Morphology	C, CD	C	R
Motility	−	−	−
Catalase activity	+	+	(+)
Oxidase activity	+	+	+
Growth on MacConkey agar	−	−	−
Acids produced from glucose	−	−	−
Growth on minimal medium containing ammonium and acetate	−	−	−
Hemolysis	(+)	(+)	+
Nitrate reduction	(+)	+	(−)
Liquefaction of gelatin	−	−	+
DNAse activity	(+/−)	(−)	−
Proteolysis on Löffler slants	(+/−)	−	+
Indole	−	−	−
Phenylalanine deaminase activity	+	−	−
Hydrolysis of Tween 80	(+)	−	+
Alkaline phosphatase activity	(−)	+	−
Esterase activity	+[b]	+	+
Acid phosphatase activity	−	−	w

Abbreviations: C, coccus; CD, diplococcus; R, rod; −, negative reaction; +, positive reaction; w, weak reaction; (+), most strains positive; (−), most strains negative; (+/−), 50% positive.
[a] Data from Kodjo A, Richard Y, Tonjum T. *Moraxella boevrei* sp. nov., a new Moraxella species found in goats. Int J Syst Bacteriol 1997;47:115–21.
[b] C4 esterase (hydrolysis of 2-naphthyl butyrate) and C8 esterase lipase (hydrolysis of 2-naphthyl caprylate).
Data from Angelos JA, Spinks PQ, Ball LM, et al. *Moraxella bovoculi* sp. nov., isolated from calves with infectious bovine keratoconjunctivitis. Int J Syst Evol Microbiol 2007;57:789–95.

The hemolytic activity associated with both *M bovoculi* and *M ovis* grown on blood agar was neutralized with rabbit polyclonal antisera against the carboxy terminus of *M bovoculi* MbvA; *M bovis* hemolytic activity was not neutralized with this antiserum.[16] However, the hemolytic activity of *M bovoculi* and *M ovis* was partially neutralized with rabbit antisera against the carboxy terminus of the *M bovis* cytotoxin. These results suggest that combining *M bovoculi* and *M bovis* antigens in vaccines against IBK may be important in developing novel vaccines against IBK.

Although the presence of an RTX toxin and an RTX operon in *M bovoculi* and laboratory evidence for neutralization of hemolytic activity associated with an RTX toxin would make a role for *M bovoculi* in the pathogenesis of IBK plausible, this role remains unproven. In some published studies, lesions consistent with IBK could not be reproduced when bacteria identified as *M ovis* or *N ovis* were used to infect bovine eyes through either direct inoculation[17] or inoculation after ultraviolet corneal irradiation.[11] The method of applying ultraviolet irradiation to corneas in the study by Pedersen[11] was previously shown to be effective for inducing IBK with *M bovis*.[18]

Other factors may be necessary for the pathogenesis of *M bovoculi* or perhaps *M bovoculi* already present in a bovine eye takes advantage of trauma (eg, from

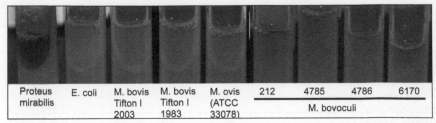

Proteus mirabilis	E. coli	M. bovis Tifton I 2003	M. bovis Tifton I 1983	M. ovis (ATCC 33078)	212	4785	4786	6170
						M. bovoculi		

Fig. 1. A phenylalanine deaminase (PD) test can differentiate *Moraxella bovoculi* that are PD-positive from *M ovis/M bovis* (PD-negative). *Proteus mirabilis* (positive control) and *Escherichia coli* (negative control) are shown in the first two tubes. Negative reactions are evident for *M bovis* and *M ovis*; positive reactions (as shown by green haziness within agar and media) are shown by four isolates of *M bovoculi*. PD-negative gram-negative cocci isolated from cattle with IBK should be further evaluated using a molecular method that involves polymerase chain reaction amplification and restriction digestion of amplified DNA. (*Data from* Angelos JA, Ball LM. Differentiation of *Moraxella bovoculi* sp. nov. from other coccoid moraxellae by the use of polymerase chain reaction and restriction endonuclease analysis of amplified DNA. J Vet Diagn Invest 2007;19:532–4.)

a foxtail) to become an established infection. In addition to foxtails or other plant awns, flies and ultraviolet radiation could also be important in ocular disease associated with *M bovoculi*.

In this author's experience, *M bovoculi* can be isolated from the eyes of completely normal dairy calves. This observation parallels the situation for *M bovis*, wherein asymptomatic *M bovis* carriers are known to exist in cattle populations. A recent investigation of an outbreak of ulcerative conjunctivitis in adult dairy cows in the California central valley identified *M bovoculi* in the absence of *M bovis* in one cow that had both conjunctivitis and corneal ulceration.[19]

M bovoculi was also associated with a February 2009 outbreak of conjunctivitis on a central California feedlot (Jim Reynolds, DVM, MPVM, and Robert Moeller, DVM, personal communication, June 2009). During this winter outbreak, 40% of 65- to 120-day old Holstein bull calves on a large feedlot developed bilateral mucopurulent conjunctivitis and epiphora approximately 1 week after being placed into group pens. These calves had been vaccinated against IBR-BVD-PI3-BRSV-Lepto at 3 and 6 weeks of age; in addition, the calves received autogenous *M bovis* and *M bovoculi* vaccines at 4 and 7 weeks of age. *Moraxella* spp were not isolated from the initial ocular swabs taken from 10 affected calves.

Necropsies on three calves showed reddened conjunctiva with periorbital conjunctival swelling; one of these calves also had corneal edema in one eye. The histology of conjunctival tissue showed lymphocytic and neutrophilic infiltrates in the submucosa, consistent with bacterial conjunctivitis. From ocular cultures taken at necropsy, *Mycoplasma bovis* was isolated in one calf and both *Mycoplasma bovis* and *Moraxella bovoculi* in one. All three calves were negative for infectious bovine rhinotracheitis.

The problem resolved after discontinued use of composted bedding and changing to fresh rice hulls/almond shells for bedding. The outbreak lasted 30 days. The mechanical irritation associated with dusty bedding is suspected to have facilitated ocular infection by *M bovoculi*.

In one field trial in which calves were vaccinated with an *M bovis* recombinant pilin–cytotoxin vaccine, *M bovoculi* tended to be isolated more frequently from calves that had been vaccinated with *M bovis* antigens than from control calves.[20] This observation might suggest that vaccination against *M bovis* and *M bovoculi* may be important when both organisms are circulating in a herd. During vaccine breaks in herds vaccinated with either commercial or autogenous *M bovis* or autogenous *M bovoculi* products, culturing eyes from IBK-affected cattle is recommended to determine whether *M bovis*, *M bovoculi*, or both organisms are present. These isolates may be useful for subsequent development of autogenous bacterins. As with IBK associated with *M bovis*, fly and weed control are presumed important along with proper nutrition, with particular attention to the adequacy of selenium and copper supplementation programs.

Although Koch's postulates have not been established for *M bovoculi* and IBK, considerable circumstantial evidence suggests that this newly characterized species of *Moraxella* plays a role in the pathogenesis of IBK. Veterinarians and producers should pay attention to laboratory diagnoses of *M ovis*, *M ovis*–like, *B ovis*, or *B ovis*–like species, because these may in fact be *M bovoculi*. Molecular and biochemical methods can help to successfully differentiate *M bovoculi* from *M ovis*/*M bovis*. Additional research is needed that helps characterize any roles for *M bovoculi* in IBK pathogenesis and should help guide future efforts to develop improved vaccines against IBK.

REFERENCES

1. Frisch JE. The relative incidence and effect of bovine infectious keratoconjunctivitis in *Bos indicus* and *Bos taurus* cattle. Anim Prod 1975;21:265–74.
2. Ward JK, Neilson MK. Pinkeye (bovine infectious keratoconjunctivitis) in beef cattle. J Anim Sci 1979;49:361–6.
3. Henson JB, Grumbles LC. Infectious bovine keratoconjunctivitis. I. Etiology. Am J Vet Res 1960;21:761–6.
4. Angelos JA, Spinks PQ, Ball LM, et al. *Moraxella bovoculi* sp. nov., isolated from calves with infectious bovine keratoconjunctivitis. Int J Syst Evol Microbiol 2007; 57:789–95.
5. Poels J. Keratitis infectiosa in cattle (*keratitis pyobacillosa*). J Am Vet Med Assoc 1917;51:526–31.
6. Fairlie G. The isolation of a haemolytic Neisseria from cattle and sheep in the North of Scotland. Vet Rec 1966;78:649–50.
7. Spradbrow PB. A microbiological study of bovine conjunctivitis and keratoconjunctivitis. Aust Vet J 1967;43:55–8.
8. Wilcox GE. Bacterial flora of the bovine eye with special reference to the Moraxella and Neisseria. Aust Vet J 1970;46:253–6.
9. Barber DM. Bacterial population of the eyes of slaughter cattle. Vet Rec 1984; 115:169.
10. Barber DM, Jones GE, Wood A. Microbial flora of the eyes of cattle. Vet Rec 1986; 118:204–6.
11. Pedersen KB. Isolation and description of a haemolytic species of Neisseria (*N. ovis*) from cattle with infectious keratoconjunctivitis. Acta Pathol Microbiol Scand B Microbiol Immunol 1972;80:135–9.
12. Dueger EL, George LW, Angelos JA, et al. Efficacy of a long-acting formulation of ceftiofur crystalline-free acid for the treatment of naturally occurring infectious bovine keratoconjunctivitis. Am J Vet Res 2004;65:1185–8.
13. Angelos JA, Ball LM. Differentiation of Moraxella bovoculi sp. nov. from other coccoid moraxellae by the use of polymerase chain reaction and restriction endonuclease analysis of amplified DNA. J Vet Diagn Invest 2007;19:532–4.

14. Angelos JA, Hess JF, George LW. Cloning and characterization of a Moraxella bovis cytotoxin gene. Am J Vet Res 2001;62:1222–8.
15. Angelos JA, Hess JF, George LW. An RTX operon in hemolytic Moraxella bovis is absent from nonhemolytic strains. Vet Microbiol 2003;92:363–77.
16. Angelos JA, Ball LM, Hess JF. Identification and characterization of complete RTX operons in *Moraxella bovoculi* and *Moraxella ovis*. Vet Microbiol 2007;125:73–9.
17. Elad D, Yeruham I, Bernstein M. Moraxella ovis in cases of infectious bovine keratoconjunctivitis (IBK) in Israel. Zentralbl Veterinarmed B 1988;35:431–4.
18. Hughes DE, Pugh DW Jr, McDonald TJ. Experimental bovine infectious keratoconjunctivitis caused by sunlamp irradiation and Moraxella bovis infection: determination of optimal irradiation. Am J Vet Res 1968;29:821–7.
19. Galvão K, Angelos JA. Ulcerative blepharitis and conjunctivitis in adult dairy cows and association with Moraxella bovoculi. Can Vet J, in press.
20. Angelos JA, Bonifacio RG, Ball LM, et al. Prevention of naturally occurring infectious bovine keratoconjunctivitis with a recombinant Moraxella bovis pilin-*Moraxella bovis* cytotoxin-ISCOM matrix adjuvanted vaccine. Vet Microbiol 2007;125:274–83.

Antimicrobial Resistance in Bovine Respiratory Disease Pathogens: Measures, Trends, and Impact on Efficacy

Jeffrey L. Watts, PhD, RM (NRCM), M(ASCP)*, Michael T. Sweeney, MS

KEYWORDS

• Antimicrobial resistance • Antimicrobial susceptibility tests
• Bovine respiratory disease • Surveillance program

Bovine respiratory disease (BRD) is one of the most costly diseases to the feedlot industry with annual global losses estimated to be over $3 billion per year.[1–3] BRD is a complex, multifactorial disease with stress, nutrition, and viral infections playing a significant role in disease development. The primary bacterial pathogens associated with BRD are *Mannheimia haemolytica*, *Pasteurella multocida*, and *Histophilus somni*.[4,5] Antibacterial therapy is essential for the effective control and treatment of BRD in feedlots. From 1988 to 2005, a variety of new antimicrobial agents were approved in the United States for the treatment of BRD including ceftiofur, tilmicosin, tulathromycin, florfenicol, enrofloxacin, and danofloxacin. These agents have transformed the treatment of BRD in feedlots by offering superior efficacy or convenience compared with older agents. Moreover, the practice of on-arrival therapy for at-risk cattle or metaphylaxis and delaying retreatment following initial therapy (posttreatment interval) was made possible because of the unique characteristics of these newer agents.[6,7]

The development of widespread resistance to the primary therapeutic antimicrobial agents by BRD pathogens would be economically devastating to the cattle industry. The detection of emerging resistance in the BRD pathogens has been hindered, however, by the lack of an annual routine surveillance program; a lack of understanding of resistance mechanisms against some classes of agents; and, until recently, the lack of BRD-specific interpretive criteria that allow the accurate detection of clinically relevant resistance. Additionally, the impact of resistance on treatment efficacy has not been well established. These factors have to be considered to

---

Veterinary Medicine Research and Development, Pfizer Animal Health, 333 Portage Road, Kalamazoo, MI 49001, USA
* Corresponding author.
E-mail address: jeffrey.l.watts@pfizer.com (J.L. Watts).

Vet Clin Food Anim 26 (2010) 79–88
doi:10.1016/j.cvfa.2009.10.009
0749-0720/10/$ – see front matter © 2010 Elsevier Inc. All rights reserved.

comprehend fully the present and future impact of resistance development in the BRD pathogens on the beef industry.

MEASURES OF ANTIMICROBIAL RESISTANCE

Antimicrobial susceptibility tests (ASTs) are the most commonly used methods for assessing the activity of a specific antimicrobial agent against a pathogen. These tests, when properly designed, provide reproducible in vitro assessments of antimicrobial potency and accurate predictions of clinical response. The most commonly used methods for conducting ASTs on veterinary pathogens are those defined by the Clinical Laboratory and Standards Institute (CLSI).[8,9]

The minimal inhibitory concentration (MIC) method is the most widely used method for determining the in vitro activity of an antimicrobial agent. Either the agar dilution or broth microdilution method may be used for MIC determinations. The microdilution broth method is most widely used because of convenience and availability of commercial systems. Generally, the microdilution method consists of doubling dilutions of the antimicrobial agent in broth, inoculation with a standardized bacterial suspension, and incubation for 18 to 24 hours.[8] The first dilution with no visible growth is considered the MIC for that strain of pathogen. Inclusion of a known quality control organism on each day of test is essential to validate test results.[8,9]

The results of the MIC test indicate the in vitro potency or activity (usually expressed in microgram per milliliter) of an antimicrobial agent against an individual bacterial strain or collection of isolates. The in vitro activity of each antimicrobial class as indicated by the MIC value is dictated by the ability of the agent to enter the bacterial cell and its interaction with the target antibacterial site (mechanism of action). Each class of agent demonstrates an inherent MIC value and direct comparisons of MIC values between antimicrobial classes are not valid. The most commonly reported summary statistics for MIC data are the MIC_{50} and MIC_{90} range. The MIC_{50} and MIC_{90} represent the MIC value at which 50% or 90% of strains in a population are inhibited. These data alone can provide substantive information regarding the prevalence of resistance mechanisms within a population of pathogens and many clinicians use these data to decide which compounds can be used empirically. For example, a low MIC_{50} and MIC_{90} value indicates that resistance has not emerged for most strains within that population, whereas a low MIC_{50} and high MIC_{90} indicate that resistance has emerged. Many clinicians select for use the agents fitting the first example for empiric use, restricting those fitting the second example only when AST results indicated susceptibility to that agent. In the BRD pathogens, this is the situation when comparing MIC data for ampicillin with the data for ceftiofur (**Fig. 1**).[10]

Clinicians should be cautioned that the MIC value alone are not to be taken as an indicator of the efficacy of a compound because other factors, such as pharmacokinetic-pharmacodynamic parameters and clinical efficacy, must be considered. The in vitro activity, associated pharmacokinetic-pharmacodynamic parameters, and currently approved dosages for the newer BRD agents that have been demonstrated to be effective in clinical efficacy studies of BRD are provided in **Table 1**.[11–13]

DEVELOPMENT OF BRD-SPECIFIC INTERPRETIVE CRITERIA

Interpretive criteria provide the means of correlating an AST result (susceptible or resistant) with a clinical outcome (cure or failure).[14] The development of veterinary-specific interpretive criteria requires a tripartite database that includes microbiologic distribution data, pharmacokinetic-pharmacodynamics information, and outcome data from clinical efficacy trials.[8,9,14] This information allows threshold values or

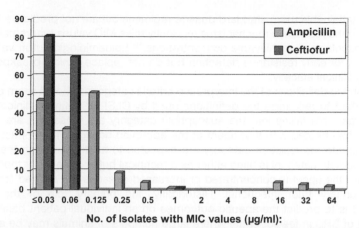

Fig. 1. Minimal inhibitory concentration (MIC) distributions for ceftiofur and ampicillin with 152 bovine strains of *Pasteurella multocida*. (*From* Catry B, Haesebrouck F, De Vliegher S, et al. Variability in acquired resistance of *Pasteurella* and *Mannheimia* isolates from the nasopharynx of calves, with particular reference to different herd types. Microb Drug Res 2005;11:387–94; with permission.)

"breakpoints" to be established for categorizing isolates as susceptible, intermediate, or resistant. It should be noted that interpretive criteria which incorporate clinical efficacy data are referred to as "clinical breakpoints" and should be differentiated from other types of categorizations, such as "microbiologic breakpoints" or "epidemiologic cutoffs."[15]

Epidemiologic cutoff values are useful in surveillance programs when detection of resistance mechanisms is important. A comparison of the MIC distributions for ampicillin and ceftiofur (see **Fig. 1**) for bovine strains of *P multocida* indicates that the population distribution is bimodal for ampicillin because of β-lactamase production in this organism.[10] In contrast, ceftiofur is not affected by β-lactamase activity and MIC values remain low. Epidemiologic cutoff values generally are predictive of clinical efficacy in those situations where the resistance mechanism raises MIC values to levels

Table 1
In vitro activity, pharmacodynamic parameters, and FDA-approved dosage for selected antimicrobial agents commonly used to treat *Mannheimia haemolytica* and *Pasteurella multocida* isolated from bovine respiratory disease

Antimicrobial Agent	MIC$_{90}$ (µg/mL)		Pharmacodynamic Parameter	FDA-approved Dose (mg/kg)
	M haemolytica	*P multocida*		
Ceftiofur	≤0.03	≤0.03	T > MIC	6.6[a]
Tulathromycin	2	1	AUC/MIC	2.5
Tilmicosin	32	32	AUC/MIC	10
Florfenicol	2	0.5	T > MIC	20
Enrofloxacin	0.06	0.125	AUC/MIC	7.5–12.5

Abbreviations: AUC, area under the curve; FDA, Food and Drug Administration; MIC, minimal inhibitory concentration; T, time.
[a] Dose is for ceftiofur crystalline free acid form.
Data from Refs.[10–13]

that are unattainable using standard dosage regimens but are not predictive in situations where the resistance mechanisms modestly raise MIC values that remain within the pharmacologically achievable concentrations.[15] Epidemiologic cutoff values are useful tools for early resistance detection but do not replace clinical breakpoints for predicting clinical efficacy.

Although the definitions of the interpretive criteria categories should seem obvious, it is important to recognize the definitions used by CLSI for defining clinical breakpoints. Organisms falling into the susceptible category are those that are likely to respond when treated with that agent at the approved dosages. In contrast, organisms falling into the resistant category are expected to fail therapy with that agent. The intermediate category is used either as a technical buffer zone or for those situations where the agent is concentrated or increased dosages are defined (eg, β-lactams in urinary tract infections). Historically, the primary role of the clinical breakpoint is to predict therapeutic outcomes on an individual patient basis. In the treatment of BRD in feedlot cattle where large numbers of animals may be at risk of developing disease, one should realize that bacterial resistance translates as a substantial reduction in clinical efficacy.

It should be recognized that although the purpose of clinical breakpoints is to predict clinical efficacy, the relationship between the AST result and outcome is imperfect.[9,14] In the best case scenario, eradication of the pathogen posttreatment is the best end point for the evaluation of efficacy. Use of this end point is generally limited to simple infections where pretreatment and posttreatment culturing of infected tissues is possible. Examples of infectious processes where this is possible include urinary tract infections and bovine mastitis.[9,14] In more complicated disease where posttreatment culturing is not possible, such as pneumonias in humans and cattle, elimination of clinical symptoms is generally used to determine efficacy.[9,14] Generally, the agreement between the AST test result and in vivo response should be at least 80% for mild to moderate disease. Other factors, such as health status, stage of infection, and bacterial virulence, may modulate overall treatment efficacy and should be considered by the clinician when evaluating treatment outcomes. The veterinary specific breakpoints for agents approved for the treatment of BRD are presented in **Table 2**.

CURRENT RESISTANCE TRENDS IN BRD PATHOGENS

Determining the current resistance trends in the BRD pathogens is problematic because the large national monitoring programs, such as the National Antimicrobial Resistance Monitoring System, are focused on zoonotic pathogens, such as *Salmonella*, and not on target animal pathogens.[16] Resistance monitoring in the BRD pathogens has been primarily limited to individual studies. To date, there have been no continuous, long-term surveillance data on the BRD pathogens reported in the literature.

The primary β-lactam antimicrobial agent used in the treatment of BRD in the United States is ceftiofur. This agent is a third-generation cephalosporin that is resistant to the β-lactamases produced by *M haemolytica* or *P multocida* that degrade older agents in this class, such as ampicillin. Based on the current data available in the literature,[10,16,17] the MIC_{90} values for ceftiofur with BRD pathogens have remained at less than or equal to 0.06 μg/mL since the introduction of the agent in 1988.

Currently, two macrolides are widely used for the treatment of BRD: tilmicosin, a 16-membered macrolide introduced in the mid-1990s in the United States; and tulathromycin, a 15-membered compound belonging to the triamilide subclass, approved for

Table 2
Veterinary-specific interpretive criteria for the newer antimicrobial agents approved for treatment of bovine respiratory disease in the United States

Antimicrobial Agent	Interpretive Category (µg/mL)		
	Susceptible	Intermediate	Resistant
Ceftiofur	≤2	4	≥8
Danofloxacin	≤0.25	NE	NE
Enrofloxacin	≤0.25	0.5–1	≥2
Tilmicosin	≤8	16	≥32
Tulathromycin	≤16	32	≥64
Florfenicol	≤2	4	≥8

Abbreviation: NE, not established.

Data from CLSI. Performance standards for antimicrobial disk and dilution susceptibility tests for bacteria isolated from animals: approved standard. 3rd edition. CLSI document M31-A3. Wayne (PA): Clinical and Laboratory Standards Institute; 2008.

use in the United States in 2005.[18,19] Surveillance data[17] indicated substantial year-to-year variation in the MIC values for tilmicosin but generally values remained below the current BRD-specific interpretive criteria for susceptibility. These data are consistent with those reported elsewhere.[17] Susceptibility data on tulathromycin indicated MIC_{90} values for *M haemolytica* and *P multocida* as 2 µg/mL and 1 µg/mL, respectively, with no changes noted between strains isolated before 2002 and those isolated from 2004 to 2006.[13,18,20] Interestingly, the precise mechanism of resistance for the macrolides in *M haemolytica* and *P multocida* has not been fully elucidated.

Florfenicol is a member of the phenicol family of antimicrobial agents that also includes chloramphenicol and thiamphenicol.[19] Chloramphenicol has been banned from use in food animals since the early 1980s. Resistance to these agents is usually associated with an enzyme that modifies the agent, such as a deacetylase.[19] The *floR* gene has been isolated from a bovine strain of *P multocida* isolated in the United Kingdom.[12] Otherwise, florfenicol resistance among the BRD pathogens has been infrequently reported.

The fluoroquinolone class of antimicrobial agents is widely used in human and veterinary medicine and approved for BRD therapy. In the United States, the two approved agents are enrofloxacin and danofloxacin. The primary target for this class of agent is DNA gyrase and topoisomerase IV, which are responsible for maintenance of DNA supercoiling.[19,21] Generally, mutations in DNA gyrase confer low-level resistance (MIC values of 0.25–1 µg/mL), whereas strains containing mutations in both DNA gyrase and topoisomerase IV demonstrate high-level resistance (MIC values ≥8 µg/mL).[19,21] Available MIC data on enrofloxacin for BRD isolates indicated that values varied between strains of *M haemolytica* (MIC_{90} >4 µg/mL) and *P multocida* (MIC_{90} = 0.12 µg/mL).[16] Catry and coworkers[10] determined that 88.9% of the MIC values for enrofloxacin with strains of *Mannheimia* and *Pasteurella* isolated from dairy, beef, and veal calves was less than or equal to 0.125 µg/mL. Of the remaining 10.1%, 9.1% demonstrated MIC values of 0.25 to 0.5 µg/mL consistent with mutations in DNA gyrase; 2% of strains demonstrated high-level resistance indicating the double mutation was present. More recently, Katsuda and colleagues[21] determined the MIC values and mutations for enrofloxacin and danofloxacin in 229 strains of *M haemolytica* isolated from pneumonia in Japanese beef cattle. Each strain represented a single isolate per herd. The MIC_{50} values for both compounds were less than or equal to 0.06 μg/mL, whereas the MIC_{90} value was 0.5 μg/mL for enrofloxacin and 1 μg/mL for danofloxacin. Of the 229 strains, there were 11 strains (4.8%) demonstrating high-level fluoroquinolone resistance indicating the presence of mutations in both DNA gyrase and topoisomerase IV. These investigators also serotyped and genotyped the resistant strains and determined that not only did all of these strains belong to the same serotype (A6), but that they were the same clone. These data indicate the broad dissemination of a single resistant clone between beef herds.

It is important for the clinician to recognize that antimicrobial resistance mechanisms can confer resistance not only to a single agent but to multiple agents within a class.[19] This type of resistance is referred to as "cross-resistance." An example of this is MLSb resistance in gram-positive bacteria, which confers resistance to macrolides, lincosamides, and B streptogramins.[19] This resistance results from the acquisition by the bacteria of the *erm* gene causing methylation of a single adenine residue at the target site. Methylation of the site confers resistance to all three classes of antimicrobial agents. Another type of resistance linkage is coresistance or associated resistance, whereby an organism acquires various resistance gene or mutations thereby becoming resistance to multiple agents.[19] This latter type of resistance is the most disconcerting because the emergence of a multidrug resistance in a pathogen dramatically limits therapeutic options. At this point in time, multidrug resistance in *M haemolytica* and *P multocida* isolated from pneumonia in feedlot cattle has not been reported. Catry and coworkers,[10] however, reported that the overall levels of resistance in *Pasteurellaceae* (*Mannheimia* spp and *P multocida*) isolates from dairy, beef, and veal calves were 17.6%, 21.9%, and 71.9%, respectively. Multidrug resistance defined as resistant to two or more agents was restricted to those organisms isolated from veal calves. These data certainly indicate the potential for multidrug resistance development in the BRD pathogens.

Dissemination of resistant bacterial clones is well recognized in bacteria, such as methicillin-resistant strains of *Staphylococcus aureus* in humans.[22] These strains can be highly adapted to their host and environment and resistant to multiple drugs. The recent report by Katsuda and colleagues[21] is the first report of a dissemination of a single antimicrobial resistant clone in *M haemolytica* isolated from bovine pneumonia. Because all the strains in the study represented single isolates from each farm, the isolation of the same clone on multiple farms indicates that transmission between farms rather than transmission of clones between animals on each farm had occurred. These data emphasize the need for systemic continuous surveillance of antimicrobial resistance in the BRD pathogens and that genotyping of strains may be important to understand the epidemiology of antimicrobial resistance in these pathogens.

THE IMPACT OF RESISTANCE ON CLINICAL EFFICACY

AST results provide information that guides the clinician in selecting the most appropriate agent for treatment of a particular disease. The overall efficacy of any antimicrobial agent is driven by multiple factors including the health status of the host, virulence of pathogen, stage of disease when therapy is initiated, and susceptibility of the organism. It is the responsibility of the clinician to incorporate this information not only in selecting an agent but also in modulating the expectations of the therapeutic success.

To properly assess the impact of resistance, the clinician must be able to assess the impact of other factors on overall efficacy for a particular disease outbreak. In BRD outbreaks, the population is stratified into those animals with mild disease that may spontaneously recover, those with moderate disease that will most likely not recover without therapeutic intervention, and those with severe or acute disease from which most will not recover regardless of intervention.

The impact of severity of disease and effect of comorbidities on overall efficacy has been well described in the literature in both human and bovine pneumonia.[1–5,23,24] Pneumonia in humans is generally categorized as either community-acquired pneumonia or hospital-acquired pneumonia. Community-acquired pneumonia is characterized by mild to moderate disease in healthy hosts and the primary agent is *Streptococcus pneumoniae*. In contrast, hospital-acquired pneumonia is usually a more severe disease in the host with significant comorbidities (ie, elderly, chemotherapy recipients, and so forth) and is often caused by *S aureus*. A comparison of the treatment efficacy for linezolid and comparator agents against susceptible isolates is provided in **Fig. 2**. These data indicate that both disease severity and comorbidities substantially reduced the overall efficacy of both linezolid and comparator agents. These effects are well understood in human medicine and are incorporated into the current therapeutic recommendations. For example, the single factor associated with survival in severe community-acquired pneumonia requiring hospitalization is whether the patient receives antimicrobial therapy within 4 hours of admission[23] and that patients' deaths occurring within 3 days of admission are not due to failure of the antibiotic therapy.[24] This effect has also been observed in cattle with BRD and it is well understood that BRD morbidity and mortality rates in treated and untreated cattle vary depending on the source and management history of the cattle.[1–5,25,26]

The effect of antimicrobial resistance in any population is to decrease overall efficacy. This effect is sufficiently profound that most clinicians select a different agent when confronted with known antimicrobial resistance. The primary goal of establishing-veterinary specific interpretive criteria is to correlate the in vitro test result with the clinical outcome data so that the clinician can select agents that are likely to be effective as indicated by a susceptible test result. For many newer agents, there is little or no antimicrobial resistance and in vitro testing is more efficient at predicting

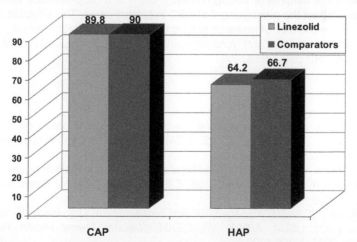

Fig. 2. The efficacy of linezolid and comparators in the treatment of community-acquired pneumonia (CAP) and hospital-acquired pneumonia (HAP) caused by susceptible isolates. (*Data from* Watts JL. The clinical relevance of susceptibility breakpoints. Proceeding of the Antimicrobial Agents in Veterinary Medicine meeting. Prague (Czech Republic); August 24–8, 2008.)

susceptibility than resistance. The understanding of the impact of resistance on clinical efficacy may only be recognized after an agent has been used for many years and sufficient resistance has emerged. Once this has occurred, the impact of resistance on clinical efficacy is readily apparent. For example, Apley[26] reported MIC data for *M haemolytica* from 12 BRD field trials with tilmicosin. Isolates were categorized as susceptible, intermediate, or resistant based on the CLSI veterinary-specific interpretive criteria for tilmicosin and *M haemolytica*.[8,26] These data indicate that the clinical success rate when treating isolates of *M haemolytica* categorized as susceptible was 84.9%. In contrast, the success rate in treating animals with isolates categorized as either intermediate or resistance was only 38.9%. These data indicate that antimicrobial resistance is linked to a substantial reduction in efficacy.[26,27] Furthermore, this reduction in efficacy is additive to any reduction associated with disease severity. These data also indicate that interpretive criteria should be periodically re-evaluated and readjusted to improve accuracy.

SUMMARY

Over the past two decades, the management of BRD has been impacted by two significant developments: the introduction of new antimicrobial agents that provide greater efficacy and convenience compared with previous agents; and the development of standardized AST methods and clinical breakpoints that are specific for the BRD pathogens. As a consequence, the clinician not only has more therapeutic options but has better tools to aid in selection of the most appropriate agent. Unfortunately, there are no long-term surveillance programs reported in the literature that provide information on the prevalence and annual rate of resistance development in the BRD pathogens. Recent information on the dissemination of a fluoroquinolone resistant clone among cattle herds in Japan indicates additional information on the epidemiology of resistance in BRD pathogens is needed.

The emergence of significant resistance to one or more agents by the BRD pathogens in individual feedlots or through dissemination of a drug-resistant clone would dramatically impact the management of BRD in feedlot cattle. This situation is further compounded by the lack of research programs in the animal health industry focused on the development of new antimicrobial agents that are active against potential emergent resistant BRD pathogens.

REFERENCES

1. USDA Part I: baseline reference of feedlot management practices, 1999. Fort Collins (CO): USDA: APHIS: VS, CEAH, National Animal Health Monitoring System; 2000: N327.0500.
2. USDA. Part II: baseline reference of feedlot health and health management, 1999. Fort Collins (CO): USDA: APHIS: VS, CEAH, National Animal Health Monitoring System; 2000. N335.1000.
3. USDA. Part III: health management and biosecurity in U.S. feedlots, 1999. Fort Collins (CO): USDA: APHIS: VS, CEAH, National Animal Health Monitoring System; 2000. N336.1200.
4. Mosier DA. Bacterial pneumonia, bovine respiratory disease update. Vet Clin North Am 1997;13:483–93.
5. Loneragan GH, Dargatz DA, Morley PS, et al. Trends in mortality ratios among cattle in US feedlots. J Am Vet Med Assoc 2001;219:1122–7.

6. Nutsch RG, Skogerboe TL, Rooney KA, et al. Comparative efficacy of tulathromycin, tilmicosin, and florfenicol in the treatment of bovine respiratory disease in stocker cattle. Vet Ther 2005;6:167–79.

7. Van Donkersgoed J, Berg J, Hendrick S. Comparison of florfenicol and tulathromycin for the treatment of undifferentiated fever in Alberta feedlot cattle. Vet Ther 2008;9:275–81.

8. CLSI. Performance standards for antimicrobial disk and dilution susceptibility tests for bacteria isolated from animals: approved standard. CLSI document M31-A3. 3rd edition. Wayne (PA): Clinical and Laboratory Standards Institute; 2008.

9. CLSI. Development of in vitro susceptibility testing criteria and quality control parameters for veterinary antimicrobial agents: approved guideline. CLSI document M37-A3. 3rd edition. Wayne (PA): Clinical and Laboratory Standards Institute; 2008.

10. Catry B, Haesebrouck F, De Vliegher S, et al. Variability in acquired resistance of Pasteurella and Mannheimia isolates from the nasopharynx of calves, with particular reference to different herd types. Microb Drug Resist 2005;11(4): 387–94.

11. Schwarz S, Kehrenberg C, Salmon S, et al. In vitro activities of spectinomycin and comparator agents against Pasteurella multocida and Mannheimia haemolytica from respiratory tract infections of cattle. J Antimicrob Chemother 2004;53: 379–82.

12. Priebe S, Schwarz S. In vitro activities of florfenicol against bovine and porcine respiratory tract pathogens. Antimicrobial Agents Chemother 2003;47(8): 2703–5.

13. Godinho KS. Susceptibility testing of tulathromycin: interpretive breakpoints and susceptibility of field isolates. Vet Microbiol 2008;129:426–32.

14. Watts JL, Yancey RJ Jr. Identification of veterinary pathogens using commercial identification systems and new trends in antimicrobial susceptibility testing of veterinary pathogens. Clin Microbiol Rev 1994;7:346–56.

15. Simjee S, Silley P, Werling HO, et al. Potential confusion regarding the term "resistance" in epidemiological studies. J Antimicrob Chemother 2008;61:228–9.

16. Kehrenberg C, Walker RD, Wu CC, et al. Antimicrobial resistance in members of the family Pasteurellaceae. In: Aarestrup FM, editor. Antimicrobial resistance in bacteria of animal origin. Washington, DC: ASM Press; 2006. p. 167–86.

17. Watts JL, Yancey RJ Jr, Salmon SA, et al. A four-year survey of antimicrobial susceptibility trends for isolates from cattle with bovine respiratory disease cases in North America. J Clin Microbiol 1994;32:725–31.

18. Evans N. Tulathromycin: an overview of a new triamilides antimicrobial for livestock respiratory disease. Vet Ther 2005;6:83–95.

19. Guardabassi L, Courvalin P. Modes of antimicrobial action and mechanisms of bacterial resistance. In: Aarestrup FM, editor. Antimicrobial resistance in bacteria of animal origin. Washington, DC: ASM press; 2006. p. 1–18.

20. Godinho KS, Keane SG, Nanjiani IA, et al. Minimum inhibitory concentrations of tulathromycin against respiratory bacterial pathogens isolated from clinical cases in European cattle and swine and variability arising from changes in in vitro methodology. Vet Ther 2005;6:113–21.

21. Katsuda K, Kohmoto M, Mikami O, et al. Antimicrobial resistance and genetic characterization of fluoroquinolone-resistant Mannheimia haemolytica isolates from cattle with bovine pneumonia. Vet Microbiol 2009, [doi: 10.1016/j.vetmic.2009.04.020].

22. Aarestrup FM, Schwarz S. Antimicrobial resistance in staphylococci and strepto-cocci of animal origin. In: Aarestrup FM, editor. Antimicrobial resistance in bacteria of animal origin. Washington, DC: ASM press; 2006. p. 187–212.
23. Blasi F, Aliberti S, Pappalettera M, et al. 100 years of respiratory medicine: pneu-monia. Respir Med 2007;101:875–81.
24. Feikin D, Schuchat A, Kolczak M, et al. Mortality from invasive pneumococcal pneumonia in the era of antibiotic resistance, 1995–1997. Am J Public Health 2000;90:223–9.
25. Kilgore WR, Spensley MS, Sun F, et al. Clinical effectiveness of tulathromycin, a novel triamilides antimicrobial, for control of respiratory disease in cattle at high risk of developing bovine respiratory disease. Vet Ther 2005;6:136–42.
26. Apley MD. Susceptibility testing for bovine respiratory and enteric disease. Vet Clin North Am Food Anim Pract 2003;19:625–46.
27. Watts JL. The clinical relevance of susceptibility breakpoints. Proceedings of the Antimicrobial Agents in Veterinary Medicine Meeting. Prague (Czech Republic); August 24–8, 2008.

Cryptosporidiosis in Neonatal Calves

Carol R. Wyatt, PhD[a],*, Michael W. Riggs, DVM, PhD[b],
Ronald Fayer, PhD[c]

KEYWORDS

- Cryptosporidiosis • Cattle • Pathophysiology
- Immunity • Diagnostics • Control

INFECTION PROCESS AND HOST CELL/PARASITE INTERACTIONS

Following ingestion of *Cryptosporidium parvum* oocysts and passage through the stomach, lectin receptors expressed on the oocyst surface mediate attachment to the intestinal mucusal lining. Exposure of oocysts to gastric acid, bile acids, pancreatic trypsin, and host-intestinal temperature facilitates their excystation and triggers expression of sporozoite-derived proteases and phospholipases involved in dissolution of the oocyst suture and sporozoite release.[1] Direct contact between *C. parvum* oocysts and terminal sialic acid residues exposed on surface glycoproteins of host cells can provide an additional key local signal for triggering excystation.[2] Following escape from oocysts, activated sporozoites secrete molecules from apical complex organelles and express surface-exposed molecules that are involved in the infection process.[3] The apical complex of *C. parvum* consists of numerous micronemes and dense granules, but only a single rhoptry.[4] In general, microneme (glyco)proteins (gp) are involved in gliding motility, and host-cell recognition and attachment by *C. parvum* zoite stages.[1,5,6] Rhoptry molecules are important in modifying the host-cell membrane in formation of the parasitophorous vacuole during invasion while dense granule molecules bind to the parasitophorous vacuole membrane and function in subsequent modification of the host-cell microenvironment.[1,5,6]

Within minutes of release from oocysts, actively motile *C. parvum* sporozoites traverse the intestinal mucus barrier by expressing mucin like surface receptors for attachment, releasing enzymes to break down mucus locally, and ultimately accessing enterocytes for attachment and invasion mediated by specific receptor-ligand

[a] Department of Diagnostic Medicine/Pathobiology, College of Veterinary Medicine, 1800 Denison Avenue, Manhattan, KS 66506, USA
[b] Department of Veterinary Science and Microbiology, University of Arizona, Tucson, AZ 85721, USA
[c] Environmental Microbiology and Food Safety Laboratory, US Department of Agriculture, 10300 Baltimore Avenue, Building 173 BARC-East, Room 100, Beltsville, MD 20705, USA
* Corresponding author.
E-mail address: cwyatt@vet.k-state.edu (C.R. Wyatt).

Vet Clin Food Anim 26 (2010) 89–103
doi:10.1016/j.cvfa.2009.10.001
0749-0720/10/$ – see front matter © 2010 Elsevier Inc. All rights reserved.
vetfood.theclinics.com

binding.[3,7,8] Multiple apical complex organelle and surface-exposed molecules of the infective sporozoite and merozoite stages that are involved in gliding motility, attachment, invasion, or intracellular development have been identified (**Table 1**).[3,7,8,10–33] These include several high molecular weight sporozoite and merozoite glycoproteins, the relationships between which are presently unclear, although distinct differences have been identified.[8,12,34] Similarly, CP15/60[15] and CP15,[16] and gp15 and gp40 derived from a gp60 precursor,[17–22] are distinct at the molecular level. Following invasion, expression of several sporozoite surface molecules follow a unique temporal pattern during subsequent intracellular development, suggesting that their functions during the life cycle are not restricted to the invasive zoite stages.[35] The molecular diversity and number of parasite molecules having established or putative roles in the pathogenesis of infection suggests that *C. parvum* has redundant mechanisms for infection or uses multiple ligand-receptor interactions during a multistep infection process. Circular and helical gliding motility of sporozoites and merozoites observed in vitro involves attachment of parasite surface molecules to host cells, followed by actin-myosin cytoskeletal motor-dependent posterior translocation and release, and forward locomotion leaving trails of parasite-derived deposits demarcating the path traversed.[1,5,7,36] Several such *C. parvum* molecules involved in gliding motility have been identified (see **Table 1**). Additionally, a cysteine protease of *C. parvum* sporozoites, designated cryptopain-1, has recently been identified.[37] This protease degrades the extracellular matrix proteins collagen and fibronectin in vitro, and is hypothesized to be involved in sporozoite invasion and exit from host cells.[37] A serine subtilisin protease has also recently been identified in *C. parvum* and is important in intracellular development of merozoites; its organellar localization, pattern of expression, and specific role in intracellular development are under investigation.[38] Similarly, the role of an acid phosphatase recently identified in *C. parvum* oocysts as a putative virulence factor is the subject of ongoing studies.[39]

Before invasion, sporozoites reorient and bind by way of their apical (anterior) end to the apical (luminal) membrane of enterocytes between microvilli. Binding is followed by host-cell actin polymerization and remodeling, a local increase in host-cell volume at the apical region, and protrusion of the host-cell microvillus membrane leading to what has been described as parasite-induced engulfment and encapsulation of the invading sporozoite.[3,40] For lack of a better term this results in an intracellular but extracytosolic, epicellular localization of the developing trophozoite, in a parasitophorous vacuole at the apical region of the host cell immediately beneath the host-cell plasma membrane.[3,41–43] A multimembranous feeder organelle subsequently forms, connecting the parasite with, and providing access to, the host-cell cytoplasm for acquisition of essential nutrients and substrates.[3,44,45] The molecular mechanisms and biochemical signaling pathways involved in these initial host cell-sporozoite interactions and subsequent life-cycle development, and gaps in existing knowledge of these processes, have been recently reviewed.[3,46,47]

PATHOPHYSIOLOGY OF DIARRHEA

C. parvum infection in young calves leads to villous atrophy and a reduction in total surface area of the small intestinal mucosa resulting from accelerated loss of mature, absorptive villous enterocytes and microvillus atrophy and increased intestinal permeability.[48–50] These lesions result in a maldigestion/malabsorption type diarrhea.[48] Although glucose or glutamine-coupled absorption of sodium and water in the crypt compartment may compensate during infection, it is limited; net absorption of all major nutrient classes is reduced, leading to malabsorption diarrhea.[50–52] In addition

Table 1
C. parvum molecules involved in the pathogenesis of host-cell infection

Molecule	Characteristics and Localization	Putative Function	References
CSL	~1300 kDa gp; dense granules, micronemes, sporozoite and merozoite surface	Ligand for intestinal epithelial cell receptor	Riggs[9]; Riggs et al[10], Langer et al[11], Riggs[12]
GP900	>900 kDa gp; micronemes, sporozoite surface	Ligand for mucus, host cells; motility	Barnes et al[13]
CP47	~47 kDa (glyco)protein; sporozoite apical sub-pellicle	Ligand for host cells	Nesterenko et al[14]
CP15/60	~15–60 kDa gps; sporozoite surface	Motility	Jenkins et al[15]
CP15	~15 kDa gp; sporozoite surface	Motility	Jenkins and Fayer[16]
gp15	~15 kDa gp; surface of sporozoites and merozoites, glycosylphosphatidyl inositol-anchored	Ligand for mucus, host cells; motility	Priest et al[17], O'Connor et al[18], Cevallos et al[19], Strong et al[20], Cevallos et al[21], Priest et al[22]
gp40	~40 kDa gp; apical complex, sporozoite/merozoite surface; reassociates with gp15 after proteolytic cleavage to form a ligand complex	Ligand for mucus, host cells; motility	Priest et al[17], O'Conner et al[18], Cevallos et al[19], Strong et al[20], Cevallos et al[21], Priest et al[22]
TRAP C1	~76 kDa (glyco)protein; sporozoite apical pole, micronemes	Motility, attachment	Spano et al[23], Putignani et al[24]
P23	~23 kDa (glyco)protein; surface of sporozoites and merozoites	Motility, attachment	Perryman et al[25], Schaefer et al[26], Yao et al[27]
GP25–200	~25–200 kDa gps; apical complex, sporozoite/ merozoite surface	Motility	Riggs et al[10], Schaefer et al[26]
Gal/GalNAc	~30 kDa lectin; apical sporozoite	Ligand for mucus, host cells	Ward and Cevallos[28], Bhat et al[29]
CP2	~82 kDa secreted or membrane (glyco)protein; sporozoite surface, parasitophorous vacuole membrane of asexual and sexual stages	Invasion, intracellular development	O'Hara et al[30]
CP12	~12 kDa (glyco)protein; sporozoite and oocyst surface	Attachment and invasion	Yao et al[27]
Cpa 135	~135 kDa (glyco)protein, part of a >200 kDa complex; sporozoite apical region, parasitophorous vacuole membrane	Motility	Tosini et al[31]
CPS-500	Glycolipid; sporozoite, and merozoite surface	Motility	Riggs et al[32], Priest et al[33]

to malabsorption, increased mucosal prostaglandin (PGI_2, PGE_2) synthesis mediates crypt secretion of Cl- and HCO_3- and inhibition of villous NaCl absorption.[48,49] These ion disturbances contribute to diarrhea and fluid loss in cryptosporidiosis, with PGE_2 acting directly on enterocytes and PGI_2 acting through the enteric nervous system.[48,49] Further, studies in macaques and immunosuppressed mice have shown that the neuropeptide substance P is elevated in the jejunum during *C. parvum* infection and contributes to villous atrophy, Cl- secretion and glucose malabsorption.[53] The role of this neuropeptide in the pathophysiology of bovine cryptosporidiosis has not yet been reported.

Direct cytotoxicity can lead to enterocyte loss and villous atrophy with several enteropathogens but is not thought to play a significant role with *C. parvum* infection in calves.[48] In vitro studies have clearly shown that host cell apoptosis is modulated during *C. parvum* infection and that apoptosis induction is ultimately involved in enterocyte loss to some extent, but is restricted to a subpopulation of 15% to 20% of the infected cells.[54,55] However, the relative roles of apoptosis in host defense, by promoting clearance of infected epithelial cells, limiting the spread of infection in a given host and thus reducing disease, *versus* parasite survival by promoting infection, life-cycle completion, and propagation, are complicated and not yet clearly defined. The apparent beneficiary of apoptosis modulation, host or parasite, largely depends on the stage of infection being examined. The ultimate beneficiary remains unclear although studies have demonstrated that *C. parvum* renders the host cell refractory to apoptosis early in infection, during trophozoite and meront development, and supports the argument that early inhibition of apoptosis promotes successful propagation and completion of the parasite's life cycle.[48,55] During the early stages of infection and trophozoite development (6–12 hours postinfection) antiapoptotic gene expression was upregulated and proapoptotic gene expression was downregulated.[55] In contrast, during the later stages of infection (24–72 hours postinfection) a shift was observed. Antiapoptotic gene expression was downregulated and proapoptotic gene expression was upregulated.[55] Although several hundred host-cell genes were regulated during *C. parvum* infection, expression of a subset of genes involved in apoptosis temporally paralleled morphologic changes indicative of apoptosis in up to approximately 20% of infected cells by approximately 24 to 48 hours postinfection, the time at which merozoites first rupture and begin egress from host cells.[55] Apoptosis was reported to be virtually absent in infected cells during early trophozoite development, up to approximately 12 hours postinfection.[55] These observations are consistent with previous studies indicating that host-cell death following *C. parvum* replication and subsequent merozoite egress occurs predominantly by non-apoptotic mechanisms.[56] Of relevance to the pathophysiology of diarrhea, enterocyte death leading to villous atrophy occurs by necrosis, not apoptosis, resulting from a defect in the host-cell plasma membrane and loss of integrity caused by physical exit of *C. parvum* stages from the infected cell.[48,56]

INNATE AND ADAPTIVE IMMUNE RESPONSES

Innate immunity consists of an array of defenses ranging from the continuous presence of inhibitory substances to immediate, short-term, responses mediated by resident cells. Several innate responses to *Cryptosporidium*, which have been characterized using mouse models, have been recently reviewed.[57] In calves, intestinal flora acquired after birth, have been suggested as important competitors for sporozoite attachment to intestinal epithelial cells.[58] A class of antimicrobial peptides called defensins can kill a broad range of microbial pathogens by disrupting bacterial cell membranes.[59] A subset of defensins, termed β-defensins, can be elevated during enteric infections, and an enteric β-defensin, made in epithelial cells, had elevated expression during *Cryptosporidium parvum* infection in cattle.[60] Innate immunity, however, is insufficient to clear *C. parvum* infection.

Adaptive immunity, generated either by vaccination or by recovery from infection, has three major characteristics: (1) it is long lasting, (2) it results in development of antigen-specific memory lymphocytes, and (3) it is specific to the pathogen that stimulated it. Adaptive immunity can include the humoral response and the cell-mediated response. After exposure to *C. parvum*, calves develop humoral and cell-mediated responses.

Humoral Response

Circulating antibodies can be found in calves after oocyst excretion terminates.[61] These antibodies can bind to several different *C. parvum* antigens that range in size from approximately 14 to more than 200 kDa, and that can be found on different parasite life-cycle stages.[62] Antigens that induce circulating neutralizing antibodies can provide protection, because they can be secreted into the gut lumen during infection. Studies in mice using monoclonal antibody reagents have identified multiple *C. parvum* antigens that can induce neutralizing antibodies. One of the proteins, termed p23, is an approximately 23 kDa, immunodominant, sporozoite antigen.[63] In carefully controlled in vivo studies, calves administered hyperimmune bovine colostrum from late-gestation cattle immunized with a recombinant p23 excreted fewer oocysts and were protected against clinical disease,[25] suggesting that neutralizing antibodies can provide protection against clinical cryptosporidiosis.

Antibodies delivered to the gut lumen can be excreted in calf feces. Studies using a recombinant p23 identified anti-p23 antibodies in calf feces.[64] Serially collected fecal samples from clinically normal, oocyst negative neonatal calves contained anti-p23 antibodies as early as 1 day after birth. Colostrum fed to the calves also had anti-p23 antibodies, at titers similar to those found in the corresponding fecal samples, suggesting that the fecal antibodies excreted from the calves were the result of passive transfer of colostral antibodies.[65] A study of fecal antibodies from *C. parvum* infected calves indicated that several antibody classes and subclasses appeared at different times after infection. Among them, IgG_1-subclass antibodies, most commonly associated with pathogen neutralization, appeared within 5 days postinfection. IgG_2-subclass antibodies, most commonly associated with cytotoxic activities, appeared beginning 7 days postinfection.[66] These time points are associated with clinical disease and recovery from clinical disease, respectively, and are consistent with the development of protective antibodies delivered to the gut lumen during *C. parvum* infection.

Cell-mediated Response

T lymphocytes are important in adaptive immune responses. A subset of T lymphocytes, termed helper T cells (CD4+), mediate responses to intracellular pathogens. The CD4+ T lymphocytes that are Th1 or Type-1 mediators stimulate differentiation of another subset of T lymphocytes (CD8+) into cytotoxic T lymphocytes (CTL), which kill infected cells. In studies of in vitro infection of neonatal calf ileal explants, resident CD4+ and CD8+ T lymphocytes accumulated around epithelial cells in oocyst inoculated explants by 24 hours after inoculation,[67] indicating that local T cells could respond to the presence of *C. parvum* infection in the gut. In ileal sections taken from calves infected 3 days previously with *C. parvum*, CD4+ and CD8+ T lymphocytes were found in various locations in the ileum, including villi, lamina propria and

Peyer's patches, in elevated proportions compared with the same tissues from uninfected calves.[68,69] Ileal intraepithelial lymphocytes (IEL) from 3-day infected calves expressed IL-10, an antiinflammatory cytokine that can downregulate Th1 responses, but they did not express IFN-γ, an important Th1-associated cytokine. Calves infected for 3 days typically had not begun to show clinical signs of cryptosporidiosis, and had not begun shedding oocysts.[69] Thus, these studies indicated that an adaptive immune response was initiated in gut tissue before the onset of diarrhea. However, that response included a downregulatory cytokine environment that could delay the development of protective immunity.

Calves develop diarrhea and shed oocysts beginning approximately 6 days post inoculation. Villous lymphoid cells taken from 6-day infected calves had elevated T lymphocyte numbers in IEL and lamina propria lymphocyte (LPL) compartments. The largest increase in IEL was accounted for by CD8$^+$ T lymphocytes. The T lymphocytes were activated, as demonstrated by expression of CD25 (an activation molecule), which is consistent with a local immune response to C. parvum. However, evidence of continued downregulation of Th1 immunity was shown by the continued absence of IFN-γ expression by infected calf IEL.[70] These observations, in conjunction with the expression of IL-10 at 3 days post inoculation, suggested early suppression of a Th1 response to C. parvum, consistent with progression of the infection within the ileum and diarrhea development.

Calves recovering from cryptosporidiosis, in which diarrhea had ended 24 to 48 hours earlier, had ileal immune responses consistent with development of protective immunity. The numbers of CD4$^+$ and CD8$^+$ IEL were elevated compared with IEL from age-matched control calves. Ileal LPL from infected calves expressed IFN-γ, and IgG$_1$, and IgG$_2$ anti-P23 antibodies were found in infected calf fecal samples.[71] These studies showed that a protective immune response in intestinal mucosa that included antibody production and a Th1 response was associated with recovery from clinical disease.

The hallmark of an adaptive immune response is the development of antigen-specific memory responses that rapidly recognize and eliminate the pathogen on re-exposure. Calves that had recovered from C. parvum infection 3 months previously had an in vitro response by blood lymphocytes to recombinant p23. CD4$^+$ and CD8$^+$ T lymphocytes proliferated, and IFN-γ was synthesized in response to p23 stimulation,[72] suggesting that a Th1 like memory response occurred in previously infected calves. Immune calves challenged with C. parvum oocysts had increased proportions of CD4$^+$ T cells, largely confined to the Peyer's patches, compared with control immune animals. Intraepithelial CD8$^+$ T cell proportions were also elevated, suggestive of a CTL response that could rapidly clear infected epithelial cells.[73]

DIAGNOSTICS

Cattle are subject to infections with four principal species of Cryptosporidium. Most data come from reports on dairy cattle in which each species presents a different prevalence pattern relative to the age of the animal. Cryptosporidium parvum is found in a high percentage of monogastric calves, especially from 1 to 3 weeks of age, but in few calves after weaning or in mature cattle. This species is often associated with diarrhea, sometimes severe, and occasionally associated with mortality. Characteristically, Cryptosporidium bovis and C. ryanae are first seen after weaning. The percentage of cattle infected with these species rises rapidly and then decreases steadily as cattle approach maturity. Neither morbidity nor mortality has been associated with infection with these species. The percentage of cattle infected with

C. andersoni is extremely low in pre-weaned calves reaching its highest levels in older heifers and mature cows, respectively. Decreased milk yield has been associated with *C. andersoni* infection but this relationship has not been well characterized. These age-related patterns of *Cryptosporidium* species in dairy cattle have been well documented from point prevalence and longitudinal studies,[74-77] and knowledge of this pattern can aid diagnosis. Few studies have been conducted with beef cattle. Most of these have been associated with cow/calf herds or farmed beef cattle and most reports have traditionally been based on microscopic identification of oocysts in fecal specimens. In very recent times, diagnosticians must consider the advantages of microscopy versus molecular methods for detection and identification.

The value of microscopic diagnosis is based on the use of simple methods to observe the small, round to slightly ovoid, colorless fecal stage named the oocyst. Oocysts of *C. parvum*, *C. bovis* and *C. ryanae* are extremely difficult to impossible to distinguish from one another. They have no discernable species-related features, they overlap in size with *C. parvum* and *C. bovis* averaging 5.4 × 4.9 μm and 4.9 × 4.6 μm, respectively, and the smaller *C. ryanae* averaging 3.7 × 3.2 μm.[78] Those of *C. andersoni* are much larger at 7.4 × 5.5 μm[79] and more easily identified. Brightfield, phase-contrast, Nomarski (differential interference contrast), and fluorescence microscopy have all been used. Fecal smears, dried and stained with a variety of stains, are the least sensitive or accurate because low numbers of oocysts or uneven distribution in feces will often yield negative findings. However, this is the most widely used method of detection because it is fast, inexpensive, and when large numbers of oocysts are present they are easy to detect. Cleaning and concentration methods are often employed to enhance detection of oocysts by microscopy and by the more sensitive molecular methods.

Typical cleaning and concentration methods employ the addition of water to feces to produce a suspension that is passed through sieves of different pore sizes, kitchen-type mesh strainers, or gauze to remove large particles followed by centrifugation to remove the smallest and lightest particles in the supernatant.[80] The remaining pellet containing the putative oocysts is usually subjected to centrifugation while suspended within or on a concentrated sugar, salt, or other solution with a final specific gravity of 1.15 to 1.2. Oocysts can then be aspirated from the surface of the supernatant. Alternatively, antibody-covered commercially available magnetizable beads such as Dynabeads (Invitrogen, Carlsbad, CA) and IMS-Grab beads (Waterborne Inc, New Orleans, LA), have been used to recover oocysts from surrounding fecal debris. Feces with a high-fat content might require additional cleaning steps with formol-ethyl acetate or diethyl ether. It is best to wash oocysts multiple times after cleaning to reduce interference with staining or other procedures.

Several stains have been helpful for identifying oocysts when using brightfield microscopy.[81] Giemsa and Gram's stains generally provide poor differentiation from background materials. Methylene blue-borax, aniline-carbol-methyl violet, and safranin-methylene blue are simple and give better differentiation. Variations on the carbol-fuchsin based acid-fast stain, such as Ziehl-Neelsen and Kinyoun are the most widely used. The latter are fast and simple and stain oocysts clear bright red.

Fluorescence microscopy is widely used by researchers and some diagnostic laboratories. Test kits are readily available from commercial sources in North America such as Meridian Diagnostics (Cincinnati, OH) and Waterborne, Inc (New Orleans, LA). Enzyme-linked immuno-assay kits are also available from several sources (Alexon Inc, Sunnyvale, CA; Dako Corp., Denmark; Diagnostic Automation Inc, Calabasas, CA; LMD Laboratories, Carlsbad CA; Techlab, Blacksbur VA; and Safepath Laboratories, Carlsbad, CA). Antibody-based products that detect the presence of *Cryptosporidium* oocysts vary in sensitivity. None appear to be species specific, therefore any relationship between a positive specimen and disease cannot be based on any of these tests alone. Diagnosis of cryptosporidiosis-related illness based on all microscopic methods requires a combination of finding large numbers of oocysts per gram of feces, clinical signs of gastrointestinal infection, and often a relationship to the age and immune status of the animal.

Molecular detection methods, used primarily for research and epidemiologic purposes, are the most sensitive and accurate. They enable identification of species and genotypes. Genotypes are genetically identifiable, unique isolates that have not received the taxonomic status of a species although several genotypes have achieved species status after sufficient data had accumulated. There is no standard gene recommended for species identification. After DNA has been extracted from oocysts recovered from feces or even from those scraped from dried stained microscope slides,[82] polymerase chain reaction-based methods are used to amplify specific genes. Fragments of the small subunit (SSU)-rDNA (18s rRNA), followed by the COWP (oocyst wall protein gene), HSP-70, and actin genes have been used most frequently. These fragments are subjected to either restriction fragment length polymorphism methods in which a collection of DNA fragments of defined length are separated by electrophoresis, with smaller fragments migrating farther than the larger fragments and creating a recognizable pattern, or by sequencing the gene fragments and comparing the base pairs with known sequences. For subtyping of *C. parvum*, primarily for epidemiologic investigations, the GP-60 gene is used.[77]

TREATMENT

There are no vaccines approved for prevention of cryptosporidiosis, and although antibodies can be found in bovine colostrum they are at levels that are not protective against cryptosporidiosis in calves that receive those colostra.[83] When cows were experimentally immunized to produce colostrum containing very high levels of IgG1, IgM, and IgA and neonatal calves were fed this colostrum and were experimentally infected with oocysts of *C. parvum*, the calves had significantly less diarrhea and shed oocysts for less time than calves fed colostrum from cows that were not hyperimmunized.[84] But because prophylaxis or the treatment of cryptosporidiosis required high titers of specific *C. parvum* antibodies in the gut lumen during a sufficiently long period, and because multiple injections of highly purified oocysts are required to elicit a strong immunoglobulin response, the production and use of this partially effective treatment is impractical and too expensive.

To stimulate a protective immune response in calves against the intracellular stages of the parasite without causing clinical illness, *C. parvum* oocysts were exposed to 400 Gy of gamma-irradiation. This level of irradiation rendered the sporozoites alive and capable of infecting gut epithelial cells but incapable of completing the life cycle. Exposure to the intracellular parasites stimulated the calves' immune systems enabling them to elicit a protective immune response after receiving a challenge exposure with fresh nonirradiated *C. parvum* oocysts.[85]

Progress in the area of chemotherapy for cryptosporidiosis has been slow, perhaps because of the uniqueness of this genus as intracellular extracytoplasmic residents of mucosal epithelial cells. There are no approved or extra-label products or other modalities with demonstrated consistent efficacy for preventing excretion of *C. parvum* oocysts or for treating associated diarrhea in dairy or beef calves. Among the drugs tested, nitazoxanide (NTZ), halofuginone, paromomycin, decoquinate, lasalocid, and sulfaquinoxaline had some demonstrable or partial activity against

C. parvum infection in ruminants. For an in-depth review see Stockdale and colleagues.[86] Although some of the following drugs are not approved for veterinary use, veterinarians are allowed to prescribe certain approved animal and human drugs in an extra-label manner under the *Animal Medicinal Drug Use and Clarification Act of 1994*.

Nitazoxanide (Alinia, Romark Laboratories, FL) has been found effective for treatment of cryptosporidiosis in immunocompromised and immunocompetent human patients by reducing oocyst excretion and diarrhea severity.[87] It is the only drug approved for treatment of cryptosporidiosis in adults and children. In experimentally infected neonatal goat kids, NTZ reduced oocyst excretion and reduced severity of diarrhea although some of the kids died from drug toxicity.[88] In one study, NTZ reduced the duration of *C. parvum* oocyst excretion and the severity of diarrhea in calves experimentally infected with *C. parvum*,[89] whereas in another study prophylactic and therapeutic use of NTZ in calves did not show a positive effect on the course of *C. parvum* infection either in reducing the clinical severity or on oocyst excretion.[90] Commercially available NTZ product is not labeled for use in cattle.

Halofuginone (Stenorol ND, Intervet, Millsboro, DE) a synthetic quinazolinone, has received positive reports from studies on treatment of veal calves,[91] dairy calves,[92–98] and lambs[99] in reducing the number of *C. parvum* oocysts excreted and in reducing the severity of diarrhea. Toxicity was reported in the lamb study. Halofuginone is available in Canada on an emergency basis only but is not available in the United States.

Paromomycin (Humatin, Pfizer, NY), an aminoglycoside antibiotic, prevented infection in kids during the period of drug administration and possibly allowed for low, undetectable, parasite development that induced a partial immunity to challenge on without symptoms or detectable oocyst excretion.[100] It reduced oocyst output and clinical signs in neonatal lambs but negative effects on growth at certain dosages levels were observed.[101] Paromomycin eliminated oocyst excretion in all but one treated dairy calf and significantly reduced the severity of diarrhea compared with untreated controls.[102]

Azithromycin (Zithromax, Pfizer, NY), a macrolide antibiotic, also decreased oocyst excretion and reduced the severity of clinical signs associated with cryptosporidiosis in naturally infected dairy calves in Turkey, but it is too expensive for use on commercial dairy farms.[103] Decoquinate (Deccox, Alpharma, NY), an approved coccidiostat, was effective in reducing oocyst excretion and reducing diarrhea in goat kids but did not allow a better weight gain.[104] Daily treatment of dairy calves with decoquinate did not affect oocyst output or clinical signs associated with cryptosporidiosis.[105]

CONTROL

Farm management goals to control cryptosporidiosis have primarily focused on cleanliness of maternity pens, calf housing, and feeding equipment and separation of cows and calves at birth, plus early detection of anorexia, diarrhea, and dehydration in neonatal calves.[106,107] Despite the apparent wisdom of such a rational approach, examination of numerous farms from Vermont to Florida with distinctly observable differences in the levels of cleanliness has not substantiated the benefits of cleanliness as a control method. Even fly control did not appear to greatly reduce the prevalence of *C. parvum* infection observed in neonatal calves among farms. Based on point-prevalence studies of multiple dairy farms combined with a 2-year long longitudinal study of one farm, it appears that virtually all calves on all farms become infected with *C. parvum*.[74–76]

SUMMARY

Cryptosporidium parvum infection poses substantial challenges for producers. The parasite is difficult to distinguish from other *Cryptosporidial* species that do not cause clinical signs, and it infects a large absorptive area of the gut, causing a malabsorption syndrome that results in diarrhea. During its complex life cycle, it produces numerous proteins that can challenge the naïve immune response of a neonatal calf. The calf gut mucosal immune system is competent to ultimately resolve the initial infection and prevent future clinical disease, but is not yet capable of responding quickly enough to prevent diarrhea. There are no licensed vaccines to prevent infection, and antibiotic treatments, although reducing oocyst output, do not prevent it; thus, infected calves remain reservoirs of infection for naïve animals. Cleanliness appears to be the best choice for reducing environmental oocyst loads. Some protection might be offered by colostrum from cattle that have already been exposed to *C. parvum*, but observation, rapid recognition, and isolation of clinically affected calves is currently the best method for minimizing spread of the disease.

REFERENCES

1. Smith HV, Nichols RAB, Grimason AM. *Cryptosporidium* excystation and invasion: getting to the guts of the matter. Trends Parasitol 2005;21(3):133–42.
2. Choudhry N, Bajaj-Elliott M, McDonald V. The terminal sialic acid of glycoconjugates on the surface of intestinal epithelial cells activates excystation of *Cryptosporidium parvum*. Infect Immun 2008;76(8):3735–41.
3. Borowski H, Clode PL, Thompson RCA. Active invasion and/or encapsulation? A reappraisal of host-cell parasitism by *Cryptosporidium*. Trends Parasitol 2008; 24(11):509–16.
4. Tetley L, Brown SMA, McDonald V, et al. Ultrastructural analysis of the sporozoite of *Cryptosporidium parvum*. Microbiology 1998;144(12):3249–55.
5. Boulter-Bitzer JI, Lee H, Trevors JT. Molecular targets for detection and immunotherapy in *Cryptosporidium parvum*. Biotechnol Adv 2007;25(1):13–44.
6. Fayer R. General biology. In: Fayer R, Xiao L, editors. *Cryptosporidium* and cryptosporidiosis. 2nd edition. Boca Raton (FL): CRC Press; 2008. p. 1–42.
7. Wanyiri J, Ward H. Molecular basis of *Cryptosporidium*-host cell interactions: recent advances and future prospects. Future Microbiol 2006;1(2):201–8.
8. Langer RC, Riggs MW. *Cryptosporidium parvum* apical complex glycoprotein CSL contains a sporozoite ligand for intestinal epithelial cells. Infect Immun 1999;67:5282–91.
9. Riggs MW. The immunobiology of cryptosporidiosis. In: Proceedings of the 27th Annual American College of Veterinary Internal Medicine Forum. Montreal; 2009, p. 69–71.
10. Riggs MW, Stone AL, Yount PA, et al. Protective monoclonal antibody defines a circumsporozoite-like glycoprotein exoantigen of *Cryptosporidium parvum* sporozoites and merozoites. J Immunol 1997;158:1787–95.
11. Langer RC, Schaefer DA, Riggs MW. Characterization of an intestinal epithelial cell receptor recognized by the *Cryptosporidium parvum* sporozoite ligand CSL. Infect Immun 2001;69:1661–70.
12. Riggs MW. Recent Advances in Cryptosporidiosis: the immune response. Microbes Infect 2002;4:1067–80.
13. Barnes DA, Bonnin A, Huang JX, et al. A novel multi-domain mucin-like glycoprotein of *Cryptosporidium parvum* mediates invasion. Mol Biochem Parasitol 1998;96:93–110.

14. Nesterenko MV, Woods K, Upton SJ. Receptor/ligand interactions between *Cryptosporidium parvum* and the surface of the host cell. Biochim Biophys Acta 1999;1454:165–73.
15. Jenkins MC, Fayer R, Tilley M, et al. Cloning and expression of a cDNA encoding epitopes shared by 15- and 60-kilodalton proteins of *Cryptosporidium parvum* sporozoites. Infect Immun 1993;61(6):2377–82.
16. Jenkins MC, Fayer R. Cloning and expression of cDNA encoding an antigenic *Cryptosporidium parvum* protein. Mol Biochem Parasitol 1995;71(1):149–52.
17. Priest JW, Kwon JP, Moss DM, et al. Detection by enzyme immunoassay of serum immunoglobulin G antibodies that recognize specific *Cryptosporidium parvum* antigens. J Clin Microbiol 1999;37(5):1385–92.
18. O'Connor RM, Wanyiri JW, Cevallos AM, et al. *Cryptosporidium parvum* glycoprotein gp40 localizes to the sporozoite surface by association with gp15. Mol Biochem Parasitol 2007;156(1):80–3.
19. Cevallos AM, Zhang X, Waldor MK, et al. Molecular cloning and expression of a gene encoding *Cryptosporidium parvum* glycoproteins gp40 and gp15. Infect Immun 2000;68:4108–16.
20. Strong WB, Gut J, Nelson RG. Cloning and sequence analysis of a highly polymorphic *Cryptosporidium parvum* gene encoding a 60-kilodalton glycoprotein and characterization of its 15- and 45-kilodalton zoite surface antigen products. Infect Immun 2000;68:4117–34.
21. Cevallos AM, Bhat N, Verdon R, et al. Mediation of *Cryptosporidium parvum* infection in vitro by mucin-like glycoproteins defined by a neutralizing monoclonal antibody. Infect Immun 2000;68:5167–75.
22. Priest JW, Kwon JP, Arrowood MJ, et al. Cloning of the immunodominant I7-kDa antigen from *Cryptosporidium parvum*. Mol Biochem Parasitol 2000;106:261–71.
23. Spano F, Putignani L, Naitza S, et al. Molecular cloning and expression analysis of a *Cryptosporidium parvum* gene encoding a new member of the thrombospondin family. Mol Biochem Parasitol 1998;92(1):147–62.
24. Putignani L, Possenti A, Cherchi S, et al. The thrombospondin-related protein CpMIC1 (CpTSP8) belongs to the repertoire of micronemal proteins of *Cryptosporidium parvum*. Mol Biochem Parasitol 2008;157(1):98–101.
25. Perryman LE, Kapil SJ, Jones ML, et al. Protection of calves against cryptosporidiosis with immune bovine colostrum induced by a *Cryptosporidium parvum* recombinant protein. Vaccine 1999;17:2142–9.
26. Schaefer DA, Auerbach-Dixon BA, Riggs MW. Characterization and formulation of multiple epitope-specific neutralizing monoclonal antibodies for passive immunization against cryptosporidiosis. Infect Immun 2000;68:2608–16.
27. Yao LQ, Yin JG, Zhang XC, et al. *Cryptosporidium parvum*: identification of a new surface adhesion protein on sporozoite and oocyst by screening of a phage-display cDNA library. Exp Parasitol 2007;115(4):333–8.
28. Ward H, Cevallos AM. *Cryptosporidium*: molecular basis of host-parasite interaction. Adv Parasitol 1998;40:151–85.
29. Bhat N, Joe A, PereiraPerrin M, et al. *Cryptosporidium* p30, a galactose/N-acetylgalactosamine-specific lectin, mediates infection in vitro. J Biol Chem 2007;282(48):34877–87.
30. O'Hara SP, Yu JR, Lin JJ. A novel *Cryptosporidium parvum* antigen, CP2, preferentially associates with membranous structures. Parasitol Res 2004;92:317–27.
31. Tosini F, Agnoli A, Mele R, et al. A new modular protein of *Cryptosporidium parvum*, with ricin B and LCCL domains, expressed in the sporozoite invasive stage. Mol Biochem Parasitol 2004;134(1):137–47.

32. Riggs MW, McNeil MR, Perryman LE, et al. *Cryptosporidium parvum* sporozoite pellicle antigen recognized by a neutralizing monoclonal antibody is a β-mannosylated glycolipid. Infect Immun 1999;67:1317–22.

33. Priest JW, Mehlert A, Arrowood MJ, et al. Characterization of a low molecular weight glycolipid antigen from *Cryptosporidium parvum*. J Biol Chem 2003; 278(52):52212–22.

34. Sturbaum GD, Schaefer DA, Jost BH, et al. Antigenic differences within the *Cryptosporidium hominis* and *Cryptosporidium parvum* surface proteins P23 and GP900 defined by monoclonal antibody reactivity. Mol Biochem Parasitol 2008;159(2):138–41.

35. Jakobi V, Petry F. Differential expression of *Cryptosporidium parvum* genes encoding sporozoite surface antigens in infected HCT-8 host cells. Microbes Infect 2006;8(8):2186–94.

36. Wetzel DM, Schmidt J, Kuhlenschmidt MS, et al. Gliding motility leads to active cellular invasion by *Cryptosporidium parvum* sporozoites. Infect Immun 2005; 73(9):5379–87.

37. Na BK, Kang JM, Cheun HI, et al. Cryptopain-1, a cysteine protease of *Cryptosporidium parvum*, does not require the pro-domain for folding. Parasitol 2009; 136(2):149–57.

38. Feng X, Akiyoshi DE, Widmer G, et al. Characterization of subtilase protease in *Cryptosporidium parvum* and *C. hominis*. J Parasitol 2007;93(3):619–26.

39. Aguirre-Garcia MM, Okhuysen PC. *Cryptosporidium parvum*: identification and characterization of an acid phosphatase. Parasitol Res 2007;101(1):85–9.

40. Chen XM, O'Hara SP, Huang BQ, et al. Localized glucose and water influx facilitates *Cryptosporidium parvum* cellular invasion by means of modulation of host-cell membrane protrusion. Proc Natl Acad Sci U S A 2005;102(18):6338–43.

41. Barta JR, Thompson RCA. What is *Cryptosporidium*? Reappraising its biology and phylogenetic affinities. Trends Parasitol 2006;22(10):463–8.

42. Valigurová A, Jirků M, Koudela B, et al. Cryptosporidia: epicellular parasites embraced by the host cell membrane. Int J Parasitol 2008;38(8–9):913–22.

43. Huang BQ, Chen X-M, LaRusso NF. *Cryptosporidium parvum* attachment to and internalization by human biliary epithelia in vitro: a morphologic study. J Parasitol 2004;90(2):212–21.

44. Hyde JE. Fine targeting of purine salvage in *Cryptosporidium* parasites. Trends Parasitol 2008;24(8):336–9.

45. Mazumdar J, Striepen B. Make it or take it: fatty acid metabolism of apicomplexan parasites. Eukaryot Cell 2007;6(10):1727–35.

46. Plattner F, Soldati-Favre D. Hijacking of host cellular functions by the apicomplexa. Annu Rev Microbiol 2008;62:471–87.

47. Pantenburg B, Dann SM, Wang HC, et al. Intestinal immune response to human *Cryptosporidium sp* infection. Infect Immun 2008;76(1):23–9.

48. Foster DM, Smith GW. Pathophysiology of diarrhea in calves. Vet Clin North Am Food Anim Pract 2009;25(1):13–36.

49. Gookin JL, Nordone SK, Argenzio RA. Host responses to *Cryptosporidium* infection. J Vet Intern Med 2002;16(1):12–21.

50. Klein P, Kleinova T, Volek Z, et al. Effect of *Cryptosporidium parvum* infection on the absorptive capacity and paracellular permeability of the small intestine in neonatal calves. Vet Parasitol 2008;152(1–2):53–9.

51. Blikslager A, Hunt E, Guerrant R, et al. Glutamine transporter in crypts compensates for loss of villus absorption in bovine cryptosporidiosis. Am J Physiol Gastrointest Liver Physiol 2001;281(3):G645–53.

52. Cole J, Blikslager A, Hunt E, et al. Cyclooxygenase blockade and exogenous glutamine enhance sodium absorption in infected bovine ileum. Am J Physiol Gastrointest Liver Physiol 2003;284(3):G516–24.
53. Robinson P, Martin P, Garza A, et al. Substance P receptor antagonism for treatment of cryptosporidiosis in immunosuppressed mice. J Parasitol 2008;94(5):1150–4.
54. Mele R, Gomez Morales MA, Tosini F, et al. *Cryptosporidium parvum* at different developmental stages modulates host cell apoptosis in vitro. Infect Immun 2004;72(10):6061–7.
55. Liu J, Deng M, Lancto CA, et al. Biphasic modulation of apoptotic pathways in *Cryptosporidium parvum*-infected human intestinal epithelial cells. Infect Immun 2009;77(2):837–49.
56. Elliott DA, Clark DP. Host cell fate on *Cryptosporidium parvum* egress from MDCK cells. Infect Immun 2003;71(9):5422–6.
57. Wyatt CR, McDonald V. Innate and T cell-mediated immune responses in cryptosporidiosis. In: Sterling CR, Adam RD, editors. World class parasites, The pathogenic enteric protozoa: *Giardia, Entamoeba, Cryptosporidium* and *Cyclospora*, vol. 8. Norwell (MA): Kluwer Academic Publishers; 2004. p. 91–102.
58. Harp J. *Cryptosporidium* and host resistance: historical perspective and some novel approaches. Anim Health Res Rev 2003;4:53–62.
59. Linde A, Ross C, Davis EG, et al. Innate immunity and host defense peptides in veterinary medicine. J Vet Intern Med 2008;2:247–65.
60. Tarver A, Clark DP, Diamond G, et al. Enteric β-defensin: molecular cloning and characterization of a gene with inducible intestinal epithelial cell expression associated with *Cryptosporidium parvum* infection. Infect Immun 1998;66:1045–56.
61. Whitmire WM, Harp JA. Characterization of bovine cellular and serum antibody responses during infection by *Cryptosporidium parvum*. Infect Immun 1991;59: 990–5.
62. Riggs MW. In: Fayer R, editor. *Cryptosporidium* and cryptosporidiosis. Boca Raton (FL): CRC Press; 1997. p. 129–61.
63. Perryman LE, Jasmer DP, Riggs MW, et al. A cloned gene of *Cryptosporidium parvum* encodes neutralization-sensitive epitopes. Mol Biochem Parasitol 1997;80:137–47.
64. Wyatt CR, Perryman LE. Detection of mucosally delivered antibody to *Cryptosporidium parvum* in infected calves. Ann N Y Acad Sci 2000;916:378–87.
65. Wang H-F, Swain JB, Besser TE, et al. Detection of antibodies to a recombinant *Cryptosporidium parvum* P23 in serum and feces from neonatal calves. J Parasitol 2003;89:918–23.
66. Wyatt CR, Brackett EJ, Mason PH, et al. Excretion patterns of mucosally delivered antibodies to p23 in *Cryptosporidium parvum* infected calves. Vet Immunol Immunopathol 2000;76:309–17.
67. Wyatt CR, Brackett EJ, Barrett WJ. Accumulation of mucosal T lymphocytes around epithelial cells after in vitro infection with *Cryptosporidium parvum*. J Parasitol 1999;85:765–8.
68. Abrahamsen MS. Bovine T cell responses to *Cryptosporidium parvum* infection. Int J Parasitol 1998;28:1083–8.
69. Wyatt CR, Barrett WJ, Brackett EJ, et al. Association of IL-10 expression by mucosal lymphocytes with increased expression of *Cryptosporidium parvum* epitopes in infected epithelium. J Parasitol 2002;88:281–6.
70. Wyatt CR, Brackett EJ, Perryman LE, et al. Activation of intestinal intraepithelial T lymphocytes in calves infected with *Cryptosporidium parvum*. Infect Immun 1997;65:185–90.

71. Wyatt CR, Brackett EJ, Savidge J. Evidence for the emergence of a type-1-like immune response in intestinal mucosa of calves recovering from cryptosporidiosis. J Parasitol 2001;87:90–5.
72. Wyatt CR, Lindahl S, Austin K, et al. Response of T lymphocytes from previously infected calves to recombinant *Cryptosporidium parvum* P23 vaccine antigen. J Parasitol 2005;91:1239–42.
73. Abrahamsen MS, Lancto CA, Walcheck B, et al. Localization of α/β and γ/δ T lymphocytes in *Cryptosporidium parvum*-infected tissues in naïve and immune calves. Infect Immun 1997;65:2428–33.
74. Fayer R, Santín M, Trout JM, et al. Prevalence of species and genotypes of *Cryptosporidium* found in 1-2-year-old dairy cattle in the eastern United States. Vet Parasitol 2006;135:105–12.
75. Fayer R, Santin M, Trout JM. Prevalence of *Cryptosporidium* species and genotypes in mature dairy cattle on farms in eastern United States compared with younger cattle from the same locations. Vet Parasitol 2007;145:260–6.
76. Santín M, Trout JM, Fayer R. A longitudinal study of cryptosporidiosis in dairy cattle from birth to 2 years of age. Vet Parasitol 2008;155:15–23.
77. Xiao L, Zhou L, Santin M, et al. Distribution of *Cryptosporidium parvum* subtypes in calves in eastern United States. Parasitol Res 2007;100:701–6.
78. Fayer R, Santin M, Trout JM. *Cryptosporidium ryanae* n. sp. (Apicomplexa: *Cryptosporidiidae*) in cattle (*Bos taurus*). Vet Parasitol 2008;156:191–8.
79. Lindsay DS, Upton SJ, Owens DS, et al. *Cryptosporidium andersoni* n. sp. (Apicomplexa: *Cryptosporidiidae*) in cattle (*Bos taurus*). J Eukaryot Microbiol 2000;47:91–5.
80. Smith H. Diagnostics. In: Fayer R, Xiao L, editors. *Cryptosporidium* and cryptosporidiosis. 2nd edition. Boca Raton (FL): CRC Press; 2008. p. 173–93.
81. Arrowood MJ. Diagnosis. In: Fayer R, editor. *Cryptosporidium* and cryptosporidiosis. Boca Raton (FL): CRC Press; 1997. p. 43–64.
82. Amar C, Pedraza-Díaz S, McLauchlin J. Extraction and genotyping of *Cryptosporidium parvum* DNA from fecal smears on glass slides stained conventionally for direct microscope examination. J Clin Microbiol 2001;39:401–3.
83. Harp JA, Woodmansee DB, Moon HW. Effects of colostral antibody on susceptibility of calves to *Cryptosporidium parvum* infection. Am J Vet Res 1989;50:117–9.
84. Fayer R, Andrews C, Ungar BL, et al. Efficacy of hyperimmune bovine colostrum for prophylaxis of cryptosporidiosis in neonatal calves. J Parasitol 1989;75:393–7.
85. Jenkins M, Higgins J, Kniel K, et al. Protection of calves against cryptosporiosis by oral inoculation with gamma-irradiated *Cryptosporidium parvum* oocysts. J Parasitol 2004;90:1178–80.
86. Stockdale H, Spencer JA, Blagburn BL. Prophylaxis and chemotherapy. In: Fayer R, Xiao L, editors. *Cryptosporidium* and cryptosporidiosis. 2nd edition. Boca Raton (FL): CRC Press; 2008. p. 255–87.
87. Rossignol JF. Nitazoxanide in the treatment of acquired immune deficiency syndrome-related cryptosporidiosis: results of the United States compassionate use program in 365 patients. Aliment Pharmacol Ther 2006;24:887–94.
88. Viel H, Rocques H, Martin J, et al. Efficacy of nitazoxanide against experimental cryptosporidiosis in goat neonates. Parasitol Res 2007;102:163–6.
89. Ollivett TL, Nydam DV, Bowman DD, et al. Effect of nitazoxanide on cryptosporidiosis in experimentally infected neonatal dairy calves. J Dairy Sci 2009;92:1643–8.

90. Schnyder M, Kohler L, Hemphill A, et al. Prophylactic and therapeutic efficacy of nitazoxanide against *Cryptosporidium parvum* in experimentally challenged neonatal calves. Vet Parasitol 2009;160:149–54.
91. Lallemond M, Villeneuve A, Belda J, et al. Field study of the efficacy of halofuginone and decoquinate in the treatment of cryptosporidiosis in veal calves. Vet Rec 2006;159:672–7.
92. Villacorta I, Peters JE, Vanopdenbosch E, et al. Efficacy of halofuginone lactate against *Cryptosporidium parvum* in calves. Antimicrobial Agents Chemother 1991;35:283–7.
93. Naciri M, Mancassola R, Yvore P, et al. The effect of halofuginone lactate on experimental *C. parvum* infections in calves. Vet Parasitol 1993;45:199–207.
94. Peters JE, Villacorta I, Naciri M, et al. Specific serum and local antibody responses against *Cryptosporidium parvum* during medication of calves with halofuginone lactate. Infect Immun 1993;61:4440–5.
95. Lefay D, Naciri M, Poirier P, et al. Efficacy of halofuginone lactate in the prevention of cryptosporidiosis in suckling calves. Vet Rec 2001;148:108–12.
96. Joachim A, Krull T, Schwarzkopf J, et al. Prevalence and control of bovine cryptosporidiosis in German dairy herds. Vet Parasitol 2003;112:277–88.
97. Jarvie BD, Trotz-Williamsm LA, McKnight DR, et al. Effect of halofuginone lactate on the occurrence of *Cryptosporidium parvum* and growth of neonatal dairy calves. J Dairy Sci 2005;88:1801–6.
98. Klein P. Preventative and therapeutic efficacy of halofuginone-lactate against *Cryptosporidium parvum* in spontaneously infected calves: a centralized, randomized, double-blind, placebo-controlled study. Vet J 2008;177:429–31.
99. Naciri M, Yvore P. Efficite du lactate d'halofuginone dans le traitment de le cryptosporidiose chez l'agneau [Efficacy of halofuginone lactate on the treatment of cryptosporidiosis of lambs]. Rec Med Vet Ec Alfort 1989;165:823.
100. Mancassola R, Reperant JM, Naciri M, et al. Chemoprophylaxis of *Cryptosporidium parvum* infection with paromomycin in kids and immunological study. Antimicrobial Agents Chemother 1995;39:75–8.
101. Viu M, Quílez J, Sánchez-Acedo C, et al. Field trial on the therapeutic efficacy of paromomycin on natural *Cryptosporidium parvum* infections in lambs. Vet Parasitol 2000;90:163–70.
102. Fayer R, Ellis W. Paromomycin is effective as prophylaxis for cryptosporidiosis in dairy calves. J Parasitol 1993;79:771–4.
103. Elitok B, Elitok OM, Pulat H. Efficacy of azithromycin dihydrate in treatment of cryptosporidiosis in naturally effected dairy calves. J Vet Intern Med 2005;19:590–3.
104. Mancassola R, Richard A, Naciri M. Evaluation of decoquinate to treat experimental cryptosporidiosis in kids. Vet Parasitol 1997;69:31–7.
105. Moore DA, Atwill ER, Kirk JH, et al. Prophylactic use of decoquinate for infections with *Cryptosporidium parvum* in experimentally challenged neonatal calves. J Am Vet Med Assoc 2003;223:839–45.
106. Harp JA, Goff JP. Strategies for the control of *Cryptosporidium parvum* infection in calves. J Dairy Sci 1998;81:289–94.
107. Nydam DV, Mohammed HO. Quantitative risk assessment of *Cryptosporidium* species infection in dairy calves. J Dairy Sci 2005;88:3932–43.

Bovine Viral Diarrhea Virus: Global Status

Julia F. Ridpath, PhD

KEYWORDS

* Bovine viral diarrhea viruses * BVDV1 * BVDV2 * Pestivirus

The term, *bovine viral diarrhea viruses (BVDVs)*, refers to a diverse group of single-stranded RNA viruses currently classified as two different species, BVDV1 and BVDV2, within the pestivirus genus. One or both species have been isolated from ruminants in all continents with the exception of Antarctica. The global status of BVDVs is in transition. Even as control programs in Scandinavia result in near eradication of BVDVs in those regions,[1] there is a growing recognition of BVDV–associated diseases in species other than cattle in North America, Southeast Asia, and Africa.[2–6] In 2007, the Office International des Epizooties added BVDV to its list of reportable diseases. It is only listed as a reportable disease of cattle, however, not as a reportable disease of multiple species. This may lead to confusion as BVDV also replicates in and causes reproductive disease in domestic species, such as pigs, goats, and sheep and in several wildlife species.

In the past decade there has been an assimilation of regional veterinary biologics companies by large international companies. This assimilation has been accompanied by removal from the market of BVDV vaccines based on strains endemic to the region. Although further research is necessary, regional variation in prevalence of BVDV subtypes (species and subgenotypes) and variation in cross-protection between BVDV subtypes suggest vaccine protection may be improved by basing vaccines on the BVDV strains prevalent in the region in which the vaccine is to be used.

In addition, a putative new member of the pestivirus genus has been identified that causes disease syndromes in cattle that are indistinguishable from clinical presentations associated with BVDV infection.[7,8] One research group has proposed that this emerging virus be called BVDV3.[9] Differentiation of this virus from BVDV1 and BVDV2 strains and restricting the expansion of this virus will be important challenges in the design of future BVDV eradication and control programs.

DISCOVERY AND CLASSIFICATION

The first recorded observation of the disease, bovine viral diarrhea (BVD), dates back to 1946 when a novel transmissible disease in cattle was observed in the state of New

Ruminant Diseases and Immunology Research Unit, National Animal Disease Center, USDA, Agricultural Research Service, 1920 Dayton Road, P.O. Box 70, Ames, IA 50010, USA
E-mail address: julia.ridpath@ars.usda.gov

Vet Clin Food Anim 26 (2010) 105–121
doi:10.1016/j.cvfa.2009.10.007
0749-0720/10/$ – see front matter. Published by Elsevier Inc.

vetfood.theclinics.com

York.[10] This disease was characterized by leukopenia, pyrexia, depression, diarrhea, anorexia, gastrointestinal erosions, and hemorrhages. The causative viral agent was isolated in 1957 and named BVDV.[11] A similar but more severe disease, termed *disease X*, was reported several years later in Canada.[12] Although similar to BVD, disease X tended to affect fewer animals per herd but had a higher mortality rate. Unlike BVD, disease X (later termed, *mucosal disease*) could not be transmitted experimentally.[13] A disease with the same clinical presentation was described by several groups in the late 1950s in Germany and termed, *Schleimhautkrankheit*.[14] Virus neutralization was used to demonstrate that the viral agents isolated from BVD and mucosal disease cases in North America and Schleimhautkrankheit in Germany and the United Kingdom were the same.[15,16] Subsequently it was demonstrated that BVDV was antigenically related to hog cholera virus (since renamed classical swine fever virus [CSFV]).[17] A decade later, immunologic similarities were also noted between BVDV, CSFV, and the causative agent of border disease in sheep (termed, *border disease virus*).[18] In 1973, the term, *pestivirus*, was coined for this antigenically related group of viruses[19] and they were classified as a genus within the family Togaviridae.[20] At that time flaviviruses were also classified as a genus within the togavirus family. Advances in the molecular characterization of flaviviruses, however, revealed fundamental differences in molecular structure, replication strategy, and genetic organization between flaviviruses and other members of the Togaviridae. These findings led to the reclassification of the flaviviruses, into a new virus family, Flaviviridae, which initially contained one genus, flavivirus.[21] The publication of the genomic sequence of the BVDV strain, NADL, the first pestivirus to be sequenced, revealed that pestiviruses had greater similarities in genomic organization, gene expression, and replication strategy to the Flaviviridae than the Togaviridae.[22] This led to the reclassification of pestiviruses, in 1991, as a new genus within the Flaviviridae family.[23] Subsequent phylogenetic analysis of isolates identified as BVDV, based on host of origin and clinical presentation, revealed two distinct genetic groups, BVDV1 and BVDV2,[24,25] which were later classified as two different species within the pestivirus genus.[26] In addition to the four recognized pestivirus species, BVDV1, BVDV2, border disease virus, and CSFV, additional species have been proposed (**Table 1**).[9,27–30] In 2004, a novel pestivirus was isolated from fetal bovine serum originating from Brazil.[31] Subsequently, other isolates from South America and Southeast Asia were identified that grouped with this virus based on phylogenetic analysis.[7,32] Some of the isolations were from fetal bovine serum, one was from a buffalo, and, significantly, some were isolated from apparently persistently infected (PI) cattle. Similarity in clinical presentation to BVDV1 and BVDV2 and the ability to establish PIs in cattle has led some researchers to suggest that this group of viruses be referred to as BVDV3.[9]

CHARACTERISTIC TRAITS
Physical Characteristics of the Viral Particle

BVDV is included as a member of the Flaviviridae because it shares many characteristics with other viruses within this family.[26,33] All Flaviviridae are spherical viruses 40 to 50 nm in diameter. The viral particle consists of an outer lipid envelope surrounding an inner protein shell or capsid that contains the viral genome. The lipid envelope, which is derived from the membranes of the infected host cell, makes these viruses susceptible to inactivation by solvents and detergents. The molecular weight of the BVDV virion has been estimated as 6.0×10^7 and the buoyant density in sucrose is 1.10 to 1.15 g/cm^3. BVDV, however, as do the other members of the pestivirus genus, differs from the rest of the Flaviviridae in that the lipid envelope that surrounds the virion is pleomorphic. The

Table 1
Species in the pestivirus genus

Recognized Species	Geographic Distribution	Host
BVDV1	Worldwide; nearing eradication in some European regions	Wild and domestic ruminants, pigs, and rabbits
BVDV2	Worldwide, although more prevalent in North and South America; nearing eradication in some European regions	Wild and domestic ruminants, pigs, and rabbits
CSFV	Eradicated in United States and Canada	Pigs, sheep, and cattle
Border disease virus	Worldwide	Sheep, goats, pigs, cattle, and wild ruminants
Putative species[a]		
Giraffe	Kenya	Giraffe
HoBi-like (BVDV3)	South America and Southeast Asia	Cattle
Pronghorn	United States	Pronghorn antelope
Bungowannah	Australia	Pigs

[a] Listed in order of increasing phylogenetic divergence from recognized pestivirus species.

resulting variation in size of enveloped particles impedes purification by banding in sucrose gradients, accurate estimation of size, and identification by electron microscopy. In addition, pestiviruses can be differentiated from other viruses within the Flaviviridae by their resistance to inactivation by low pH. Although most flaviviruses and hepaciviruses are inactivated by low pH, pestiviruses are stable over a broad pH range. Infectivity is not affected by freezing but decreases at temperatures above 40°C. As discussed previously, BVDVs are inactivated by organic solvents and detergents. Other methods of inactivation include trypsin treatment (0.5 mg/mL at 37°C for 60 minutes), ethylenimine (reduction of 5 log10 units using 10 mmol/L at 37°C for 2 hours), electron beam irradiation (4.9 and 2.5 kGy needed to reduce virus infectivity 1 log10 unit for frozen and liquid samples, respectively), and gamma irradiation (20–30 kGy).

The Viral Genome and Gene Products

The genomes of all Flaviviridae consist of a single strand of positive-sense RNA, between 9 and 12.3 kilobases long, that codes for a single open reading frame (ORF). There is no subgenomic mRNA associated with Flaviviridae infections. The viral structural proteins are encoded at the 5′ end and the nonstructural proteins are encoded in the remaining 3′ end. The ORF is translated as one long polyprotein that is cleaved after translation into individual proteins. The nonstructural proteins assist in this cleavage and in replication of positive and negative-strand RNA.

The genome of a pestiviruses, in the absence of insertions, is approximately 12.3 kilobases long with an ORF that contains approximately 4000 codons. The ORF is preceded and followed by 5′ and 3′ untranslated regions of 360 to 390 nucleotides and 200 to 240 nucleotides, respectively. The 5′ terminus does not contain a cap structure.[34] Although there is no poly(A) tract present at the 3′ end, pestiviruses genomes terminate with a short poly(C) tract. Although the genome is made up of single-stranded RNA, there is considerable secondary structure inherent as evidenced by its ability to bind CF-11 cellulose in the presence of 15% ethanol,[35] solubility in 2 mol/L LiCl,[22] and resistance to hydrolysis by low concentrations of RNase A.[36] It is thought that stem and loop structures found in the 5' untranslated region are integral to the formation of an internal ribosomal entry site that functions to direct the attachment of assembly of the ribosome at the first codon of the ORF (for review, see Neill[37]). The order of the individual viral proteins within the polyprotein is as follows: Npro-C-Erns-E1-E2-p7-NS2/3-NS4a-NS4b-NS5a-NS5b. The attributes and functions of each viral protein are listed in **Table 2**. In comparison to the other genera within Flaviviridae, pestiviruses encode two unique proteins. The first is the nonstructural protein, N^{pro}, which is encoded at the beginning of the ORF (preceding the region coding for the structural proteins). The N^{pro} is a proteinase, which cleaves itself from the viral polypeptide. This protein also functions in the suppression of the host's innate immune system. Studies suggest N^{pro} prevents the production of type I interferon by blocking the activity of interferon regulatory factor 3.[38,39] The second unique gene product is the envelope glycoprotein, E^{rns}, which possesses an intrinsic RNase activity. This protein is found in the infectious viral particle and secreted in soluble form. It is thought that the secreted E^{rns} prevents the induction of beta interferon by binding to and degrading double-stranded RNA.[40]

Variations in Genotype (Species), Subgenotype, Biotype, and Virulence

The viruses grouped under the heading of BVDV are highly heterogeneous and encompass viruses belonging to two different species. Viruses of either species may exist as two different biotypes, cytopathic and noncytopathic, and are of varying virulence from avirulent to highly virulent. The two recognized species of BVDV are BVDV1 and BVDV2. Although this segregation was first based on phylogenetic analysis,[24,25] subsequent characterization of viral strains from the two species demonstrated antigenic differences.[41] The practical significance of the observed antigenic differences was evidenced by the failure of vaccines and diagnostics based on BVDV1 strains to control and detect BVDV2 strains.[42] Although BVDV1 and BVDV2 viruses are cross-reactive, they can be differentiated based on antigenic differences. Neutralizing antibody titers found in convalescent sera are typically severalfold higher against viruses from the same species compared with viruses from the other species,[43,44] and monoclonal antibody binding patterns are distinct.[25,45]

Although antigenic differences may be used to differentiate the species, nucleotide sequence relatedness is the most reliable criteria. Differences between BVDV1 and BVDV2 genomes are not relegated to any one region and differences may be found throughout the entire genome.[46] Differences between BVDV1 and BVDV2 in some genomic regions, however, are more amenable to comparison or have greater biologic significance. The 5' untranslated region is the most commonly used region for detection and characterization because of highly conserved motifs that are favorable to PCR amplification. Because the N^{pro} region is unique to pestiviruses, however, comparison of this region is gaining favor for characterization of putative pestivirus species.

Phylogenetic analysis has also revealed subgenotype groupings within the BVDV1 and BVDV2 species, 12 in BVDV1 viruses (BVDV1a, BVDV1b, BVDV1c, BVDV1d, BVDV1e, BVDV1f, BVDV1g, BVDV1h, BVDV1i, BVDV1j, BVDV1k, and BVDV1l)[47] and two in BVDV2 viruses (BVDV2a and BVDV2b).[48] Furthermore, additional subgenotypes of BVDV1 have been identified in isolations of BVDV from cattle in South Africa and Switzerland but have not yet been assigned names.[49–51] The clinical significance of segregation into subgenotypes is a matter of discussion. Different BVDV subgenotypes predominate in different geographic locations[24,49,51–69] and studies have shown antigenic differences between subgenotypes as demonstrated by differences in cross-neutralization,[49,61] monoclonal antibody binding,[45] and response of PI animals

Table 2
Bovine viral diarrhea viruses proteins

Protein	Size (kd)	Structural	Attributes	Function
N^{pro}	20	N	Unique to pestivirus genus Highly conserved Sequence frequently used in phylogenetic comparisons	Autoprotease Suppresses host immune response
C (Capsid)	14	Y	Conserved	Forms nucleocapsid of virion
E^{rns}	48	Y	Unique to pestivirus genus Glycosylated Found in the infectious viral particle and secreted in soluble form Detection target for antigen-based tests	Integral viral membrane protein Ribonuclease activity of soluble form suppresses host immune response Possesses minor neutralizing epitope
E1	25	Y	Glycosylated	Integral viral membrane protein
E2	53	Y	Glycosylated Immune system–generated antibodies against E2 after vaccination with killed or modified live vaccine Sequence displays most variability of all viral proteins	Integral viral membrane protein Possesses dominant neutralizing epitopes
p7	7	N	Required for production of infectious virus but not RNA replication	Unknown
NS2/3	80	N	Highly conserved Detection target for antigen-based tests Immunodominant nonstructural protein Antibodies generated against protein after modified live vaccination but not killed vaccination Cytopathic viruses cleave to NS2 and NS3	RNA helicase Serine protease Cleaves itself and downstream nonstructural proteins from viral polyprotein
NS4a	7.2	N	Hydrophobic	Serine protease cofactor
NS4b	38	N	Hydrophobic	Replicase component
NS5a	55	N	Phosphorylated	Replicase component
NS5b	81	N		RNA-dependent RNA polymerase

to vaccination.[70] It is not known, however, if variations in subgenotypes are significant enough to have an impact on the detection or the protection afforded by vaccination.

BVDV strains may exist as one of two biotypes, cytopathic and noncytopathic. Segregation into biotype is based on activity in cultured epithelial cells.[11,71] Noncytopathic viruses predominate in nature. Cytopathic viruses are rare and usually found in association with outbreaks of mucosal disease, a rare highly fatal form of BVDV infection. It is believed that cytopathic strains arise from noncytopathic strains through a mutational event that results in the cleavage of the NS2/3 viral protein to the NS2 and NS3 proteins. The most frequently observed mutational event resulting in BVDV biotype change is recombination, in which short pieces of genetic code are inserted into the genome of a noncytopathic BVDV strain.[72] The inserted code may originate from another BVDV or from the infected host cell. Not all recombination events are associated with biotype change, however, as some noncytopathic viruses have insertions[46,73] and some cytopathic viruses do not have insertions.[74] Cytopathology in vitro does not correlate with virulence in vivo. The most clinically severe form of acute BVDV infection is associated with noncytopathic viruses.[24,73,75–77] The significance of BVDV biotypes to control programs lies in that noncytopathic BVDV, but not cytopathic BVDV, may establish a PI in a fetus that persists throughout its lifetime. For this reason most modified live BVDV vaccines use cytopathic BVDV.

High and low virulence BVDV2 strains have been characterized.[41,75,78–82] In the United States, low virulence BVDV2 strains have been selected for use in modified live vaccines[43] and high virulence BVDV2 strains have been used as challenge strains to assess the efficacy of protection induced by vaccination.[83,84] Although there is variation in virulence in BVDV1 strains[85] there is little information available in the literature. To date, the most virulent BVDV strains characterized belong to the BVDV2 species.

Clinical Presentation

Clinical presentation varies depending on strain of virus, species of host, immune status of host, reproductive status of host, age of host, and concurrent infections with other pathogens. Although the term, *diarrhea*, is prominent in the name, respiratory and reproductive disease associated with BVDV infection are more commonly reported.[86,87] The clinical presentation of reproductive disease is due to the direct infection of the fetus and the outcome depends on the stage of gestation in which the fetal infection occurs.[88] Although abortions and weak calves have been attributed to BVDV infection in late gestation,[89] infections occurring earlier in gestation generally have greater impact on reproduction. Fetal infections in cattle, occurring between 42 and 125 days of gestation, result in fetal reabsorption, mummification, abortion, congenital malformations, or the establishment of PI animals. PI animals shed BVDV throughout their lifetimes and are important carriers in the introduction of BVDV into naive populations. If a PI animal becomes infected with a cytopathic BVDV it may succumb to a relatively rare but invariably fatal form of BVD, called mucosal disease.[90]

Although the PI animal is frequently the source of BVDV entering a herd, subsequent spread of the virus and observed clinical disease are the result of acute infection. The severity of acute infections is dependent on the viral strain, immune status of host, and presence of secondary pathogens. BVDVs are lymphotrophic and acute infections result in the reduction of circulating lymphocytes[41] and the suppression of innate immune functions.[91–93] The resulting immunosuppression results in reduced resistance to secondary pathogens and increased severity of clinical disease after secondary infections.[94] The interaction of BVDV with secondary pathogens is thought to be one of the contributing factors in bovine respiratory disease complex (BRD).

Emerging Recognition of Bovine Viral Diarrhea Virus–Associated Disease in Nonbovine Hosts

Although BVDV infections are most commonly associated with cattle, there is evidence, based on virus isolation and serology, that BVDVs replicate in a wide variety of domesticated and wild ruminants. Losses to food and fiber producers due to infection of nonbovine domesticated species are usually associated with reproductive disease. It has been demonstrated that BVDVs are the causative agents of reproductive disease in goats,[95] sheep,[96,97] and pigs.[98–102] It seems that infection of pregnant animals belonging to these species results in clinical presentation similar to that seen in cattle. The primary consequences are due to the direct infection of the fetus and the outcome of infection depends on the stage of gestation in which the fetal infection occurs. One of the resulting outcomes is the birth of PI animals. Recently the emergence of BVDV-associated abortions and congenital defects (including PI) in New World camelids has led to renewed interest in BVDV in nonbovine hosts. Before 2002, prevalence in New World camelid populations was reported to be low and no clinical disease was associated with exposure.[103] The conventional wisdom was that although infections in New World camelids might occasionally occur, they were rare and resulted from contact with cattle. These assumptions were called into question by the isolation of BVDV from a stillborn alpaca[104] and the subsequent identification of crias PI with BVDV.[105–107] In a 2008 survey conducted among members of the (US-based) Alpaca Owner and Breeder Association, 25.4% of herds had been exposed to BVDV, based on serology, and 6.3% had PI crias in residence.[108] The PI crias may be unthrifty and suffer from congenital defects, such as stunting or abnormal coat properties, or they may seem normal. Just as PI cattle are considered the main vector for introduction of BVDV to naive herds, it seems that PI alpacas shed virus that readily infects naive cohorts. In contrast to BVDV infections in cattle in which there is extensive heterogeneity in infecting BVDV strains, BVDV isolated from PI alpaca belong to one subgroup of one species and seem to be relatively similar based on phylogenetic analysis.[3,107] These reports indicate that a limited number of BVDV strains have adapted to improved replication in alpaca, that these strains circulate between alpaca populations in the absence of contact with cattle, and that PI alpacas are a source for the introduction of BVDV into naive alpaca herds. The comparatively low incidence of exposure, homogeneity of BVDV strains, and limited use of vaccines suggest that eradication of BVDV from commercial alpaca herds in the United States is achievable via testing and elimination of PI animals followed by surveillance via serology to rapidly detect and control any reintroduction of BVDV into alpaca herds.

Although there is evidence of BVDV replication in wild ruminants based on serology and virus isolation, including antelope, giraffe, African buffalo, bison (European and American), big horn sheep, mountain goats, and various *Cervidae* (reindeer, kudu, roe deer, red deer, fallow deer, mule deer, white-tailed deer, and caribou),[2,5,6,28,50,109–113] the level of exposure and prevalence of PI animals is largely unknown. Regional surveillance based on serology varies significantly depending on method of sampling. In serologic surveys of white-tailed deer populations residing in the United States, sampled deer collected by net gunning[114–117] reported higher BVDV exposure rates than surveys that sampled deer harvested by hunters.[118] The difference in exposure rate may be related to differences in populations sampled. Net gunning results in sampling of animals of both genders and all age groups whereas hunter-harvested animals tend to be predominantly adult males.

Recently, several studies have focused on BVDV infections in white-tailed deer. PI white-tailed deer have been harvested from the field[6,118] and generated under experimental conditions.[119,120] The clinical progression of acute disease after inoculation of fawns was similar to that seen in BVDV infections in cattle and included fever and reduction of circulating lymphocytes.[121] Similarly, the clinical presentation of BVDV-associated reproductive disease in white-tailed deer is similar to that observed in cattle and includes readsorption, abortion, mummification, and birth of PI fawns.[122] The presence of neutralizing antibody titers in pregnant does seem to protect against BVDV infection in the fawns they carried. Transmission of BVDV between PI cattle and pregnant deer resulting in the birth of PI fawns has been confirmed under experimental conditions.[123]

Because free-ranging wild ruminant populations are frequently in contact with domestic cattle, possible transfer of BVDV between cattle and wild ruminants has significant implication for proposed BVDV control programs. Furthermore, reintroduction of endangered species to ecosystems that include domestic cattle may fail due to BVDV transmission from cattle to the newly introduced, BVDV naive species.

DETECTION AND CONTROL

BVDV diagnostics have focused on the detection of PI animals. Historically, virus isolation in cultured bovine cells has been the standard against which other tests were evaluated. Because of ease and lower expense, however, antigen detection by immunohistochemistry or antigen capture ELISA (ACE) and nucleic acid detection by reverse transcriptase–polymerase chain reaction are gaining favor. In contrast to virus isolation, these methods do not differentiate between deposited nonreplicating viral remnants and biologically active virus. No one-time test can reliably differentiate between acute and PIs. For that reason, two positive tests from samples collected 3 weeks apart are necessary to diagnose PI. Antigen-based testing methods, such as immunohistochemistry and ACE, are robust and results are highly reproducible between laboratories. These tests frequently depend, however, on one or two monoclonal antibodies, which target viral proteins. A viral variant has been identified that escapes detection by immunohistochemistry and ACE tests based on the binding of a monoclonal antibody against the viral protein E^{rns}.[124] Prevalance of such BVDV variants is unstudied. Multiple testing strategies, including polyclonal or pooled monoclonal antibodies that detect more than one viral glycoprotein, may be necessary to detect all PI calves and facilitate eradication of BVDV.

In addition to tests that recognize all BVDV species and subgenotypes in circulation, there is a need for tests that differentiate between BVDV1 and BVDV2 and other species of pestiviruses. Until the early 1990s, there were only three recognized species in the pestivirus genus, BVDV, border disease virus, and CSFV. Subsequently, BVDV were divided into two different species, BVDV1 and BVDV2.[24,25] Four additional putative pestivirus species have been identified, based on phylogenetic analysis. In chronologic order they are Giraffe[125] (isolated from one of several giraffes in the Nanyuki District of Kenya suffering from mucosal disease-like symptoms),[126] HoBi (first isolated from fetal bovine serum originating in Brazil and later from samples originating in Southeast Asia),[31] Pronghorn (isolated from an emaciated blind pronghorn antelope in the United States),[29] and Bungowannah (isolated after an outbreak in pigs, resulting in stillbirth and neonatal death, in Australia).[127] Three of these putative new species have been isolated from only one geographic region. In contrast, infection with the HoBi species has been isolated from cattle samples originating in South America and Southeast Asia.[31,128] The clinical presentation (reproductive disease and PI) in dairies in Thailand mimics that of BVDV1 or BVDV2 and has led to the suggestion that this group of viruses be called BVDV3.[9] Based on phylogenetic and antigenic differences it is probable that diagnostics and vaccines designed to detect and prevent BVDV1 and BVDV2 infection will not be effective against the HoBi species.[31] Introduction of the HoBi species into new geographic regions would have serious consequences for BVDV control programs.

Vaccination is effective in reducing the spread of BVDV but cannot on its own eliminate BVDV from populations. This is because control by vaccination is compromised by the heterogeneity observed in BVDV strains, by the lack of complete fetal protection afforded by vaccination, and, most significantly, by the failure to remove PI animals from cattle populations. Killed and modified live vaccines are available for the prevention of BVD. There are two different goals for BVDV vaccination that are reflected in two different label claims that may be pursued in licensing US BVDV vaccines.[129–131] One goal is to prevent clinical disease after exposure to BVDV. The corresponding label claim for licensure would be, "Aids in prevention and/or reduction of BVD disease." The "BVD disease" referred to in this label claim is not defined as respiratory, enteric, or reproductive disease. In practice, clinical presentation (pyrexia, diarrhea, and nasal discharge) or factors associated with immunosuppression (leukopenia) or hemorrhaging (thrombocytopenia) are used as criteria for reduction in animal health after BVDV exposure.[84,132] Another goal is to prevent the fetal infection that leads to PI. The label claim for this goal would be, "Aids in prevention of fetal infection including PI calves." The level of protection that is required to prevent acute disease or fetal infection is largely unknown. It has been shown that a titer of 16 is required for reduction of clinical disease whereas a titer greater than 256 is required to prevent systemic shed.[133] The level of neutralizing titer required for fetal protection is unknown. Although protective B-cell immune responses have been studied more frequently, it has been demonstrated that T-cell–based immune responses are protective on their own.[134–136] Licensing requirements for validation of BVDV vaccine efficacy are currently based on clinical trials involving the challenge of vaccinates with a single intranasal inoculation of a BVDV field strain. Under field conditions, however, animals are more likely to be exposed over an extended period of time by cohousing with a PI animal. The importance of including prolonged viral exposure in evaluating the efficacy of vaccines is suggested by studies demonstrating fetal exposure to BVDV after contact between pregnant vaccinated cattle and PI cohorts.[137]

Design of vaccination programs need to take into account stressors that reduce an animal's ability to respond to vaccination, differences in immune response related to age, and pregnancy status and periods of greatest vulnerability to infection and negative outcomes of infection. Thus, different strategies may need to be devised for establishing programs for neonates, breeding herds, stocker calves, replacement heifers, and dairy or feedlot production.

BOVINE VIRAL DIARRHEA VIRUSES ERADICATION PROGRAMS

The success of control efforts in Scandinavia[138–140] demonstrates BVDV eradication is possible and has led to the development of other regional control programs.[141–145] It is not possible, however, to take a one-size-fits-all approach to the design of eradication programs for different regions.[145] Program design will vary based on the incidence of BVDV, density of animal populations, animal movement, contact with wildlife populations, level of producer compliance, variation in circulating BVDV strains, and prevalent type of production unit or industry. Although the details of program design may differ by region, to be most effective, a control program must provide for biosecurity aimed at the development of management practices that prevent BVDV from being introduced into a herd, surveillance (to detect and remove PI animals), and means, such as vaccination, to limit BVDV spread if it is introduced into a herd.

SUMMARY

Despite eradication efforts, BVDV infections remain a source of economic loss for producers worldwide. The clinical presentation, pathogenesis, and basic biology of BVDV are complex. There are two states of infection (acute infection and PI), a continuum of virulence, two biotypes (cytopathic and noncytopathic), two species (BVDV1 and BVDV2), and many subgenotypes. The prevalence of BVDV species and subgenotypes varies by geographic region. Although infections are most commonly associated with cattle, they also occur in a wide variety of domesticated and wild ruminants. The circulation of BVDV in nonbovine species has economic, ecologic, and control implications. Although the economic impact of BVDV is largely due to the effects of acute infections, PI animals are the most common sources of virus and the most frequent vectors for introduction of virus into naive herds. Vaccines are effective in limiting the spread of BVDV in populations but are insufficient as a stand-alone tool for eradication. Recent advances in BVDV research and diagnostics have led to the development of improved and expanded testing aimed at the detection and removal of PI animals. This in turn has contributed to rapidly increasing number of regional eradication and control programs. The most efficacious of these are built around a three-pronged attack, consisting of biosecurity, surveillance, and control.

REFERENCES

1. Lindberg A, Brownlie J, Gunn GJ, et al. The control of bovine viral diarrhoea virus in Europe: today and in the future. Rev Sci Tech 2006;25(3):961–79.
2. Nelson DD, Dark MJ, Bradway DS, et al. Evidence for persistent bovine viral diarrhea virus infection in a captive mountain goat (*Oreamnos americanus*). J Vet Diagn Invest 2008;20(6):752–9.
3. Kim SG, Anderson RR, Yu J, et al. Genotyping and phylogenetic analysis of bovine viral diarrhea virus isolates from BVDV infected alpacas in North America. Veterinary Microbiology 2009;136(3):209–16.
4. Mingala CN, Konnai S, Tajima M, et al. Classification of new BVDV isolates from Philippine water buffalo using the viral E2 region. J Basic Microbiol 2009;49(5): 495–500.
5. Depner K, Hubschle OJ, Liess B. Prevalence of ruminant pestivirus infections in Namibia. Onderstepoort J Vet Res 1991;58(2):107–9.
6. Chase CC, Braun LJ, Leslie-Steen P, et al. Bovine viral diarrhea virus multiorgan infection in two white-tailed deer in southeastern South Dakota. J Wildl Dis 2008; 44(3):753–9.
7. Stahl K, Kampa J, Alenius S, et al. Natural infection of cattle with an atypical 'HoBi'-like pestivirus–implications for BVD control and for the safety of biological products. Vet Res 2007;38(3):517–23.
8. Kampa J, Alenius S, Emanuelson U, et al. Bovine herpesvirus type 1 (BHV-1) and bovine viral diarrhoea virus (BVDV) infections in dairy herds: self clearance and the detection of seroconversions against a new atypical pestivirus. Vet J 2009;182(2):223–30.
9. Liu L, Xia H, Wahlberg N, et al. Phylogeny, classification and evolutionary insights into pestiviruses. Virology 2009;385(2):351–7.
10. Olafson P, McCallum A, Fox F. An apparently new transmissible disease of cattle. Cornell Vet 1946;36:205–13.

11. Lee KM, Gillespie JH. Propagation of virus diarrhea virus of cattle in tissue culture. Am J Vet Res 1957;18:952–3.
12. Childs TX. Disease of cattle. Can J Vet Res 1946;10:316–9.
13. Ramsey F, Chivers W. Mucosal disease of cattle. North Am Vet 1953;34:629–33.
14. Liess B. Cytopathogenicity discovery and impact in BVD research. Paper presented at International Symposium Bovine Viral Diarrhea Virus A 50 Year Review 1996; Cornell University, Ithaca, NY.
15. Gillespie J, Coggins L, Thompson J, et al. Comparison by neutralization tests of strains of virus isolated from virus diarrhea and mucosal disease. Cornell Vet 1961;51:155–9.
16. Kniazeff A, Huck R, Jarrett W, et al. Antigenic relationship of some bovine viral diarrhoea-mucosal disease viruses from the United States, Great Britain and West Germany. Vet Rec 1961;73:768–9.
17. Darbyshire J. Agar gel diffusion studies with a mucosal disease of cattle. II. A serological relationship between a mucosal disease and swine fever. Res Vet Sci 1962;3:123–8.
18. Plant JW, Littlejohns IE, Gardiner AC, et al. Immunological relationship between border disease, mucosal disease and swine fever. Vet Rec 1973;92(17):455.
19. Horzinek MC. The structure of togaviruses. Prog Med Virol 1973;16:109–56.
20. Fenner F. Classification and nomenclature of viruses. Second report of the International Committee on Taxonomy of Viruses. Intervirology 1976;7(1–2):1–115.
21. Westaway EG, Brinton MA, Gaidamovich S, et al. Flaviviridae. Intervirology 1985;24(4):183–92.
22. Collett MS, Anderson DK, Retzel E. Comparisons of the pestivirus bovine viral diarrhoea virus with members of the flaviviridae. J Gen Virol 1988;69(Pt 10): 2637–43.
23. Francki R, Fauquet CM, Knudson D, et al. The fifth report of the International Committee on Taxonomy of Viruses. New York: Springer Verlag; 1991.
24. Pellerin C, van den Hurk J, Lecomte J, et al. Identification of a new group of bovine viral diarrhea virus strains associated with severe outbreaks and high mortalities. Virology 1994;203(2):260–8.
25. Ridpath JF, Bolin SR, Dubovi EJ. Segregation of bovine viral diarrhea virus into genotypes. Virology 1994;205(1):66–74.
26. Thiel HJ, Collett MS, Gould EA, et al. Family Flaviviridae. In: Fauquet CM, Mayo MA, Maniloff J, et al, editors. Eighth report of the International Committee on Taxonomy of Viruses. San Diego (CA): Elsevier Academic Press; 2005. 981-9980-9912-249951-249954.
27. Avalos-Ramirez R, Orlich M, Thiel HJ, et al. Evidence for the presence of two novel pestivirus species. Virology 2001;286(2):456–65.
28. Becher P, Orlich M, Kosmidou A, et al. Genetic diversity of pestiviruses: identification of novel groups and implications for classification. Virology 1999;262(1):64–71.
29. Vilcek S, Ridpath JF, Van Campen H, et al. Characterization of a novel pestivirus originating from a pronghorn antelope. Virus Res 2005;108(1–2):187–93.
30. Kirkland PD, Frost MJ, Finlaison DS, et al. Identification of a novel virus in pigs—Bungowannah virus: a possible new species of pestivirus. Virus Res 2007; 129(1):26–34.
31. Schirrmeier H, Strebelow G, Depner K, et al. Genetic and antigenic characterization of an atypical pestivirus isolate, a putative member of a novel pestivirus species. J Gen Virol 2004;85(Pt 12):3647–52.
32. Stalder HP, Meier P, Pfaffen G, et al. Genetic heterogeneity of pestiviruses of ruminants in Switzerland. Prev Vet Med 2005;72(1–2):37–41 [discussion: 215–9].

33. Ridpath JF. Bovine viral diarrhea virus. In: Mahy BWJ, Regenmortel MHV, editors. Encyclopedia of virology, vol. 1. Oxford (UK): Elsevier; 2008. p. 374–80.
34. Brock KV, Deng R, Riblet SM. Nucleotide sequencing of 5′ and 3′ termini of bovine viral diarrhea virus by RNA ligation and PCR. J Virol Methods 1992; 38(1):39–46.
35. Purchio AF, Larson R, Torborg LL, et al. Cell-free translation of bovine viral diarrhea virus RNA. J Virol 1984;52(3):973–5.
36. Purchio AF, Larson R, Collett MS. Characterization of virus-specific RNA synthesized in bovine cells infected with bovine viral diarrhea virus. J Virol 1983;48(1): 320–4.
37. Neill JD. Interactions of virus and host. In: Goyal SM, Ridpath JF, editors. Bovine viral diarrhea virus diagnosis, management and control. Ames (IA): Blackwell Publishing; 2005. p. 177–95.
38. Hilton L, Moganeradj K, Zhang G, et al. The NPro product of bovine viral diarrhea virus inhibits DNA binding by interferon regulatory factor 3 and targets it for proteasomal degradation. J Virol 2006;80(23):11723–32.
39. Seago J, Hilton L, Reid E, et al. The Npro product of classical swine fever virus and bovine viral diarrhea virus uses a conserved mechanism to target interferon regulatory factor-3. J Gen Virol 2007;88(Pt 11):3002–6.
40. Iqbal M, Poole E, Goodbourn S, et al. Role for bovine viral diarrhea virus Erns glycoprotein in the control of activation of beta interferon by double-stranded RNA. J Virol 2004;78(1):136–45.
41. Ridpath JF, Neill JD, Frey M, et al. Phylogenetic, antigenic and clinical characterization of type 2 BVDV from North America. Vet Microbiol 2000;77(1–2):145–55.
42. Deregt D. Introduction and history. In: Goyal SM, Ridpath JF, editors. Bovine viral diarrhea virus: diagnosis, management and control. Ames (IA): Blackwell Publishing; 2005. p. 3–34.
43. Fulton RW, Ridpath JF, Confer AW, et al. Bovine viral diarrhoea virus antigenic diversity: impact on disease and vaccination programmes. Biologicals 2003; 31(2):89–95.
44. Ridpath JF. Practical significance of heterogeneity among BVDV strains: impact of biotype and genotype on U.S. control programs. Prev Vet Med 2005;72(1–2): 17–30 [discussion: 215–9].
45. Bolin SR, Ridpath JF. Prevalence of bovine viral diarrhea virus genotypes and antibody against those viral genotypes in fetal bovine serum. J Vet Diagn Invest 1998;10(2):135–9.
46. Ridpath JF, Bolin SR. The genomic sequence of a virulent bovine viral diarrhea virus (BVDV) from the type 2 genotype: detection of a large genomic insertion in a noncytopathic BVDV. Virology 1995;212(1):39–46.
47. Vilcek S, Paton DJ, Durkovic B, et al. Bovine viral diarrhoea virus genotype 1 can be separated into at least eleven genetic groups. Arch Virol 2001;146(1): 99–115.
48. Flores EF, Ridpath JF, Weiblen R, et al. Phylogenetic analysis of Brazilian bovine viral diarrhea virus type 2 (BVDV-2) isolates: evidence for a subgenotype within BVDV-2. Virus Res 2002;87(1):51–60.
49. Bachofen C, Stalder H, Braun U, et al. Co-existence of genetically and antigenically diverse bovine viral diarrhoea viruses in an endemic situation. Vet Microbiol 2008;131(1–2):93–102.
50. Kabongo N, Van Vuuren M. Detection of bovine viral diarrhoea virus in specimens from cattle in South Africa and possible association with clinical disease. J S Afr Vet Assoc 2004;75(2):90–3.

51. Kabongo N, Baule C, Van Vuuren M. Molecular analysis of bovine viral diarrhoea virus isolates from South Africa. Onderstepoort J Vet Res 2003;70(4): 273–9.
52. Hornberg A, Fernandez SR, Vogl C, et al. Genetic diversity of pestivirus isolates in cattle from Western Austria. Vet Microbiol 2009;135(3–4):205–13.
53. Tajima M, Frey HR, Yamato O, et al. Prevalence of genotypes 1 and 2 of bovine viral diarrhea virus in Lower Saxony, Germany. Virus Res 2001;76(1):31–42.
54. Giammarioli M, Pellegrini C, Casciari C, et al. Genetic diversity of bovine viral diarrhea virus 1: Italian isolates clustered in at least seven subgenotypes. J Vet Diagn Invest 2008;20(6):783–8.
55. Jackova A, Novackova M, Pelletier C, et al. The extended genetic diversity of BVDV-1: typing of BVDV isolates from France. Vet Res Commun 2008;32(1): 7–11.
56. Arias P, Orlich M, Prieto M, et al. Genetic heterogeneity of bovine viral diarrhoea viruses from Spain. Vet Microbiol 2003;96(4):327–36.
57. Toplak I, Sandvik T, Barlic-Maganja D, et al. Genetic typing of bovine viral diarrhoea virus: most Slovenian isolates are of genotypes 1d and 1f. Vet Microbiol 2004;99(3–4):175–85.
58. Vilcek S, Durkovic B, Kolesarova M, et al. Genetic diversity of international bovine viral diarrhoea virus (BVDV) isolates: identification of a new BVDV-1 genetic group. Vet Res 2004;35(5):609–15.
59. Vilcek S, Drew TW, McGoldrick A, et al. Genetic typing of bovine pestiviruses from England and Wales. Vet Microbiol 1999;69(4):227–37.
60. Jones LR, Zandomeni R, Weber EL. Genetic typing of bovine viral diarrhea virus isolates from Argentina. Vet Microbiol 2001;81(4):367–75.
61. Pizarro-Lucero J, Celedon MO, Aguilera M, et al. Molecular characterization of pestiviruses isolated from bovines in Chile. Vet Microbiol 2006;115(1–3):208–17.
62. Evermann JF, Ridpath JF. Clinical and epidemiologic observations of bovine viral diarrhea virus in the northwestern United States. Vet Microbiol 2002; 89(2–3):129–39.
63. Fulton RW, Ridpath JF, Ore S, et al. Bovine viral diarrhoea virus (BVDV) subgenotypes in diagnostic laboratory accessions: distribution of BVDV1a, 1b, and 2a subgenotypes. Vet Microbiol 2005;111(1–2):35–40.
64. Mishra N, Pattnaik B, Vilcek S, et al. Genetic typing of bovine viral diarrhoea virus isolates from India. Vet Microbiol 2004;104(3–4):207–12.
65. Mishra N, Dubey R, Rajukumar K, et al. Genetic and antigenic characterization of bovine viral diarrhea virus type 2 isolated from Indian goats (*Capra hircus*). Vet Microbiol 2007;124(3–4):340–7.
66. Drew TW, Sandvik T, Wakeley P, et al. BVD virus genotype 2 detected in British cattle. Vet Rec 2002;151(18):551.
67. Matsuno K, Sakoda Y, Kameyama K, et al. Genetic and pathobiological characterization of bovine viral diarrhea viruses recently isolated from cattle in Japan. J Vet Med Sci 2007;69(5):515–20.
68. Mahony TJ, McCarthy FM, Gravel JL, et al. Genetic analysis of bovine viral diarrhoea viruses from Australia. Vet Microbiol 2005;106(1–2):1–6.
69. Stahl K, Benito A, Felmer R, et al. Genetic diversity of bovine viral diarrhoea virus (BVDV) from Peru and Chile. Pesqui Vet Bras 2009;29:41–4.
70. Fulton RW, Step DL, Ridpath JF, et al. Response of calves persistently infected with noncytopathic bovine viral diarrhea virus (BVDV) subtype 1b after vaccination with heterologous BVDV strains in modified live virus vaccines and Mannheimia haemolytica bacterin-toxoid. Vaccine 2003;21(21–22):2980–5.

71. Gillespie J, Baker J, McEntee K. A cytopathogenic strains of virus diarrhea virus. Cornell Vet 1960;50:73–9.
72. Becker Y. Evolution of viruses by acquisition of cellular RNA or DNA nucleotide sequences and genes: an introduction. Virus Genes 2000;21(1–2):7–12.
73. Ridpath JF, Neill JD, Vilcek S, et al. Multiple outbreaks of severe acute BVDV in North America occurring between 1993 and 1995 linked to the same BVDV2 strain. Vet Microbiol 2006;114(3–4):196–204.
74. Quadros VL, Mayer SV, Vogel FS, et al. A search for RNA insertions and NS3 gene duplication in the genome of cytopathic isolates of bovine viral diarrhea virus. Braz J Med Biol Res 2006;39(7):935–44.
75. Carman S, van Dreumel T, Ridpath J, et al. Severe acute bovine viral diarrhea in Ontario, 1993–1995. J Vet Diagn Invest 1998;10(1):27–35.
76. Corapi WV, French TW, Dubovi EJ. Severe thrombocytopenia in young calves experimentally infected with noncytopathic bovine viral diarrhea virus. J Virol 1989;63(9):3934–43.
77. Corapi WV, Elliott RD, French TW, et al. Thrombocytopenia and hemorrhages in veal calves infected with bovine viral diarrhea virus. J Am Vet Med Assoc 1990; 196(4):590–6.
78. Liebler-Tenorio EM, Ridpath JE, Neill JD. Distribution of viral antigen and development of lesions after experimental infection with highly virulent bovine viral diarrhea virus type 2 in calves. Am J Vet Res 2002;63(11):1575–84.
79. Liebler-Tenorio EM, Ridpath JF, Neill JD. Lesions and tissue distribution of viral antigen in severe acute versus subclinical acute infection with BVDV2. Biologicals 2003;31(2):119–22.
80. Liebler-Tenorio EM, Ridpath JF, Neill JD. Distribution of viral antigen and development of lesions after experimental infection of calves with a BVDV 2 strain of low virulence. J Vet Diagn Invest 2003;15(3):221–32.
81. Odeon AC, Kelling CL, Marshall DJ, et al. Experimental infection of calves with bovine viral diarrhea virus genotype II (NY-93). J Vet Diagn Invest 1999;11(3): 221–8.
82. Kelling CL, Steffen DJ, Topliff CL, et al. Comparative virulence of isolates of bovine viral diarrhea virus type II in experimentally inoculated six- to nine-month-old calves. Am J Vet Res 2002;63(10):1379–84.
83. Cortese VS, West KH, Hassard LE, et al. Clinical and immunologic responses of vaccinated and unvaccinated calves to infection with a virulent type-II isolate of bovine viral diarrhea virus. J Am Vet Med Assoc 1998;213(9):1312–9.
84. Fairbanks K, Schnackel J, Chase CC. Evaluation of a modified live virus type-1a bovine viral diarrhea virus vaccine (Singer strain) against a type-2 (strain 890) challenge. Vet Ther 2003;4(1):24–34.
85. Ridpath JF, Neill JD, Peterhans E. Impact of variation in acute virulence of BVDV1 strains on design of better vaccine efficacy challenge models. Vaccine 2007;25(47):8058–66.
86. Moerman A, Straver PJ, de Jong MC, et al. Clinical consequences of a bovine virus diarrhoea virus infection in a dairy herd: a longitudinal study. Vet Q 1994; 16(2):115–9.
87. Evermann JF, Barrington GM. Clinical features. In: Goyal SM, Ridpath JF, editors. Bovine viral diarrhea virus: diagnosis, management and control. Ames (IA): Blackwell Publishing; 2005. p. 105–20.
88. Brock KV, Grooms DL, Givens MD. Reproductive disease and persistent infections. In: Goyal SM, Ridpath JF, editors. Bovine viral diarrhea virus: diagnossis, management and control. Ames (IA): Blackwell Publishing; 2005. p. 145–56.

89. Ward GM, Roberts SJ, McEntee K, et al. A study of experimentally induced bovine viral diarrhea-mucosal disease in pregnant cows and their progeny. Cornell Vet 1969;59(4):525–38.
90. Liebler-Tenorio E. Pathogenesis. In: Goyal SM, Ridpath JF, editors. Bovine viral diarrhea virus: diagnosis, Management and Control. Ames (IA): Blackwell Publishing; 2005. p. 121–44.
91. Brackenbury LS, Carr BV, Charleston B. Aspects of the innate and adaptive immune responses to acute infections with BVDV. Vet Microbiol 2003;96(4):337–44.
92. Peterhans E, Jungi TW, Schweizer M. BVDV and innate immunity. Biologicals 2003;31(2):107–12.
93. Al-Haddawi M, Mitchell GB, Clark ME, et al. Impairment of innate immune responses of airway epithelium by infection with bovine viral diarrhea virus. Vet Immunol Immunopathol 2007;116(3–4):153–62.
94. Bolin SR. Bovine viral diarrhea viruses in mixed infections. In: Brogden KM, Guthmiller JM, editors. Polymicrobial diseases. Washington, DC: ASM Press; 2002. p. 33–50.
95. Lamm CG, Broaddus CC, Holyoak GR. Distribution of bovine viral diarrhea virus antigen in aborted fetal and neonatal goats by immunohistochemistry. Vet Pathol 2009;46(1):54–8.
96. Becher P, Konig M, Paton DJ, et al. Further characterization of border disease virus isolates: evidence for the presence of more than three species within the genus pestivirus. Virology 1995;209(1):200–6.
97. Carlsson U. Border disease in sheep caused by transmission of virus from cattle persistently infected with bovine virus diarrhoea virus. Vet Rec 1991;128(7):145–7.
98. Kulcsar G, Soos P, Kucsera L, et al. Pathogenicity of a bovine viral diarrhoea virus strain in pregnant sows: short communication. Acta Vet Hung 2001; 49(1):117–20.
99. Liess B, Moennig V. Ruminant pestivirus infection in pigs. Rev Sci Tech 1990; 9(1):151–61.
100. Terpstra C, Wensvoort G. A congenital persistent infection of bovine virus diarrhoea virus in pigs: clinical, virological and immunological observations. Vet Q 1997;19(3):97–101.
101. Walz PH, Baker JC, Mullaney TP, et al. Experimental inoculation of pregnant swine with type 1 bovine viral diarrhoea virus. J Vet Med B Infect Dis Vet Public Health 2004;51(4):191–3.
102. Wensvoort G, Terpstra C. Bovine viral diarrhoea virus infections in piglets born to sows vaccinated against swine fever with contaminated vaccine. Res Vet Sci 1988;45(2):143–8.
103. Wentz PA, Belknap EB, Brock KV, et al. Evaluation of bovine viral diarrhea virus in New World camelids. J Am Vet Med Assoc 2003;223(2):223–8.
104. Goyal SM, Bouljihad M, Haugerud S, et al. Isolation of bovine viral diarrhea virus from an alpaca. J Vet Diagn Invest 2002;14(6):523–5.
105. Carman S, Carr N, DeLay J, et al. Bovine viral diarrhea virus in alpaca: abortion and persistent infection. J Vet Diagn Invest 2005;17(6):589–93.
106. Evermann JF. Pestiviral infection of llamans and alpacas. Small Rumin Res 2006; 61:201–6.
107. Foster AP, Houlihan MG, Holmes JP, et al. Bovine viral diarrhoea virus infection of alpacas (*Vicugna pacos*) in the UK. Vet Rec 2007;161(3):94–9.
108. Topliff CL, Smith DR, Clowser SL, et al. Prevalence of bovine viral diarrhea virus infections in alpacas in the United States. J Am Vet Med Assoc 2009;234(4): 519–29.

109. Hamblin C, Hedger RS. The prevalence of antibodies to bovine viral diarrhoea/mucosal disease virus in African wildlife. Comp Immunol Microbiol Infect Dis 1979;2(2–3):295–303.

110. Hamblin C, Anderson EC, Jago M, et al. Antibodies to some pathogenic agents in free-living wild species in Tanzania. Epidemiol Infect 1990;105(3):585–94.

111. Zarnke RL. Serologic survey for selected microbial pathogens in Alaskan wildlife. J Wildl Dis 1983;19(4):324–9.

112. Taylor SK, Lane VM, Hunter DL, et al. Serologic survey for infectious pathogens in free-ranging American bison. J Wildl Dis 1997;33(2):308–11.

113. Frolich K, Flach EJ. Long-term viral serology of semi-free-living and captive ungulates. J Zoo Wildl Med 1998;29(2):165–70.

114. Couvillion CE, Jenney EW, Pearson JE, et al. Survey for antibodies to viruses of bovine virus diarrhea, bluetongue, and epizootic hemorrhagic disease in hunter-killed mule deer in New Mexico. J Am Vet Med Assoc 1980;177(9):790–1.

115. Van Campen H, Ridpath J, Williams E, et al. Isolation of bovine viral diarrhea virus from a free-ranging mule deer in Wyoming. J Wildl Dis 2001;37(2):306–11.

116. Cantu A, Ortega SJ, Mosqueda J, et al. Prevalence of infectious agents in free-ranging white-tailed deer in northeastern Mexico. J Wildl Dis 2008;44(4):1002–7.

117. Wolf KN, DePerno CS, Jenks JA, et al. Selenium status and antibodies to selected pathogens in white-tailed deer (Odocoileus virginianus) in Southern Minnesota. J Wildl Dis 2008;44(1):181–7.

118. Passler T, Walz PH, Ditchkoff SS, et al. Evaluation of hunter-harvested white-tailed deer for evidence of bovine viral diarrhea virus infection in Alabama. J Vet Diagn Invest 2008;20(1):79–82.

119. Duncan C, Ridpath J, Palmer MV, et al. Histopathologic and immunohistochemical findings in two white-tailed deer fawns persistently infected with Bovine viral diarrhea virus. J Vet Diagn Invest 2008;20(3):289–96.

120. Passler T, Walz PH, Ditchkoff SS, et al. Experimental persistent infection with bovine viral diarrhea virus in white-tailed deer. Vet Microbiol 2007;122(3–4):350–6.

121. Ridpath JF, Mark CS, Chase CC, et al. Febrile response and decrease in circulating lymphocytes following acute infection of white-tailed deer fawns with either a BVDV1 or a BVDV2 strain. J Wildl Dis 2007;43(4):653–9.

122. Ridpath JF, Driskell EA, Chase CC, et al. Reproductive tract disease associated with inoculation of pregnant white-tailed deer with bovine viral diarrhea virus. Am J Vet Res 2008;69(12):1630–6.

123. Passler T, Walz PH, Ditchkoff SS, et al. Cohabitation of pregnant white-tailed deer and cattle persistently infected with Bovine viral diarrhea virus results in persistently infected fawns. Vet Microbiol 2009;134(3–4):362–7.

124. Gripshover EM, Givens MD, Ridpath JF, et al. Variation in E(rns) viral glycoprotein associated with failure of immunohistochemistry and commercial antigen capture ELISA to detect a field strain of bovine viral diarrhea virus. Vet Microbiol 2007;125(1–2):11–21.

125. van Rijn PA, van Gennip HG, Leendertse CH, et al. Subdivision of the pestivirus genus based on envelope glycoprotein E2. Virology 1997;237(2):337–48.

126. Plowright W. Other virus diseases in relation to the JP15 programme. Paper presented at Joint Campaign Against Rinderpest, Proceedings of the First Technical Review Meeting, Phase IV1969; Mogadiscio, Kenya.

127. Finlaison DS, King KR, Frost MJ, et al. Field and laboratory evidence that Bungowannah virus, a recently recognised pestivirus, is the causative agent of the porcine myocarditis syndrome (PMC). Vet Microbiol 2009;136(3–4):259–65.

128. Liu L, Kampa J, Belák S, et al. Virus recovery and full-length sequence analysis of atypical bovine pestivirus Th/04_KhonKaen. Vet Microbiol 2009;138(1–2):62–8.
129. Title 9 Code of Federal Regulations (9CFR) Killed BVD vaccine. In: Biologics/APHIS/USDA CfV, ed1974, ammended 1991.
130. Title 9 Code of Federal Regulations (9CFR) Modified live BVD vaccine. In: Biologics/APHIS/USDA CfV, ed1990.
131. CVB Notice 02CVB Notice 02–1919 Vaccine claims for protection of the fetus against BVDV. In: Biologics/APHIS/USDA CfV, ed2002.
132. Hamers C, Couvreur B, Dehan P, et al. Assessment of the clinical and virological protection provided by a commercial inactivated bovine viral diarrhoea virus genotype 1 vaccine against a BVDV genotype 2 challenge. Vet Rec 2003; 153(8):236–40.
133. Bolin SR, Ridpath JF. Assessment of protection from systemic infection or disease afforded by low to intermediate titers of passively acquired neutralizing antibody against bovine viral diarrhea virus in calves. Am J Vet Res 1995;56(6):755–9.
134. Endsley JJ, Roth JA, Ridpath J, et al. Maternal antibody blocks humoral but not T cell responses to BVDV. Biologicals 2003;31(2):123–5.
135. Ridpath JE, Neill JD, Endsley J, et al. Effect of passive immunity on the development of a protective immune response against bovine viral diarrhea virus in calves. Am J Vet Res 2003;64(1):65–9.
136. Bolin SR. Immunogens of bovine viral diarrhea virus. Vet Microbiol 1993;37(3–4): 263–71.
137. Rodning SP, Givens MD, Zhang Y, et al. Evaluating the efficacy of vaccination for bovine viral diarrhea virus. Paper presented at 7th ESVV Pestivirus Symposium. Uppsala, Sweden, September 16–19, 2008.
138. Stahl K, Kampa J, Baule C, et al. Molecular epidemiology of bovine viral diarrhoea during the final phase of the Swedish BVD-eradication programme. Prev Vet Med 2005;72(1–2):103–8 [discussion: 215–9].
139. Valle PS, Skjerve E, Martin SW, et al. Ten years of bovine virus diarrhoea virus (BVDV) control in Norway: a cost-benefit analysis. Prev Vet Med 2005;72(1–2): 189–207 [discussion: 215–9].
140. Uttenthal A, Stadejek T, Nylin B. Genetic diversity of bovine viral diarrhoea viruses (BVDV) in Denmark during a 10-year eradication period. APMIS 2005; 113(7–8):536–41.
141. Lindberg AL, Alenius S. Principles for eradication of bovine viral diarrhoea virus (BVDV) infections in cattle populations. Vet Microbiol 1999;64(2–3):197–222.
142. Greiser-Wilke I, Grummer B, Moennig V. Bovine viral diarrhoea eradication and control programmes in Europe. Biologicals 2003;31(2):113–8.
143. Lindberg AL. Bovine viral diarrhoea virus infections and its control. A review. Vet Q 2003;25(1):1–16.
144. Sandvik T. Progress of control and prevention programs for bovine viral diarrhea virus in Europe. Vet clin North Am 2004;20(1):151–69.
145. Houe H, Lindberg A, Moennig V. Test strategies in bovine viral diarrhea virus control and eradication campaigns in Europe. J Vet Diagn Invest 2006;18(5): 427–36.

Bovine Coronavirus Associated Syndromes

Mélanie J. Boileau, DVM, MS[a],*, Sanjay Kapil, DVM, MS, PhD[b,c]

KEYWORDS

- Bovine respiratory coronavirus
- Bovine enteropathogenic coronavirus
- Calf diarrhea • Winter dysentery

IMPACT OF BOVINE RESPIRATORY DISEASE COMPLEX

Bovine respiratory disease complex (BRDC) represents a major cause of economic loss in the beef and dairy cattle industries worldwide. In North America especially, this complex represents the leading cause of morbidity and mortality in 6- to 10-month-old beef cattle after entry into feedlots (United States Department of Agriculture, 2000).[1] The financial losses are in part due to mortality, which can reach up to 69% in beef calves during first 2 months of arrival.[2] Reduced growth performance and overall treatment costs (eg, metaphylactic and therapeutic use of antibiotics) for BRDC in a 1000-cattle feedlot has been estimated to be $13.90 per animal, assuming calves are slaughtered after 200 days on feed; labor and handling costs excluded.[3]

The BRDC is a multifactorial disease arising from a combination of environmental, host, management, viral, and bacterial factors. The disease often develops along with stressful conditions such as weaning, shipping, commingling, dietary changes, and adjustments to the feed yard environment. These conditions favor viral infections of the lower respiratory tract that may become further complicated by *Mannheimia haemolytica* serotype 1[4] and *Pasteurella multocida*, both commensal bacteria of the nasal cavity. Viral infections well known to play an important role in the development of BRDC include bovine herpesvirus 1 (BHV-1), bovine respiratory syncytial virus (BRSV), bovine viral diarrhea virus (BVDV), and parainfluenza virus type 3 (PI-3). Most cattle arriving at feedlot are routinely vaccinated against these viruses, which

[a] Food Animal Medicine and Surgery, Department of Veterinary Clinical Sciences, Oklahoma State University Center for Veterinary Health Sciences, 1 BVMTH, Farm Road, Stillwater, OK 74078, USA
[b] Oklahoma Animal Disease Diagnostic Laboratory, Center for Veterinary Health Sciences, Farm & Ridge Road, Stillwater, OK 74078-2046, USA
[c] Department of Veterinary Pathology, Oklahoma State University, 250 McElroy Hall, Stillwater, OK, USA
* Corresponding author.
E-mail address: melanie.boileau@okstate.edu (M.J. Boileau).

Vet Clin Food Anim 26 (2010) 123–146
doi:10.1016/j.cvfa.2009.10.003
0749-0720/10/$ – see front matter © 2010 Elsevier Inc. All rights reserved.

has led to a decrease in incidence of these primary pathogens. However, other viral agents continue to cause substantial losses due to BRDC (Sanjay Kapil, unpublished data, 2008). There is currently a growing body of evidence[1,4-9] showing that bovine coronavirus (BCoV) may be involved in the development of BRDC.

BOVINE CORONAVIRUS

Animal coronaviruses are divided into 3 antigenic groups: Group 1 has no hemagglutinin-esterase (HE), and important members of this group are feline infectious peritonitis and transmissible gastroenteritis virus in swine; Group 2 has HE and contains BCoV[10]; and Group 3 contains avian virus–like infectious bronchitis virus. There are only a few studies on molecular epidemiology of BCoV.[11-13] These studies have targeted the spike gene of BCoV for phylogenetic analysis because it is the most critical surface protein that binds to the receptor N-acetyl-9-O-acetylneuraminic acid of the virus.[14] The Japanese BCoV isolates (1999–2008) cluster in 4 phylogenic groups. Japanese isolates collected after 2005 were included in antigenic Group 4.[11] In another study from South America, the Brazilian BCoV isolates were genetically divided into 2 groups.[12] At present, there are no large-scale studies that have compared the BCoV isolates from America and other parts of the world.

Epidemiology of Bovine Coronaviruses

Bovine coronavirus is widespread in the cattle population, resulting in economic losses to the beef and dairy industry throughout the world. The virus has been detected on all continents and there is serologic incidence (>90%) that suggests most cattle become exposed to BCoV in their lifetime. In a recent study, the presence of BCoV in lungs was second in incidence after bovine herpesvirus.[15] Both in beef and dairy herds, BCoV can be associated with calf diarrhea, calf respiratory disease, winter dysentery, respiratory disease in adult cattle, and combined pneumonia and diarrhea in calves and adults.[16,17] The coronavirus strains isolated from nasal secretions and lung tissues of cattle with fatal cases of pneumonia have been classified as bovine respiratory coronaviruses (BRCoV). The coronavirus strains isolated from neonatal calves and adult cattle with diarrhea are referred to as bovine enteric or enteropathogenic coronaviruses (BECoV).[18] Furthermore, for clinical purposes, BECoV can be further subdivided into BCoV- induced calf diarrhea (BCoV-CD) and winter dysentery (BCoV-WD). The clinical manifestation of the disease syndromes are not solely related to the virus itself but also to host and environmental factors; for example, the immunologic status of the animal, environmental temperature, and secondary coinfections with other pathogens.[19]

Researchers have debated over last several years whether BCoV isolated from the gastrointestinal and respiratory tracts of affected cattle are the same virus or are dissimilar, perhaps altered in biologic, antigenic, and genetic (sequence) properties. Several publications have supported the hypothesis that enteric and respiratory BCoV may be the same virus detected at different stages of its infectious life cycle.[20-29] Early reports[28,29] suggested antigenic and genomic similarity between isolates of BCoV from the respiratory and enteric tracts of cattle. Later studies[5,25,30,31] identified differences in antigenic, genomic, and culture characteristics between the 2 groups of BCoV isolates. At present, it is still unclear whether isolates of BRCoV and BECoV can be distinguished antigenically.[30,32] Specific factors associated with their respective tropism for the respiratory or digestive tracts are also undefined. The reasons for scientific uncertainties[33] include that BCoV RNA genome is the longest (approximately 32,000 bases) compared with other animal viruses and is capable of further evolution. In addition, the number of complete sequences published on this virus is scarce, for example, 4 isolates comprising Mebus (U00735), Québec (AF220295), and Louisiana (NC_003045) enteric and respiratory BCoV. Due to the insufficient number of BCoV isolates sequenced, an accurate comparison of BECoV and BRCoV origin is therefore difficult to establish. Moreover, there are temporal changes and geographic differences that further confound the conclusions.[34]

Coronaviruses within the antigenic group 2 are known to cross between species. Beyond cattle, other domestic animals (horses, water buffalo,[35] camel,[36] New World camelids[37]), and wildlife (deer, elk[38]) and zoo animals (giraffe[39]) also have BCoV-like viruses that can infect calves because these viruses are genetically related to BCoV. The infection of small ruminants with coronavirus is less common. There is seasonal variation in the incidence of BCoV diarrhea. Stressors, including inclement weather[40] and shipping, are important contributing factors that may exacerbate disease from BCoV and BRCoV infections.

TRANSMISSION AND PATHOGENESIS

Infection is primarily via feco-oral and to a lesser extent, respiratory (aerosol) routes.[20,23,41–43] Bovine enteropathogenic coronavirus is shed in mucosal secretions from the upper respiratory tract and excretions from the gastrointestinal tract.[43–45] Bovine coronavirus is ubiquitous in the cattle population and persists in adults as subclinical infections.[44,46] However, under stressful conditions adult cattle can shed BCoV in feces and nasal secretions.[46] Most often, transmission of BECoV is horizontal, and occurs from carrier dam to offspring postpartum[47] or from clinically or chronically infected calves housed in proximity to naïve ones. Evidence of vertical transmission has not been reported.[47] In close herds, respiratory tract infections constitute a source of BCoV transmission to cows or young calves.[26] Experimental inoculation of BCoV-CD and BCoV-WD strains of BCoV in adult dairy cows has been associated with development of clinical signs and viral shedding in the feces.[48]

Bovine coronavirus is a pneumoenteric virus that replicates in the enterocytes of the intestinal tract and the epithelium of the upper respiratory tract.[34,43] More specifically, the virus has been shown to replicate in the respiratory tract of calves, with viral antigen detected in the epithelium of the lung, trachea, and nasal turbinates.[7,23] Park and colleagues[34] have suggested that BCoV infections of the respiratory tract may occur via inhalation, via monocyte-associated viremia that may originate from the intestines after ingestion of BCoV, or via cell-free viremia. In one study, peak of BCoV shedding in nasal secretions occurred at 3 days before arrival and in feces, at 3 days following entry to feedlot, under field conditions.[20] Researchers have proposed that replication and shedding of BCoV in nasal secretions is first initiated through the respiratory tract (oropharynx) then spreads to the gastrointestinal tract through the swallowing of large quantities of virus with subsequent shedding in the feces.[20,49] Other reports have documented BCoV shedding in both nasal passages and feces within the same animal concurrently.[20–22] Respiratory disease can be consistently reproduced experimentally in young calves using a pneumoenteric BCoV, Minnesota-1988 (MN-1988).[50,51]

Coronavirus is an enveloped single-stranded RNA virus, and is not as stable in the environment as rotavirus.[47] However, in the presence of organic material, these viruses may remain infectious for up to 3 days. Of note, coronaviruses can bind extremely well to clay, clay minerals, and charcoal in vitro, with an adsorption of 99%.[52] These findings suggest that clay soils can concentrate BCoV on its surface, which can be clinically relevant, as the animals grazing on these types of soils could get exposed to infectious doses of BCoV.

Dogs may play a role in BCoV infection; canine respiratory coronavirus is genetically related to BCoV and has been found in kennel cough cases in Europe and the United States.[53] Dogs may represent a passenger of the BCoV on farms.[54]

ROLE OF BOVINE CORONAVIRUS IN BOVINE RESPIRATORY DISEASE COMPLEX

Within the last 2 decades, BRCoV has been associated, either alone or along with other respiratory pathogens, with the emergence of shipping fever pneumonia of beef cattle after transport to feedlot[5] and enzootic calf pneumonia.[55–57]

However, there is still conflicting information in the literature regarding the true role of BCoV as a pathogen of the respiratory tract in calves[7,58] and feedlot cattle. Several investigators have shown that BCoV may represent one important pathogen involved in the development of BRDC,[1,4–6,8,9,59,60] whereas others could not detect any correlation between BCoV shedding and respiratory tract disease under field conditions.[21,32,61] At least 3 studies failed to reproduce clinical signs of BRDC in calves after experimental inoculation with BCoV,[22,23,62] which may be due to choice of the viral isolate used to experimentally reproduce the infection. In contrast, 2 research groups reported that BCoV can be isolated from clinically healthy cattle,[24,31] whereas others have failed to detect the presence of BCoV in feedlot calves experiencing respiratory tract disease.[6,8,59]

In 1995, it was reported that all 4 of Koch's postulates to associate BCoV with upper and lower respiratory tract disease in neonatal calves were fulfilled.[45] However, these postulates do have limitations when being applied to complex diseases such as BRDC in adult cattle.[9,63] Investigators recently supported BRCoV as the primary inciting cause of the 2 epizootics of shipping fever pneumonia they investigated,[4] based on Thomson's modification[64] of Evans' criteria of causation.[9,65]

There is evidence that BRCoV can be repeatedly isolated in the majority of calves sampled soon after feedlot entry.[32,59,60] Cattle shedding BCoV nasally and seroconverting within the first month after entering the feedlot are at increased risk for respiratory disease[60] and 1.6 times more likely to require subsequent treatment for BRDC.[8] Reported rates of nasal BCoV isolation in several studies have ranged from 8.1% to 60%.[8,20,21,31,60] In one report, cattle that shed BCoV in their nasal secretions during the first 28 days after feedlot arrival were 2.2 times more likely to have pulmonary lesions at slaughter compared with nonshedders.[8] Although there was no statistical association between clinical signs and virus shedding, another trial reported that feedlot cattle shedding BCoV nasally were 2.7 times more likely to show respiratory signs, and those shedding BCoV fecally were 2.5 times more likely to develop diarrhea.[32]

Most of the calves shedding BCoV nasally at arrival have low but detectable antibody titers at arrival and typically seroconvert within the first 3 to 4 weeks after feedlot entry, suggesting that they are often infected with BRCoV at times when respiratory tract disease is likely to occur.[32,59,61] Two published seroepidemiologic studies found that although higher antibody titers against BCoV at feedlot arrival were significantly associated with a decreased subsequent risk of treatment for BRDC within cattle groups, there was no association between evidence of recent infection (titer increase) and the incidence of BRDC.[1,61] In contrast, several investigators have shown that high antibody titers against BCoV at feedlot arrival have consistently been associated with a decrease in BCoV infection, shedding, or both, under field conditions[20,21,32] or in experimental challenge studies.[26,62] Decreased BCoV shedding in nasal secretions and protection against BCoV infection have been associated with high serum antibody titers (geometric mean: GMT) ranging from 1600 to 2,262[20,21,26,32] at feed yards entry. Moreover, cattle entering feedlots with high antibody titers against BCoV appeared less likely to seroconvert to BCoV than cattle without detectable BCoV titers at arrival.[1,59,62]

Depending on the feedlot, active immunity was reported to be associated with moderate to high seroconversion (4-fold increase in BRCoV antibody titers) in the face of clinical respiratory tract infection in 58% of 814 cattle,[59] 61% of 604 cattle,[1] 91% of 85 cattle,[32] and 90% in 852 cattle spread among 3 different feed yards, and in 95% of 57 cattle.[21]

Economic Impact of Bovine Respiratory Coronavirus

Several investigators have shown that BCoV-associated BRDC is correlated with decreased performance in feedlot cattle.[1,21,32] According to a published report,[1] shedding of BRCoV correlated with a reduction in weight gain. One study involving 837 calves in 4 feedlots from 2 states (Ohio, Texas) showed that the BCoV shedding or seroconversion status did not affect the average daily gain.[8] However, shedding of BCoV in feces of 6- to 7-month-old cross-bred feedlot steers was associated with a reduced weight gain of 8.17 kg (17.9 lb) during a period of 21 days.[21] In an Ohio feedlot,[32] calves that seroconverted to BCoV gained 5.9 kg (13 lb) (26%) less than the nonseroconverted group during the first 21 days after arrival to the feedlot. Seroconversion to BCoV was almost associated significantly ($P<.06$) with reduction in weight gain but not with clinical signs. In one report involving 203 feedlot calves from New Mexico and Arkansas, animals shedding BCoV in nasal secretions, feces, or both, gained on average 8 kg (17.64 lb) less than calves that were not shedding the virus over a 35-day period following entry.[20] Therefore, BCoV infections may contribute directly to economic losses in feedlot cattle by impacting weight gains or, similar to other respiratory viruses, by predisposing cattle to secondary bacterial infection.

Clinical Manifestation of Bovine Respiratory Coronavirus

Under experimental conditions, neonatal, colostrum-deprived calves inoculated with BCoV can develop respiratory distress, such as wheezing and open-mouth breathing.[51] Under natural conditions, calf pneumonia caused by BRCoV can be observed in calves aged 6 to 9 months. Affected animals may develop fever,[23] serous to mucopurulent nasal discharge,[66] coughing, tachypnea, and dyspnea.[5,7]

Respiratory illness caused by BRCoV in an Ohio feedlot was characterized by coughing and nasal discharge along with diarrhea, and was observed in 62% and 77% of cattle.[32] Diagnostic investigation of 214 BRDC outbreaks in Italy was associated with an 85% morbidity rate in those due to BRCoV infection.[67] The mortality rate due to BCoV infection can be high.[4,67]

In another study,[2] viral respiratory disease was seen in 19% of the animals and accounted for 20% of the mortality in feedlot cattle. Bovine respiratory coronavirus was detected in approximately 2% of the cases based on virus isolation in cell culture. If fluorescent antibody testing or reverse transcriptase-polymerase chain reaction (RT-PCR) were used for detection of BRCoV, the actual incidence may have been higher. The reason RT-PCR gives higher estimates of BCoV infection in lungs is because, at core body temperature, the replication of BCoV may be diminished. However, in the upper cooler parts of the respiratory tract, replication of the virus is abundant and can become the source of the virus for the lower respiratory tract.

OTHER CLINICAL SYNDROMES ASSOCIATED WITH BOVINE CORONAVIRUS
Bovine Enteropathogenic Coronavirus Associated with Diarrhea in Calves

Pathogenesis and pathology

Enteropathogenic bovine coronavirus is widely recognized as an important primary pathogen causing neonatal calf diarrhea (BCoV-CD).[68,69] The pathology of BCoV-CD is often more severe than that of rotavirus, resulting in a mucohemorrhagic enterocolitis.[70] Infection leads to destruction of the absorptive intestinal villous epithelial cells.[69,71,72] Virus replication is cytocidal and initially occurs throughout the length of the villi in all levels of the small intestine, eventually spreading throughout the large intestine up to the end of the large colon and rectum, causing a malabsorptive diarrhea. Large concentration of BCoV can be typically found in the spiral colon. Infected epithelial cells die, slough off, and are replaced by immature cells. Stunting and fusion of adjacent villi and atrophy of colonic ridges may be seen on microscopic examination of BCoV-infected small and large intestine, respectively.[69,71,73–75] In case of malabsorptive diarrhea caused by BCoV, the fluid load in the gut lumen can be further exacerbated by the compensatory hyperplasia and secretions from the crypt epithelial cells.[76] The absorptive and digestive capacity of the intestinal tract is therefore compromised by loss of surface area and presence of immature cells, which are unable to secrete the normal digestive enzymes.[76–78] Lesions and consequences are most severe in younger animals.[47]

Continual enteral feeding may result in more nutrients presented to the small intestine than the damaged villi can absorb.[79] Undigested nutrients are fermented in the large intestine, promoting bacterial overgrowth and production of organic acids, especially D-lactate.[80] The osmotic effects of the unabsorbed nutrients draw water into the gut lumen and contribute to the diarrhea.[76] Over time, if fluid losses exceed intake, extensive water (mainly from the extracellular space), sodium, chloride, potassium, and bicarbonate loss occurs.[81] Dehydration and metabolic acidosis subsequently develops. The acidosis has several causes including fecal bicarbonate loss, endogenous L-lactic acid production in response to dehydration and poor tissue perfusion, and local D-lactic acid production within the gastrointestinal tract.[80,81]

Epidemiology

Bovine coronavirus causes enteritis in both dairy and beef herds, with naturally occurring cases showing clinical signs of disease between 5 and 30 days of life.[82–85] According to the BCoV enzyme-linked immunosorbent assay (ELISA) database from Kansas State University, Manhattan, KS, 1 in 3 case of calf diarrhea in the age group of 1 to 9 weeks can be due to BCoV. Clinical disease may occur as young as 24 hours of age in colostrum-deprived calves, and as late as 5 months of age.[42,73,85,86] The incidence of BCoV-CD in naturally occurring outbreaks has been reported to vary from 15% to 70%.[73,87,88]

Once infected, a calf can excrete high levels of virus (eg, 1 billion virus particles per ml of feces) within 48 hours after experimental infection, and this may persist up to 14 days.[50] Clinically recovered calves may continue to shed low levels of virus for weeks.[50] Of note, BECoV may be detected in the feces of both diarrheic and healthy calves, with clinically diarrheic calves more commonly tested positive (incidence: 8%–69%) compared with healthy calves (incidence: 0%–24%).[73,76,82,85,88,89]

BECoV has been detected intermittently at very low levels in the feces of more than 70% of clinically normal cows, despite the presence of specific antibodies in serum and feces.[46,87] In one study involving 132 cows and heifers with no previous BCoV vaccination history, all were found to have substantial levels of antibodies.[90] In nonvaccinated cows, the rate of virus excretion has been reported to increase by 50% to 60% during the winter months, by 65% at parturition, and by 71% 2 weeks postpartum.[44] This virus is more stable in the colder climates, due to lower ambient temperature and reduced ultraviolet light levels,[47] and has been reported to cause winter dysentery in adult cattle[91] especially after snow storms or sudden changes in ambient temperatures. Calves born to BCoV carrier dams have a significantly higher risk of developing BCoV diarrhea[92] due to periparturient exposure from fecal contamination of the perineum, teats, and the calving area.

Economic impact
Diarrhea remains an important cause of illness and death in young beef calves. Economic losses associated with the disease include decreased performance, mortality, and the expenses of medication and labor to treat sick animals. Annually, beef cattle herds may experience death rates of 5% to 10% or greater, and sometimes up to 100% morbidity.

Clinical signs
The severity of the BECoV enteritis depends on the age of the calf at time of infection, its immunologic status, the size of the infective dose, and the virulence of the BECoV strain in question. As a general rule, the severity of the disease is increased and the incubation period is shortened in younger compared with older calves, especially those with failure of passive transfer. A yellow to blood-stained mucus-containing diarrhea initially develops, which then progresses to a profuse watery diarrhea.[23,51] When the fluid intake is insufficient to meet the losses, affected animals become clinically dehydrated, depressed, weak, and hypothermic, and their suckle reflex is loosened. The majority of calves recover, but a few may develop pyrexia, recumbency, and progression to cardiovascular collapse (from dehydration, acidosis, and associated hyperkalemia), coma, and death if the diarrhea is particularly severe and left untreated.[22,23,69,70,74,81] Some of the BECoV-infected calves may develop a pneumoenteritis syndrome in which both diarrhea and mild signs of respiratory tract disease are present.[17] Affected calves shed the virus not only in their feces but also in their nasal secretions.[16,51]

Differential diagnosis
Other enteropathogens, such as rotavirus, are frequently detected in feces from BECoV-infected calves.[83,88] Rotaviruses are the leading cause and coronaviruses are a major contributor of calf diarrhea; however, infections with BCoV are more severe because they affect both the small and large intestines. In most outbreaks of acute undifferentiated BCoV-CD, calves frequently shed 1, 2, or multiple agents simultaneously.[85,93] Mixed infections are typically associated with more severe disease.[85] Researchers have reported that calves shedding 2 or more pathogens were 6 times more likely to develop clinical diarrhea compared with the ones that shed only one or no pathogen.[84] Besides rotavirus and coronavirus, *Cryptosporidium parvum*, enterotoxigenic *Escherichia coli*, and *Salmonella* spp are recognized as the major infectious agents associated with diarrhea in calves.[82,84,89,94,95] Without specific testing, it is usually impossible to make a definitive etiologic diagnosis solely based on clinical signs.[70,95] Signs of colitis in calves including tenesmus and presence of frank blood and mucus in the feces may be present with *Salmonella* spp, coronavirus, BVDV, enteropathogenic *E. coli*, or coccidian infection.[70]

Bovine Enteropathogenic Coronavirus Associated with Winter Dysentery in Adult Cattle

Etiology, pathogenesis, and pathology
During the past 2 decades, evidence has accumulated implicating BCoV as a cause of winter dysentery (BCoV-WD).[63,96–106] Winter dysentery is a sporadic acute,

contagious hemorrhagic enterocolitis of cattle that occurs in epizootic fashion in a herd.[105] The pathophysiological characteristics of BCoV infection can be attributed to lesions of the colonic mucosa.[102] The intestinal lesions are comparable with those observed in calves with BECoV-induced diarrhea. Epithelial cells of colonic crypts are destroyed by viral action, leading to degeneration, necrosis of crypt epithelium, and petechial hemorrhage, without involvement of the Peyer patches. Fine streak of frank blood or large blood clots may be present in the lumen of the spiral colon, distal colon, and rectum.[91,104] Even though histologic changes have been observed predominantly in the colonic mucosa, blood from the distal duodenum was observed aborally in cattle that died of winter dysentery.[104] Loss of intestinal mucosal epithelium from colonic crypts leads to transudation of extracellular fluid and blood. The respiratory tract of BCoV-WD affected animals may show hyperemia of the tracheal mucosa and localized foci of pneumonia.[107]

Epidemiology

In the United States, BCoV-WD is more common in the northern states; however, it has been reported throughout the world including Australia, Sweden, the United Kingdom, Israel, France, Belgium, Italy, Japan, Cuba, and Canada.[40,63,97,103,104,108] The disease occurs usually during the colder months of the year[63] and often coincides with close confinement of cattle. Only seldom have reports described BCoV-WD occurring during the warmer season.[34,40,108] The disease is characterized by a high morbidity rate ranging from 50% to 100%.[63,91] In contrast, mortality rate is usually low, typically less than 2%, with only a few reports describing case fatality associated with this virus.[91,99,107] Winter dysentery outbreaks are predominantly seen in young postpartum adult dairy cows, which then experience a marked drop in milk production, resulting in 25% to 95% milk losses.[66,100,104,109–111] In the acute stage of the disease, this may last 3 to 6 days. When it persists for a few days to a week or more after the outbreak terminates, economic loss can be substantial.[112]

Though infrequent, BCoV-WD has been also observed in adult beef cattle[97] and in 6- to 9-month-old feedlot calves.[91] Although most reports indicate this to be a disease of adult cattle, in a herd outbreaks of mild diarrhea may be observed in heifers and calves as young as 4 months old.[40,113]

The incubation period for BCoV-WD ranges from 2 to 8 days. In small housed herds, the incidence of diarrhea during an outbreak begins with the explosive appearance of signs in 10% to 15% of animals on the first day.[113] By the second day, another 20% to 40% are affected; morbidity reaches 100% by the fourth day.[104] By the end of the week the first affected animals are completely recovered, and only a small number of new cases occur.[113] Within 2 to 3 weeks of the onset of diarrhea, all animals have recovered. In large herds the outbreak may be prolonged for 6 to 8 weeks.[63] This scenario is typical of a herd that had not experienced an epizootic of winter dysentery during the preceding few years.

Epidemiologic studies of BCoV-WD have suggested that various host and environmental factors may contribute to the appearance of the disease.[48,63,101,106,114] These factors include the age and reproductive status of the animal, with recently calved 2- to 6-year-olds being the most susceptible,[112] and previous history of a BCoV disease outbreak in herds comprising more than 60 cows.[114] Environmental risk factors for BCoV-WD include drop in atmospheric temperature, close confinement, poor ventilation, and using manure-handling equipment to handle feed. Although nonspecific, historical findings associated with BCoV-WD outbreak may include recent stressors (eg, inclement weather), incoming farm visitors who have had close contact with cattle, or introduction of a newly purchased animal.[112]

Clinical signs

Winter dysentery is an acute diarrheic disease of predominantly dairy and infrequently beef cattle characterized by an acute onset of dark brown, often hemorrhagic, watery, and commonly profuse diarrhea accompanied by some degree of anorexia and depression.[63,66,102,114] The diarrhea may contain a slight to copious amount of mucus. The amount of blood varies from case to case and ranges from just visible flecks or streaks to large clots, or it may be uniformly mixed into the feces.[113] Pyrexia is usually not present during the diarrheal phase of the disease, although it has been reported to precede it by 24 to 48 hours[107,112] or have no consistent relationship.[115] Mild to moderate signs of respiratory disease (eg, cough, nasal discharge)[40,91,107,116] have been inconsistently observed preceding or concurrent with the diarrhea.[26,113] As mentioned previously, milk production can be significantly reduced in affected lactating cows. A few cases may show mild colic signs while other animals appear weak.[113] If the diarrhea is severe or persists longer than 1 or 2 days, dehydration and secondary polydipsia may develop. Ruminal motility is commonly reduced and intestinal borborygmi may be increased.

The odor in a barn during an outbreak of BCoV-WD has been described as musty, fetid, and unpleasantly sweet.[66,109] The period of illness in an individual is brief, and within a herd the outbreak usually lasts less than 2 weeks.[113] According to most reports the shorter and less severe the diarrhea, the more rapid the recovery and return to normal condition ensues.[109]

Differential diagnosis

Winter dysentery is usually recognized by the clinical syndrome described here and by exclusion of other causes of acute and contagious diarrhea of adult cattle.[107] Diarrhea caused by BVDV, coccidiosis, and salmonellosis must be considered in the differential diagnosis of BCoV-WD. PCR, virus isolation or immunohistochemistry (ear notch), fecal floatation, and fecal bacterial culture should be performed to rule out BVDV, coccidiosis, and salmonellosis, respectively. Specific hematologic changes that would be consistent with a diagnosis of BCoV-WD have not been reported.[113] If significant dysentery persists for longer than a day, anemia may develop due to significant blood loss.

The disease syndrome is more often than not diagnosed on the basis of history of acute onset of diarrhea and dysentery affecting at least 15% of the adult cattle herd; rapid spread causing a drop in milk production of 10% or more; resulting in less than 2% fatalities.[101] The rapid occurrence of multiple cases within a herd combined with spontaneous recovery over a few days and absent oral mucous membranes erosions suggests BCoV-WD.

DIAGNOSIS OF BOVINE CORONAVIRUSES

Because of similarity of clinical signs induced by various infectious agents, physical examination of calves or adult cattle with respiratory tract disease or diarrhea is not sufficient for diagnosis of BRCoV infection. Bovine respiratory coronavirus can only be identified through laboratory confirmation of appropriate specimens submitted. Suggested antemortem samples for BRCoV infection in calves and adult cattle include nasal swabs submitted in phosphate-buffered saline (pH 7.2) or normal saline in red-top tubes. Oropharyngeal fluid collected with a probang cup can be used to diagnose BRCoV in adult cattle. Trachea (upper one-third), and lungs can be collected at necropsy. However, the distribution of BCoV in the lungs is focal and thus, it is critical that multiple pieces are submitted for virus detection. Viral antigen has been detected in the apical and middle lung lobes of calves infected experimentally with BCoV (MN-1998) whereby 5% to 10% of the macrophages were positive for BCoV (**Fig. 1**) (Tawfik Aboellail, and Sanjay Kapil, unpublished data, 2000). Other suitable respiratory tissues include nasal turbinates, but these may be difficult to sample. Nasal turbinates and nasal glands have been found to be strongly positive for BCoV antigen using immunohistochemistry and immunofluorescence (**Figs. 2** and **3**).[117] Spiral colon is the sample of choice for detection of BECoV at necropsy because the virus persists in that specific location for the longest time after oral infection.[50] A fresh fecal sample collected directly from the rectum can be also included, as cattle with respiratory disease commonly shed the virus in the feces concomitantly. Approximately 2 to 5 g of fresh feces can be sent to the laboratory in wide-mouth jars. It is important to submit all tissue and fecal samples over ice-packs using overnight delivery to increase the likelihood of BCoV detection.

Diagnostic tests of choice for BCoV are antigen-capture ELISA[118] using Z3A5 monoclonal as capture antibody. Another useful diagnostic reagent is 8F2 monoclonal antibody (MoAb), which binds to nucleocapsid protein of BCoV, the most predominant protein of the virus (www.ruraltechinc.com).[119] The 8F2 reacts with the viral antigen in formalin-fixed intestines (see **Fig. 3**) and lungs. The 8F2 MoAb reacts with a conserved epitope of the antigenic group 2 coronaviruses such as alpaca, equine, camel, and elk coronavirus. Other laboratory-based methods for detection of BCoV include hemag-glutination assay using mouse erythrocytes; this method, with modification (such as slide agglutination test), can be used in developing countries and for animal-side testing. RT-PCR assays can be used for sensitive detection of BCoV in clinical samples. The targets are the conserved nucleocapsid gene for detection of the virus and spike gene for epidemiologic investigation and strain differentiation. At present, there is no commercial test available for BCoV antigen detection in the United States. However, lateral flow immunoassays (LFT) are useful cow and calf-side tests, and are available in European Union for BCoV antigen detection in the feces.[120]

Based on experimental infection with a pneumoenteric isolate of BRCoV, neonatal colostrum-deprived calves develop interstitial pneumonia (**Fig. 4**) and emphysema, pulmonary congestion and hemorrhage (**Fig. 5**), and edema of the interlobular septa, with the ventrolateral areas of the lungs being mainly affected.[45] Most of these calves showed cryptitis in the spiral colon on histologic examination (**Fig. 6**).

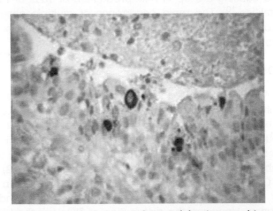

Fig. 1. BCoV antigen in macrophages was detected by immunohistochemistry (8F2) in formalin-fixed section of lungs from an adult cow showing clinical signs of lower respiratory tract infection.

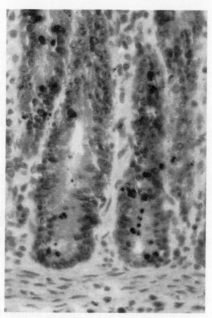

Fig. 2. Immunohistochemistry on formalin-fixed section of the intestine submitted from a calf stained with 8F2 anti nucleoprotein antigen of BCoV. Brown staining in the crypts indicates positivity for BCoV.

TREATMENT OF BOVINE CORONAVIRUS INFECTION
Bovine Respiratory Coronavirus

There are no specific antiviral treatments for BCoV infection in beef or dairy cattle. However, because viral infection can predispose to development of secondary bacterial infection in the lungs and the fact that BCoV cannot be differentiated clinically from other important viral or bacterial pathogens involved in BRDC, parenteral antibiotic therapy administered early in the disease process, at sufficient dosage and duration, is recommended to prevent or limit the development of bacterial pneumonia in cattle with viral respiratory tract infection.[55] The use of nonsteroidal anti-inflammatory drugs

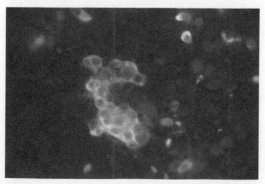

Fig. 3. Nasal cells positive for BCoV by direct fluorescent antibody test using anti-BCoV fluorescein isothiocyanate conjugate. Swab was collected from a calf experimentally infected with a pneumoenteric BCoV (MN-1988).

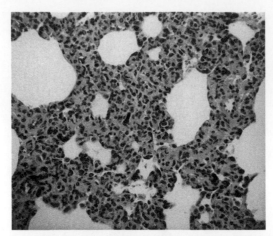

Fig. 4. Interstitial pneumonia in a calf experimentally infected with MN-1988 pneumoenteric BCoV isolate.

(NSAIDs) such as flunixin meglumine (Banamine), currently labeled specifically for the control of pyrexia associated with BRDC in the United States, has been shown to be useful in other viral pneumonias (eg, PI-3) by improving clinical signs and reducing lung consolidation.[121] However, flunixin meglumine may not be cost-effective when used in large feedlots and can potentially lead to renal toxicity or abomasal ulceration if overdosed, used for prolonged periods of time, or used in severely dehydrated animals. Approved in the European Union for use in food animals, a single injection of the long-acting NSAID meloxicam (Metacam) administered as an adjunct therapy for BRDC in feedlot cattle resulted in substantial pharmacoeconomic benefit.[122] Based on a limited number of publications[123,124] and due to its impairment of immune function, it is usually not recommended to use corticosteroids as an adjunct therapy for the treatment of undifferentiated pneumonia in feedlot cattle. Other ancillary therapies suggested for treatment of BRDC have included Vitamin C or B injection, bovine

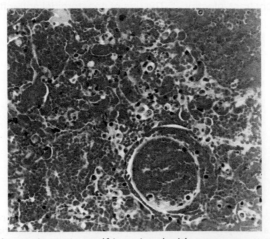

Fig. 5. Pulmonary hemorrhages in a calf inoculated with a pneumoenteric isolate of BCoV.

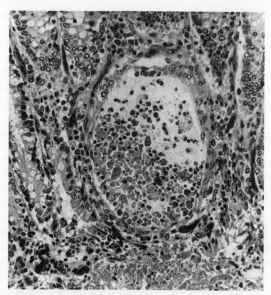

Fig. 6. Crypt dilation after experimental infection of a calf with MN-1988 BCoV isolate.

respiratory vaccine (IBR, BVDV, BRSV, PI-3) at the time of BRDC therapy, antihistamines, anthelmintics (eg, levamisole), probiotics, and oral electrolytes; however, no published data are available to support their use.[123,124]

Supportive therapy represents an important component of BRDC treatment, and is aimed at relieving stress and allowing time for the sick animal to foster its own resistance.[55] All sick cattle should be provided shelter to avoid adverse weather conditions and not be crowded while isolated in designated hospital pens. These cattle should be provided best-quality, highly palatable feed, and easy access to fresh drinking water and mineral mixes.

Bovine Enteropathogenic Coronavirus

Calf diarrhea

Treatment of calves suffering from BECoV enteritis is entirely supportive and should be instituted based on clinical signs and, if possible, laboratory data including blood gas analysis, to determine the extent of metabolic acidosis, blood glucose and electrolyte abnormalities, and testing for the presence of BECoV in feces. Treatment goals should follow the same general guidelines as those recommended for diarrhea caused by other enteropathogens. In brief, treatment should include correction of fluid loss and dehydration, electrolyte imbalance, acidosis, hypoglycemia, and hypothermia. This correction is achieved primarily through administration of oral electrolytes or intravenous polyionic isotonic crystalloid fluid therapy, and provision of a warm and dry environment. Selection of the type of fluids, the amount to provide, and rate and route of administration is based on the age and weight of the animal(s), severity and duration of clinical signs, level of metabolic acidosis, and whether the affected calf has a suckle reflex. The authors refer the reader to other in-depth reviews on the treatment and management of diarrhea caused by BCoV in calves.[70,93,125,126]

Winter dysentery

Most animals with BCoV-WD recover spontaneously in a few days without specific treatment, but in some cases supportive therapy may be indicated.[113] Many palliative treatments have been recommended and used over the years, including intestinal astringents, protectants, adsorbents, and antibiotics. Based on 30 years of observations, Roberts[112] considered none of these treatments altered the course of the disease. Abundant provision of fresh drinking water, palatable feed, and free-choice salt is the most useful nonspecific therapy. Oral or intravenous fluid therapy may be indicated, depending on the extent of dehydration. The occasional animal with prolonged or severe dysentery may necessitate a whole blood transfusion.

STRATEGY FOR CONTROL AND PREVENTION OF BOVINE CORONAVIRUS

There are no specific and effective methods to control or prevent disease caused by BCoV. Identification and isolation of carrier cows and calves should in theory decrease the pathogen load in the environment; however, in practice this approach may be unattainable as BCoV infections are typically widespread, even in close herds.[42,87,92] Therefore, management procedures must emphasize enhancing passive and active immunity to prevent clinical disease, minimizing stressors, and reducing the exposure of young susceptible calves. Protection relies on continual presence of a protective antibody within the gut lumen, which is passively acquired from the dam in the form of specific neutralizing antibodies (predominantly immunoglobulin type 1 [IgG1]) ingested in the colostrum or milk.[78,90] This IgG isotype has activity against the spike protein of BCoV.

Lactogenic immunity will vary depending on the levels of maternal BECoV antibodies present in the serum and colostrum.[43] Ingestion of colostrum from an immune cow prevents the shedding of BCoV in the feces, and reduces the risk of spread to other herd mates (including calves) and environmental contamination. However, when colostral antibody wanes, calves become susceptible to BCoV infections, especially the ones born to primiparous cows.[46]

In problem herds, the immune status of susceptible calves may be raised either via vaccination of pregnant cows to increase the level of passively acquired immunity, or via oral vaccination of newborn calves to stimulate active immunity.[78] Oral administration of spray-dried bovine serum supplemented calf milk replacer (from Land-O-Lakes, Kansas City, MO) has been associated with a decrease in the severity of the clinical signs in calves experimentally inoculated with BCoV (Sanjay Kapil, unpublished data, 1999).[127] This protection may vary and is dependent largely on the total amount of antibody titer against BCoV present.

Factors that can have an adverse effect on the calf's immune status include dystocia, exposure to environmental extremes such as hot, cold, wet, or windy conditions, overcrowding, excessive handling in the postnatal period, and direct exposure to pathogens.[82,128,129] As a result, newborn calves should be placed in sheltered environments, ideally on dry bedding, while trying to keep the concentration of enteric pathogens present at a minimum. Management strategies or husbandry practices to reduce exposure of the neonate to infected fecal material or aerosol primarily include thorough cleaning and disinfection of calving or nursery areas, adequate ventilation, physical isolation of clinically affected animals,[130,131] and noncommingling between younger and older calves, as described in the Sandhills calving system.[132] The authors refer the reader to other review articles for more specific biosecurity and biocontainment recommendations to minimize gastrointestinal pathogen exposure for both dairy or beef herds calving in confined areas or at pastures.[70,93,133]

Disinfection

As with any infectious disease, isolation and segregation of affected animals in quarantine, sanitation, and disinfection of footwear and equipment may help limit the spread of the disease. Bovine coronavirus is an enveloped RNA virus and is more sensitive to soaps, lipid solvents such as ether or chloroform, and common disinfectants such as formalin, phenol, and quaternary ammonium compounds, compared with nonenveloped viruses.[47] Removal of organic material is critical before application of disinfectant for maximal effectiveness. Bovine coronavirus can remain infectious for up to 3 days in soil, feces, and bedding materials.

Bovine Coronavirus Vaccines

Vaccines for bovine enteropathogenic coronavirus

There are 2 types of vaccines commercially available for the prevention of enteric disease caused by BCoV in neonatal calves. One is a killed vaccine (Scour-Guard 3(K), Pfizer Animal Health, NY; Guardian, Intervet/Schering-Plough Animal Health, NE; Scour-Bos, Novartis Animal Health, IA) administered to late pregnant cows for passive maternal immunization of their calves. The other is a modified-live BCoV (Calf-Guard, Pfizer Animal Health, NY) administered orally to calves at birth to provide active immunization. However, in a field study conducted in Austria, the efficacy of such immunization was questioned.[134] Passive immunization via colostrum has been found to be a reliable mode of vaccinating calves against BCoV, even though antibodies present locally within the gastrointestinal tract, an open-ended system, are typically short lived. Immunizing the pregnant cattle to produce a high colostral IgG1 level will protect the newborn calf against BCoV infection only if there is transfer of passive colostral antibodies within 24 hours after birth. Calves immunized after 24 hours of age may not be protected.

Vaccines differ in injection site reactions, and this can be an important consideration before use. In a preliminary study, the attenuated respiratory strain of the virus was found to be safe for intramuscular administration in cattle.[135] In another trial, about 50% of cows vaccinated with inactivated BCoV and bacterial component vaccine became lame and developed myositis.[136]

Antigenic variation among bovine enteropathogenic and respiratory coronaviruses

Previous reports have demonstrated that BCoV replicates in the upper respiratory tract of gnotobiotic calves following experimental inoculation.[23,41] Moreover, Hasoksuz and colleagues[31] reported that most (9 of 10) BRCoV strains isolated from the nasal passages of cattle entering feedlots in Ohio were similar to reference strains of BECoV previously isolated from calves with diarrhea and adult cattle with winter dysentery. This finding suggests that BRCoV and BECoV are antigenically related and cross-reactive, therefore vaccines developed to protect against enteric strains may also protect against respiratory tract strains of BCoV if administered intranasally.[31,60,62] However, BECoV isolates are antigenically classified among 3 subgroups 1–3 using a polyclonal antiserum against the Mebus strain of BCoV. Antigenic Group 3 is the predominant BECoV presently circulating in the United States.[137] Recent calf diarrhea isolates of BECoV are not blocked in hemagglutination-inhibition test by polyclonal antiserum prepared against antigenic Group 1 (Mebus isolate of BECoV). From the list of commercially available BECoV vaccines listed previously, only one (Guardian, Intervet/Schering-Plough Animal Health, NE) contains both antigenic variants of BECoV.

Vaccine for bovine respiratory coronaviruses

Modern vaccination programs using multivalent killed or modified-live viral vaccines and attenuated bacterial antigen have been associated with a decrease in BRDC incidence and prevalence; however, none of the commercially available vaccines are labeled for prevention of BRCoV. Protection of the respiratory tract from BRCoV has not been well studied except for one trial[60] in which extralabel use of the modified-live coronavirus and rotavirus vaccine in feedlot calves administered intranasally significantly decreased the subsequent rate of treatment for respiratory disease in cattle that had relatively low serum antibody titers against BCoV at arrival.[60] More specifically, there was an overall reduction of 26% among vaccinated calves treated for BRDC on entry to the feedlot. Furthermore, BCoV vaccinated calves with detectable intranasal BCoV had a 36% reduction in treatment for BRDC, and those with low antibody titers at arrival had 42% reduction, compared with unvaccinated calves. Although the 26% and 36% reduction was not statistically significant, it was considered clinically significant. The association between antibody titers against BCoV at feedlot arrival seems to correlate with protection from respiratory tract infection, and may promote higher weight gains[1] and reduce virus shedding in nasal secretions.[138] In one study, feedlot cattle that had BCoV antibody titers of greater than 1600 did not shed BCoV fecally or nasally.[32]

In the future, BCoV vaccines may be needed to decrease the economic losses due to BCoV infection in feedlot cattle. It has been suggested recently that feedlot calves should be vaccinated against BCoV at least 3 weeks before shipping to induce a serum IgG GMT of 1860 or more, to provide protection from BCoV infection and its direct or combined effects with other pathogens of BRDC.[20] Plummer and colleagues[60] suggested that development of an intranasally administered vaccine against BCoV, either by itself or combined with BHV-1, may have an added or synergistic effect in reducing incidence and subsequent treatment for BRDC in feedlot cattle.

SUMMARY

Bovine coronavirus is widespread in the cattle industry and is associated with significant economic losses. Clinical syndromes associated with BCoV (calf diarrhea, pneumonia in calves and adult cattle, winter dysentery, and combined pneumonia and diarrhea in young and adult cattle) are due to the virus tropism for the intestinal tract, nasal passages, proximal trachea, and lungs.

Only 4 BCoV isolates have been completely sequenced and thus, the information about the genetics of the virus is still limited. The coronaviruses responsible for enteric and respiratory syndromes in adult cattle and calves are closely related antigenically and genetically, and can be reproduced experimentally. From a vaccination point of view, the enteropathogenic and respiratory BCoV have not been clearly differentiated; however, they do cross-react to a great extent.

It is likely that BCoV work synergistically with other pathogens of the bovine respiratory tract in combination with various stressors to allow bacterial or viral colonization of the lungs, thus leading to development of BRDC. In calves, lack of colostral immunity is an important predisposing factor in the development of most infectious diseases, including diarrhea and respiratory tract infection caused by BCoV. Inclement weather is an important environmental stressor contributing to outbreaks of winter dysentery in dairy cattle.

There is a growing body of evidence in support of a causal relationship between BCoV and BRDC by predisposing or directly inducing lower respiratory tract disease, leading to poor growth performance in feedlot cattle and calves. This issue must be considered in disease prevention or preconditioning programs in the near future. The emergence of the respiratory tract infections caused by BRCoV in the cattle industry warrants timed, active immunization with appropriate antigens (antigenic Groups 1 and 3) to prevent this infection in stocker and feedlot cattle. Current strategies to prevent BCoV-induced enteritis in calves consist in vaccinating the late pregnant cows to provide passive colostral protection.

REFERENCES

1. Martin SW, Nagy E, Shewen PE, et al. The association of titers to bovine coronavirus with treatment for bovine respiratory disease and weight gain in feedlot calves. Can J Vet Res 1998;62(4):257–61.
2. Gagea MI, Bateman KG, Dreumel TV, et al. Diseases and pathogens associated with mortality in Ontario feedlots. J Vet Diagn Invest 2006;18(1):18–28.
3. Snowder GD, Van Vleck LD, Cundiff LV, et al. Bovine respiratory disease in feedlot cattle: environmental, genetic, and economic factors. J Anim Sci 2006; 84:1999–2008.
4. Storz J, Purdy CW, Lin X, et al. Isolation of respiratory coronaviruses, other cytocidal viruses and *Pasteurella* spp. from cattle involved in two natural outbreaks of shipping fever. J Am Vet Med Assoc 2000;216(10):1599–604.
5. Storz J, Stine L, Liem A, et al. Coronavirus isolations from nasal swabs samples in cattle with signs of respiratory tract disease after shipping. J Am Vet Med Assoc 1996;208(9):1452–5.
6. Lin XQ, O eilly KL, Storz J, et al. Antibody responses to respiratory coronavirus infections of cattle during shipping fever pathogenesis. Arch Virol 2000;145(11): 2335–49.
7. McNulty MS, Bryson DG, Allan GM, et al. Coronavirus infection of the bovine respiratory tract. Vet Microbiol 1984;9(5):425–34.
8. Lathrop SL, Wittum TE, Brock KV, et al. Association between infection of the respiratory tract attributable to bovine coronavirus and health and growth performance of cattle in feedlots. Am J Vet Res 2000;61(9):1062–6.
9. Storz J, Lin X, Purdy CW, et al. Coronavirus and *Pasteurella* infections in bovine shipping fever pneumonia and Evans' criteria for causation. J Clin Microbiol 2000;38(9):3291–8.
10. Hasoksuz M, Vlasova A, Saif LJ. Detection of group 2a coronaviruses with emphasis on bovine and wild ruminant strains. Virus isolation and detection of antibody, antigen, and nucleic acid. Methods Mol Biol 2008;454:43–59.
11. Kanno T, Kamivoshi T, Ishihara R, et al. Phylogenic studies of bovine coronaviruses isolated in Japan. J Vet Med Sci 2009;71(1):83–6.
12. Takiuchi E, Alfieri AF, Alfieri AA. Molecular analysis of the bovine coronavirus S1 gene by direct sequencing of diarrheic fecal specimens. Braz J Med Biol Res 2008;41(4):277–82.
13. Liu L, Hägglund S, Hakhverdan M, et al. Molecular epidemiology of bovine coronavirus on the basis of comparative analysis of the S gene. J Clin Microbiol 2006;44(3):957–60.
14. Popova R, Zhang X. The spike but not the hemagglutinin/esterase protein of bovine coronavirus is necessary and sufficient for viral infection. Virology 2002;294(1):222–36.
15. Kapil S, Lamm CG, McVey DS, et al. Detection of bovine respiratory coronavirus in beef cattle. In: Proceedings of the 27th annual meeting of the American Society of Virologists. Cornell University, Ithaca, NY, July 15, 2008. p. 9–1.
16. Carman PS, Hazlett MJ. Bovine coronavirus infection in Ontario, 1990-1991. Can Vet J 1992;33(12):812–4.
17. Storz J. Respiratory disease of cattle associated with coronavirus infections. In: Howard JL, Smith RA, editors. Current veterinary therapy: food animal practice 4. Philadelphia: WB Saunders; 1998. p. 291–3.
18. Lin XQ, O'Reilly KL, Storz J. Antibody responses of cattle with respiratory coronavirus infections during pathogenesis of shipping fever pneumonia are lower

with antigens of enteric strains than with those of a respiratory strain. Clin Diagn Lab Immunol 2002;9(5):1010–3.

19. Tsunemitsu H, Saif LJ. Antigenic and biologic comparisons of bovine coronavirus derived from neonatal calf diarrhea and winter dysentery of adult cattle. Arch Virol 1995;140(7):1303–11.

20. Thomas CJ, Hoet AE, Sreevatsan S, et al. Transmission of bovine coronavirus and serologic responses in feedlot calves under field conditions. Am J Vet Res 2006;67(8):1412–20.

21. Cho KO, Hoet AE, Loerch SC, et al. Evaluation of concurrent shedding of bovine coronavirus via the respiratory tract and enteric route. Am J Vet Res 2001;62(9): 1436–41.

22. Reynolds DJ, Debney TG, Hall GA, et al. Studies on the relationship between coronaviruses from the intestinal and respiratory tracts in calves. Arch Virol 1985;85(1–2):71–83.

23. Saif LJ, Redman DR, Moorhead PD, et al. Experimentally induced coronavirus infections in calves: viral replication in the respiratory and intestinal tracts. Am J Vet Res 1986;47(7):1426–32.

24. Tsunemitsu H, Yonemichi H, Hirai T, et al. Isolation of bovine coronavirus from feces and nasal swabs of calves with diarrhea. J Vet Med Sci 1991;53(3):433–7.

25. Hasoksuz M, Lathrop S, Al-dubaib MA, et al. Antigenic variation among bovine enteric coronaviruses (BEVC) and bovine respiratory coronaviruses (BRCV) detected using monoclonal antibodies. Arch Virol 1999;144(12): 2441–7.

26. El-Kanawati ZR, Tsunemitsu H, Smith DR, et al. Infection and cross-protection studies of winter dysentery and calf diarrhea bovine coronavirus strains in colostrum-deprived and gnotobiotic calves. Am J Vet Res 1996;57(1): 48–53.

27. Hasoksuz M, Sreevatsan S, Cho KO, et al. Molecular analysis of the S1 subunit of the spike glycoprotein of respiratory and enteric bovine coronavirus isolates. Virus Res 2002;84(1–2):101–9.

28. Reynolds DJ. Coronavirus replication in the intestinal and respiratory tracts during infection of calves. Ann Rech Vet 1983;14(4):445–6.

29. Zhang X, Herbst W, Kousoulas KG, et al. Comparison of the S genes and the biological properties of respiratory and enteropathogenic bovine coronaviruses. Arch Virol 1994;134(3–4):421–6.

30. Gelinas A-M, Boutin M, Sasseville AM-J, et al. Bovine coronaviruses associated with enteric and respiratory diseases in Canadian dairy cattle display different reactivities to anti-HE monoclonal antibodies and distinct amino acid changes in their HE, S and ns4.9 protein. Virus Res 2001;76(1):43–57.

31. Hasoksuz M, Lathrop SL, Gadfiled KL, et al. Isolation of bovine respiratory coronaviruses from feedlot cattle and comparison of their biological and antigenic properties with bovine enteric coronaviruses. Am J Vet Res 1999;60(10): 1227–33.

32. Hasoksuz M, Hoet AE, Loerch SC, et al. Detection of respiratory and enteric shedding of bovine coronaviruses in cattle at an Ohio feedlot. J Vet Diagn Invest 2002;14(4):308–13.

33. Kanno T, Hatama S, Ishihara R, et al. Molecular analysis of the S glycoprotein gene of bovine coronaviruses isolated in Japan from 1999-2006. J Gen Virol 2007;88(Pt 4):1218–24.

34. Park SJ, Kim GY, Choy HE, et al. Dual enteric and respiratory tropisms of winter dysentery bovine coronavirus in calves. Arch Virol 2007;152(10):1885–900.

35. Decaro N, Martella V, Elia G, et al. Biological and genetic analysis of a bovine-like coronavirus isolated from water buffalo (*Bubalus bubalis*) calves. Virology 2008;370(1):213–22.
36. Wunschman A, Frank R, Pomeroy K, et al. Enteric coronavirus infection in a juvenile dromadery (*Camelus dromaderius*). J Vet Diagn Invest 2002;14(5):441–4.
37. Genova SG, Streeter RN, Simpson KM, et al. Detection of an antigenic group 2 coronavirus in an adult alpaca with enteritis. Clin Vaccine Immunol 2008;15(10): 1629–32.
38. Majhdi F, Minocha HC, Kapil S. Isolation and characterization of a coronavirus from elk calves with diarrhea. J Clin Microbiol 1997;35(11):2937–42.
39. Hasoksuz M, Alekseev K, Vlasova A, et al. Biologic, antigenic, and full-length genomic characterization of a bovine-like coronavirus isolated from a giraffe. J Virol 2007;81(10):4981–90.
40. Decaro N, Mari V, Desario C, et al. Severe outbreak of bovine coronavirus infection in dairy cattle during the warmer season. Vet Microbiol 2008;126(1–3):30–9.
41. Saif LJ. Development of nasal, fecal and serum isotype-specific antibodies in calves challenged with bovine coronavirus or rotavirus. Vet Immunol Immunopathol 1987;17(1–4):425–39.
42. Heckert RA, Saif LJ, Hoblet KH, et al. A longitudinal study of bovine coronavirus enteric and respiratory infections in dairy calves in two herds in Ohio. Vet Microbiol 1990;22(2–3):187–201.
43. Heckert RA, Saif LJ, Myers GW, et al. Epidemiologic factors and isotype-specific antibody responses in serum and mucosal secretions of dairy calves with bovine coronavirus respiratory tract and enteric tract infections. Am J Vet Res 1991;52(6):845–51.
44. Collins JK, Riegel CA, Olson JD, et al. Shedding of enteric coronavirus in adult cattle. Am J Vet Res 1987;48(3):361–5.
45. Kapil S, Goyal SM. Bovine coronavirus-associated respiratory disease. Comp Cont Educ Pract Vet 1995;17(9):1179–81.
46. Crouch CF, Bielefeldt Ohmann H, Watts TC, et al. Chronic shedding of bovine enteric coronavirus antigen-antibody complexes by clinically normal cows. J Gen Virol 1985;66(Pt 7):1489–500.
47. Evermann JF, Benfield DA. Coronaviral infections. In: Williams ES, Barber IK, editors. Infectious diseases of wild mammals. 3rd edition. Ames (IA): Iowa State University Press; 2001. p. 245–53.
48. Tsunemitsu H, Smith DR, Saif LJ. Experimental inoculation of adult dairy cows with bovine coronavirus and detection of coronavirus in feces by RT-PCR. Arch Virol 1999;144(1):167–75.
49. Saif LJ, Smith KL. Enteric viral infections of calves and passive immunity. J Dairy Sci 1985;68(1):206–28.
50. Kapil S, Trent AM, Goyal SM. Excretion and persistence of bovine coronavirus in neonatal calves. Arch Virol 1990;115(1–2):127–32.
51. Kapil S, Pomeroy KA, Goyal SM, et al. Experimental infection with a virulent pneumoenteric isolate of bovine coronavirus. J Vet Diagn Invest 1991;3(1):88–9.
52. Clark KJ, Sarr AB, Grant PG, et al. In vitro studies on the use of clay, clay minerals and charcoal to adsorb bovine rotavirus and bovine coronavirus. Vet Microbiol 1998;63(2–4):137–46.
53. Lorusso A, Desario C, Mari V, et al. Molecular characterization of a canine respiratory coronavirus strain detected in Italy. Virus Res 2009;141(1):96–100.
54. Kaneshima T, Hohdatsu T, Hagino R, et al. The infectivity and pathogenicity of a group 2 bovine coronavirus in pups. J Vet Med Sci 2007;69(3):301–3.

55. Woolums AR, Ames TR, Baker JC. The bronchopneumonias (respiratory disease complex of cattle, sheep, and goats). In: Smith BP, editor. Large animal internal medicine. 4th edition. St. Louis (MO): Mosby Elsevier; 2009. p. 602–43.
56. Thomas LH, Gourlay RN, Stott EJ, et al. A search for new microorganisms in calf pneumonia by the inoculation of gnotobiotic calves. Res Vet Sci 1982;33(2): 170–82.
57. Busato A, Steiner L, Tontis A, et al. Frequency and etiology of calf losses and calf diseases in cow-calf farms. I. Methods of data collection, calf mortality, and calf morbidity. Dtsch Tierarztl Wochenschr 1997;104(4):131–5.
58. Ganaba R, Belanger D, Dea S, et al. A seroepidemiological study of the importance in cow-calf pairs of respiratory and enteric viruses in beef operations from northwestern Quebec. Can J Vet Res 1995;59(1):26–33.
59. Lathrop SL, Wittum TE, Loerch SC, et al. Antibody titers against bovine coronavirus and shedding of the virus via the respiratory tract in feedlot cattle. Am J Vet Res 2000;61(9):1057–61.
60. Plummer PJ, Rohrbach BW, Daugherty RA, et al. Effect of intranasal vaccination against bovine enteric coronavirus on the occurrence of respiratory tract disease in a commercial backgrounding feedlot. J Am Vet Med Assoc 2004; 225(5):726–31.
61. O'Connor A, Martin SW, Nagy E, et al. The relationship between the occurrence of undifferentiated bovine respiratory disease and titer changes to bovine coronavirus and bovine viral diarrhea virus in 3 Ontario feedlots. Can J Vet Res 2001; 65(3):137–42.
62. Cho KO, Hasoksuz M, Nielsen PR, et al. Cross-protection studies between respiratory and calf diarrhea and winter dysentery coronavirus strains in calves and RT-PCR and nested PCR for their detection. Arch Virol 2001; 146(12):2401–9.
63. Saif LJ. A review of evidence implicating bovine coronavirus in the etiology of winter dysentery in cows: an enigma resolved? Cornell Vet 1990;80(4):303–11.
64. Thomson RG. A perspective on respiratory disease in feedlot cattle. Can Vet J 1980;21(6):181–5.
65. Evans AS. Causation and disease: the Henle-Koch postulates revisited. Yale J Biol Med 1976;49(9):175–95.
66. Traven M, Naslund K, Linde N, et al. Experimental reproduction of winter dysentery in lactating cows using BCV-comparison with BCV infection in milk-fed calves. Vet Microbiol 2001;81(2):127–51.
67. Cavirani S, Galvani G, Taddei S, et al. Involvement of coronavirus in acute bovine respiratory disease (BRD) of cattle. In: Proceedings of the X International Symposium of Veterinary Laboratory Diagnosticians. Salsomaggiore (PR), Italy, July 4–7, 2001. p. 395–6.
68. Lavazza A, Boldini M, Lombardi G, et al. Identification of rotavirus and coronavirus in neonatal diarrhoea of calves submitted to the Brescia laboratory in 1991-1992. Atti della Societa Italiana di Buiatria 1993;25:249–58.
69. Mebus CA, Stair EL, Rhodes MB, et al. Pathology of neonatal calf diarrhea induced by a coronavirus-like agent. Vet Pathol 1973;10(1):45–64.
70. Gunn AA, Naylor JA, House JK. Diarrhea. In: Smith BP, editor. Large animal internal medicine. 4th edition. St. Louis (MO): Mosby Elsevier; 2009. p. 340–63.
71. Mebus CA, Newman LE, Stair EL. Scanning electron, light, and immunofluorescent microscopy of intestine of gnotobiotic calf infected with calf diarrheal coronavirus. Am J Vet Res 1975;36(12):1719–25.

72. Mebus CA, Stair EL, Rhodes MB, et al. Neonatal calf diarrhea: propagation, attenuation, and characteristics of a coronavirus-like agent. Am J Vet Res 1973;34(2):145–50.
73. Langpap TJ, Bergeland ME, Reed DE. Coronaviral enteritis of young calves: virologic and pathologic findings in naturally occurring infections. Am J Vet Res 1979;40(10):1476–8.
74. Bridger JC, Woode GN, Meyling A. Isolation of coronavirus from neonatal calf diarrhea in great Britain and Denmark. Vet Microbiol 1978;3(2):101–13.
75. Babiuk LA, Sabara M, Hudson GR. Rotavirus and coronavirus infections in animals. Prog Vet Microbiol Immunol 1985;1:80–120.
76. Moon HW. Mechanisms in the pathogenesis of diarrhea: a review. J Am Vet Med Assoc 1978;172(4):443–8.
77. Woode GN, Smith GN, Dennis MJ. Intestinal damage in rotavirus infected calves assessed by D-xylose malabsorption. Vet Rec 1978;102(15):340–1.
78. Clark MA. Bovine coronavirus. Br Vet J 1993;149(1):51–70.
79. Nappert G, Hamilton D, Petrie L, et al. Determination of lactose and xylose malabsorption in preruminant diarrheic calves. Can J Vet Res 1993;57(3): 152–8.
80. Ewaschuk JB, Naylor JM, Palmer R, et al. D-Lactate production and excretion in diarrheic calves. J Vet Intern Med 2004;18(5):744–7.
81. Lewis LD, Phillips RW. Pathophysiologic changes due to coronavirus-induced diarrhea in the calf. J Am Vet Med Assoc 1978;173(5 Pt 2):636–42.
82. Bendali F, Bichet H, Schelcher F, et al. Pattern of diarrhoea in newborn beef calves in south-west France. Vet Res 1999;30(1):61–74.
83. Durham PJK, Farquharson BC, Stevenson BJ. Rotavirus and coronavirus associated diarrhoea in calves. N Z Vet J 1979;27(12):271–2.
84. Hoet AE, Smiley J, Thomas C, et al. Association of enteric shedding of bovine torovirus (Breda virus) and other enteropathogens with diarrhea in veal calves. Am J Vet Res 2003;64(4):485–90.
85. Reynolds DJ, Morgan JH, Chanter N, et al. Microbiology of calf diarrhoea in southern Britain. Vet Rec 1986;119(2):34–9.
86. Mostl K, Burki F. Incidence of diarrhea and of rotavirus- and coronavirus-shedding in calves, whose dams had been vaccinated with an experimental oil-adjuvanted vaccine containing bovine rotavirus and bovine coronavirus. Zentralbl Veterinarmed B 1988;35(3):186–96.
87. Crouch CF, Acres SD. Prevalence of rotavirus and coronavirus antigens in the feces of normal cows. Can J Comp Med 1984;48(3):340–2.
88. Marsolais G, Assaf R, Montpetit C, et al. Diagnosis of viral agents associated with neonatal calf diarrhea. Can J Comp Med 1978;42(2):168–71.
89. Snodgrass DR, Terzolo HR, Sherwood D, et al. Aetiology of diarrhea in young calves. Vet Rec 1986;119(2):31–4.
90. Crouch CF, Oliver S, Hearle DC, et al. Lactogenic immunity following vaccination of cattle with bovine coronavirus. Vaccine 2000;19(2-3):189–96.
91. Cho KO, Halbur PG, Bruna JD, et al. Detection and isolation of coronavirus from feces of three herds of feedlot cattle during outbreaks of winter dysentery-like diseases. J Am Vet Med Assoc 2000;217(8):1191–4.
92. Bulgin MS, Ward A, Barrett DP, et al. Detection of rotavirus and coronavirus shedding in two beef cow herds in Idaho. Can Vet J 1989;30(3):235–9.
93. Barrington GM, Gay JM, Evermann JF. Biosecurity for neonatal gastrointestinal diseases. Vet Clin North Am Food Anim Pract 2002;18(1):7–34.

94. Moon HW, McClurkin AW, Isaacson RE, et al. Pathogenic relationships of rotavirus, *Escherichia coli*, and other agents in mixed infections in calves. J Am Vet Med Assoc 1978;173(5 Pt 2):577–83.

95. Acres SD, Saunders JR, Radostits OM. Acute undifferentiated neonatal diarrhea of beef calves: the prevalence of enterotoxigenic *E. coli*, reo-like (rota) virus and other enteropathogens in cow-calf herds. Can Vet J 1977;18(5):113–21.

96. Benfield DA, Saif LJ. Cell culture propagation of a coronavirus isolated from cows with winter dysentery. J Clin Microbiol 1990;28(6):1454–7.

97. Espinasse J, Viso M, Laval A, et al. Winter dysentery: a coronavirus-like agent in the faeces of beef and dairy cattle with diarrhoea. Vet Rec 1982;110(16): 385.

98. Broes A, Van Opdenbosch E, Wellemans G. Isolement d'un coronavirus chez des bovins atteints d'enterite hemorragique hivernale (winter dysentery) en Belgique [Isolation of a coronavirus from Belgian cattle with winter haemorrhagic enteritis]. Ann Med Vet 1984;128(4):299–303.

99. Natsuaki S, Goto K, Nakamura K, et al. Fatal winter dysentery with severe anemia in an adult cow. J Vet Med Sci 2007;69(9):957–60.

100. Saif LJ, Redman DR, Brock KV, et al. Winter dysentery in adult dairy cattle: detection of coronavirus in the faeces. Vet Rec 1988;123(11):300–1.

101. Smith DR, Fedorka-Cray PJ, Mohan R, et al. Epidemiologic herd-level assessment of causative agents and risk factors for winter dysentery in dairy cattle. Am J Vet Res 1998;59(8):994–1001.

102. van Kruiningen HJ, Khairallah LH, Sasseville VG, et al. Calfhood coronavirus enterocolitis: a clue to the etiology of winter dysentery. Vet Pathol 1987;24(6): 564–7.

103. Takahashi E, Inaba Y, Sato K, et al. Epizootic diarrhoea of adult cattle associated with a coronavirus-like agent. Vet Microbiol 1980;5(2):151–4.

104. Kruiningenvan HJ, Hiestand L, Hill DL, et al. Winter dysentery in dairy cattle: recent findings. Comp Cont Educ Pract Vet 1985;7(10):S591–9, S598–9.

105. Tsunemitsu H, El-Kanawati ZR, Smith DR, et al. Isolation of coronaviruses antigenically indistinguishable from bovine coronavirus from wild ruminants with diarrhea. J Clin Microbiol 1995;33(12):3264–9.

106. Smith DR, Fedorka-Cray PJ, Mohan R, et al. Evaluation of cow-level risk factors for the development of winter dysentery in dairy cattle. Am J Vet Res 1998;59(8): 986–93.

107. MacPherson LW. Bovine virus enteritis (winter dysentery). Can J Comp Med Vet Sci 1957;21(6):184–92.

108. Barrera Valle M, Rodriguez Batista E, Betancourt Martell A, et al. Short communication. First report in Cuba of bovine coronavirus detection in a winter dysentery outbreak. Spanish J Agr Res 2006;4(3):221–4.

109. Campbell SG, Cookingham CA. The enigma of winter dysentery. Cornell Vet 1978;68(4):423–41.

110. Fleetwood AJ, Edwards S, Foxell PW, et al. Winter dysentery in adult dairy cattle. Vet Rec 1989;125(22):553–4.

111. Durham PJ, Hassard LE, Armstrong KR, et al. Coronavirus-associated diarrhea (winter dysentery) in adult cattle. Can Vet J 1989;30(10):825–7.

112. Roberts SJ. Winter dysentery in dairy cattle. Cornell Vet 1957;47(3):372–88.

113. Guard CL, Fecteau G. Winter dysentery in cattle. In: Smith BP, editor. Large animal internal medicine. 4th edition. St. Louis (MO): Mosby Elsevier; 2009. p. 876–7.

114. White ME, Schukken Hein Y, Tanksley B. Space-time clustering of, and risk factors for, farmer-diagnosed winter dysentery in dairy cattle. Can Vet J 1989; 30(12):948–51.
115. Kahrs RF, Scott FW, Hillman RB. Epidemiologic observations on bovine winter dysentery. Bovine Practitioner 1973;8:36–9.
116. Traven M, Silvan A, Larsson B, et al. Experimental infection with bovine coronavirus (BCV) in lactating cows: clinical disease, viral excretion, interferon-alpha and antibody response. Bovine Pract 1995;29:64–5.
117. Dar AM, Kapil S, Goyal SM. Comparison of immunohistochemistry, electron microscopy, and direct fluorescent antibody test for the detection of bovine coronavirus. J Vet Diagn Invest 1998;10(2):152–7.
118. Schoenthaler SL, Kapil S. Development and applications of a bovine coronavirus antigen detection enzyme-linked immunoassay. Clin Diagn Lab Immunol 1999;6(1):130–2.
119. Daginakatte GC, Chard-Bergstrom C, Andrews GA, et al. Production, characterization, and uses of monoclonal antibodies against recombinant nucleoprotein of elk coronavirus. Clin Diagn Lab Immunol 1999;6(3):341–4.
120. Luginbuhl A, Reitt K, Metzler A, et al. Field study of the prevalence and diagnosis of diarrhea-causing agents in the newborn calf in a Swiss veterinary practice area. Schweiz Arch Tierheilkd 2005;147(6):245–52.
121. Selman IE, Allan EM, Gibbs HA, et al. Effect of anti-prostaglandin therapy in experimental parainfluenza type 3 pneumonia in weaned, conventional calves. Vet Rec 1984;115(5):101–5.
122. Friton G, Cajal C, Leemann R, et al. Pharmaco-economic benefit of meloxicam (Metacam) in the treatment of respiratory disease in feedlot cattle. In: Proceedings of the 23rd World Buiatrics Conference. Quebec, Canada, July 11–16, 2004.
123. Apley M. Ancillary therapy in food animal infectious disease with a focus on steroids and NSAIDS in bovine respiratory disease and toxic mastitis: what should (and shouldn't we be doing?). In: Proceedings of the Ontario Veterinary Medical Association (OVMA). Ontario; 2008. p. 203–10.
124. Apley M. Ancillary therapy of bovine respiratory disease. Vet Clin North Am Food Anim Pract 1997;13(3):575–92.
125. Naylor JM. Oral electrolyte therapy. Vet Clin North Am Food Anim Pract 1999; 15(3):487–504.
126. Berchtold J. Intravenous fluid therapy of calves. Vet Clin North Am Food Anim Pract 1999;15(3):505–31.
127. Arthington JD, Jaynes CA, Tyler HD, et al. The use of bovine serum protein as an oral support therapy following coronavirus challenge in calves. J Dairy Sci 2002; 85(5):1249–54.
128. Bendali F, Sanaa M, Bichet H, et al. Risk factors associated with diarrhoea in newborn calves. Vet Res 1999;30(5):509–22.
129. Kasari TR, Wikse SE. Perinatal mortality in beef herds. Vet Clin North Am Food Anim Pract 1994;10(1):1–185.
130. Heath SE. Neonatal diarrhea in calves: investigation of herd management practices. Comp Cont Educ Pract Vet 1992;14(3):385–93.
131. Heath SE. Neonatal diarrhea in calves: diagnosis and intervention in problem herds. Comp Cont Educ Pract Vet 1992;14(7):995–1002.
132. Smith DR, Grotelueschen DM, Knott T, et al. Prevention of neonatal diarrhea with the Sandhills calving system. In: Proceedings of the 37th Annual

Conference of American Association of Bovine Practitioners. Forth Worth, TX, September 23–25, 2004. p. 23–5.

133. Pence M, Robbe S, Thomson J. Reducing the incidence of neonatal calf diarrhea through evidence-based management. Comp Cont Educ Pract Vet 2001; 23:S73–5.

134. de Leeuw PW, Tiessink JW. Laboratory experiments on oral vaccination of calves against rotavirus or coronavirus induced diarrhea. Zentralbl Veterinarmed B 1985;31(1):55–64.

135. Decaro N, Campolo M, Mari V, et al. A candidate modified-live bovine coronavirus vaccine: safety and immunogenicity evaluation. New Microbiol 2009;32(1): 109–13.

136. O'Toole D, Steadman L, Raisbeck M, et al. Myositis, lameness, and recumbency after use of water-in-oil adjuvanted vaccines in near-term beef cattle. J Vet Diagn Invest 2005;17(1):23–31.

137. Kapil S, Richardson KL, Maag TR, et al. Characterization of bovine coronavirus isolates from eight different states in the USA. Vet Microbiol 1999;67:221–30.

138. Lin X, O'Reilly KL, Burrel ML, et al. Infectivity-neutralizing and hemagglutinin-inhibiting antibody responses to respiratory coronavirus infections of cattle in pathogenesis of shipping fever pneumonia. Clin Diagn Lab Immunol 2001;8(2):357–62.

The Role of Wildlife in Diseases of Cattle

Hana Van Campen, DVM, PhD[a],*, Jack Rhyan, DVM, MS[b]

KEYWORDS

- Wildlife • Disease • Cattle • TB • Tuberculosis
- Brucellosis • BVD

The opportunities for transmission of infectious agents between cattle and wildlife are dependent on specific behaviors, management practices, physiologic events, and environmental circumstances in the life of domestic and wild species and attributes of the infectious organisms. These factors include an agent's ability to infect a new host, the portals of entry and exit from a new host, the course of a disease and its morbidity (rapid recovery or death vs prolonged shedding), behavior and density of host species, climatic conditions, time interval for shedding, and overlap of host range with other susceptible species. Depending on these factors, a new host may be a "dead-end" host, that is, unable to maintain the infection without continuing transmission from other species, thereby resulting in no long-term consequence to the resident populations; or it may become a "maintenance" host, able to maintain infection without continual introduction from other species. Dead-end and maintenance hosts may be able to transmit infection to other species[1]; however, the maintenance host that is also capable of interspecies transmission is the most significant in terms of disease epidemiology. This article discusses how various factors contribute to the introduction, maintenance, and spread of infectious agents within wildlife and between wildlife and cattle.

BASIC BEHAVIORAL AND MANAGEMENT CONSIDERATIONS

Animals are often classified into categories of domestic, wildlife, captive wildlife, zoo, and so forth, and certain biases accompany those labels. It can be helpful, instead, to consider them as animal populations with differing, and sometimes overlapping, behaviors, ecologies, pathogens, and types of management. It is also important to remember that the addition of one or more components of an intensive management system (increasing density of animals by supplemental feeding or fencing) may tip the

[a] Veterinary Diagnostic Laboratory, Department of Microbiology, Immunology and Pathology, Colorado State University, 300 West Drake Road, Fort Collins, CO 80523-1644, USA
[b] US Department of Agriculture, Animal and Plant Health Inspection Service, Veterinary Services, 4101 LaPorte Avenue, Fort Collins, CO 80521, USA
* Corresponding author.
E-mail address: hvancamp@lamar.colostate.edu (H. Van Campen).

Vet Clin Food Anim 26 (2010) 147–161
doi:10.1016/j.cvfa.2009.10.008
0749-0720/10/$ – see front matter © 2010 Elsevier Inc. All rights reserved.

ecologic balance toward increased diseases and parasites in a population and their transmission to other populations. Current North American examples include brucellosis, caused by *Brucella abortus*, in elk (*Cervus elaphus nelsoni*) on winter feedgrounds in the Greater Yellowstone Area (GYA); tuberculosis (TB), caused by *Mycobacterium bovis*, in white-tailed deer (*Odocoileus virginianus*) in the northeastern portion of lower Michigan, where supplemental feeding and baiting were longstanding practices; and recently, evidence for bovine viral diarrhea virus (BVDV) infections in several free-ranging species.

Related considerations are the effect of a species' behavior on the epidemiology of a disease in that species and the impact of changes in management on the behavior and, consequently, the disease. Again, GYA elk exemplify this concept. In areas of the GYA remote from feedgrounds, brucellosis prevalence is low, yet on feedgrounds, prevalence is high.[2,3] Outside of the GYA, brucellosis prevalence in elk is most likely zero,[4,5] and elk herds translocated from the GYA to other sites have no brucellosis. This difference in prevalence is likely due to the species' reclusive calving behavior, which keeps the elk cow and calf away from the herd for several days after calving. This behavior normally minimizes risk of *B abortus* transmission to other animals and, in less intensively managed settings, almost certainly relegates elk to the role of a dead-end host. When a nearby feedground is added to the equation, however, the risk of infection increases dramatically. Besides increasing animal density, this practice increases the animals' risk of exposure to an infectious abortion near feedlines, postaborting dams on feedlines, and resultant feed contamination by infectious vaginal discharge. This management practice, then, changes the behavior and density of free-ranging elk, likely converting what in nature is a dead-end host to a maintenance host of the infection.

In North America, the most problematic wildlife/cattle interface diseases probably were originally transmitted from livestock to wildlife. Currently, these include brucellosis in GYA bison (*Bison bison*) and elk and TB in Michigan white-tailed deer (*O virginianus*) and in elk in Riding Mountain National Park (RMNP), Manitoba, Canada.[6] In recent years these diseases have become especially troublesome because, after near eradication of the diseases in cattle, wildlife have maintained and transmitted the infection back to adjacent cattle populations.

Finally, it should be emphasized that each population interface (wildlife/wildlife or wildlife/cattle) should be regarded as unique when considering risk of interspecies disease transmission. The same disease at the interface of the same two species may behave differently in different areas or situations. This can be for a variety of reasons, including different climatic environments; different management of one or both species; shared food, water, and mineral sources; population densities; predation variables; concurrent diseases; and so forth. An example of this concept is a comparison of *M bovis* infection in feral swine/wild boar (*Sus scofa*) in four different situations: Australia, the Hawaiian island of Molokai, southern Spain, and France. In the Northern Territory of Australia, the prevalence of *M bovis* in feral swine decreased from 40% in some areas[7] to 0.25%[8] after the disease was essentially eradicated from cattle and water buffalo. On the island of Molokai, a survey for TB in 1980 of feral swine in proximity to a recently discovered *M bovis*–infected cattle herd found an estimated prevalence based on culture and histopathology of 20%.[9] In 1983, after the cattle herd was removed, a survey found *M bovis* infection in 3.2% of swine collected from the same area.[10] The decreased prevalence was attributed to removal of the infected cattle herd and to intense hunting pressure that had decreased density of feral swine. In 1997, after complete depopulation and restocking of cattle on the island, bovine TB reappeared in cattle in proximity to the original infected premises. Subsequent hunter-kill sampling has shown the infection has persisted in feral swine at a low prevalence (Robert Meyer, DVM, MS, unpublished data, 2009). *M bovis* is maintained in wild boar and red deer in southern Spain with prevalence in boars ranging from 40% to 100% in various areas[11]; it is present at high prevalence in boar populations with no contact with cattle. Similarly in France, after the country was declared free of bovine TB in 2000, wildlife surveys conducted in 2001–2002 and 2005–2006 showed increasing prevalence of *M bovis* infection in wild boar (29% and 42%) and red deer (13% and 24%).[12] The Australian feral swine had primarily gastrointestinal lesions indicative of exposure by ingestion whereas the Molokai swine and wild boar in Spain had thoracic lymph node and lung involvement, suggesting an aerosol route of transmission. In the French studies in 2005–2006, the disease was not found in a sample of 55 European badgers (*Meles meles*), collected from the endemic area, in contrast to in the United Kingdom, where badgers are the wildlife reservoir host of *M bovis*.

The main opportunity for transmission of infectious agents between wildlife and cattle occurs on pasture. Access to pasture varies with the different cattle management systems. Grazing is used by a minority of US dairies; however, heifers are commonly pastured from the postweaning period until entrance into the lactating herd and cows in late gestation from dry-off to calving. Approximately 50% of dairy operators observe contact between deer and cattle with some regional variation.[13] In addition to contact on pasture, transmission of infectious agents from deer to dairy cattle is possible where deer have access to feed in haystacks, open silage pits, feed bunks, mineral blocks, and water sources. Deer may also acquire infections from cattle through contact with waste from cow pens or milking parlors and calf facilities or on pastures fertilized with manure. Gestational status may be immaterial for the transmission of some infections, whereas, the transmission of others, such as *B abortus* and BVDV to pregnant females, may be clinically and epidemiologically important. Most dairies in the United States breed cows year round so that cows in all stages of pregnancy are present in a lactating herd throughout the year, a breeding scheme distinct from the synchronous, seasonal breeding of beef cattle, and wild ruminant species. Asynchronous breeding reduces the proportion of cows in early gestation at each point in time, thus reducing the potential number of persistently infected (PI) calves that potentially could be generated per BVDV exposure.

The physical layout and management of cattle feedlots largely preclude direct contact between wildlife and cattle. In conventional feedyards, feed is the most likely source of infectious agents. Access to water and mineral sources is more limited with little chance for use or contamination by animals residing outside individual pens. The risk of transmission to other animals leading to the continuation of infection is low in conventional feedlots because the cattle go to slaughter; however, potential transmission of infectious agents to humans and other species via ingestion of contaminated meat and by-products can occur. The presence of some agents (eg, BVDV) in some by-products, such as bovine serum, can still serve as a source of infection if the contaminated material makes its way into biologic products, such as vaccines.

Not all feedlots are dead ends for infectious agents. An important trend in dairy and beef heifer management is the increased use of development feedlots in which heifers are grown and bred. Animals and their waste are highly concentrated and the source of feed and water centralized, creating an ideal environment for the spread of some infections after introduction by contact, aerosol, or ingestion.

The highest probability of contact and transmission of infectious agents between wildlife and cattle occurs in the extensive management systems used to raise beef cattle in North America. Wildlife and cattle ranges overlap, and feed, water, and mineral sources are shared between species on many farms and ranches. More than 70% of beef operations report contact between their cattle and wild cervids.[14] Under these circumstances, the transmission of infections by direct contact, ingestion, or aerosol between livestock and free-ranging species is not surprising.

BRUCELLOSIS: HISTORY AND CURRENT SITUATION

In 1887, *B mellitensis* was isolated and described by David Bruce from the spleen of a dead sailor who had contracted Malta fever, now known as brucellosis, by drinking unpasteurized goat's milk. Ten years later Bernard Bang isolated and described *B abortus*, which was associated with infectious abortions in cattle. Subsequently, *B suis* was associated with abortions in swine; *B ovis* was associated with epididymitis and occasional abortions in sheep; *B canis* caused reproductive and bone lesions in canids; *B neotomae* caused no apparent disease in wood rats in Utah; and a group of brucellae, with recently proposed names of *B ceti* and *B pinnipedialis*, was isolated from marine mammals.[15] Of these, all but *B ovis* and possibly *B neotomae*, of which little is known, are infectious to humans.

Worldwide, *Brucella* spp are associated with wildlife reservoirs at several interfaces with livestock. The better-known interface brucellosis situations include *B abortus* in bison (*Bison bison*), elk, and cattle in the GYA; *B suis* in feral swine and wild boars, domestic swine, and cattle in several locations worldwide; *B suis* biovar 2 in European hares (*Lepus europaeus*) and domestic swine in Europe; and *B suis* biovar 4 in caribou (*Rangifer tarandus*) and reindeer in the Arctic. Bison in Wood Buffalo National Park in Alberta and the Northwest Territories in Canada are maintenance hosts for *B abortus* and *M bovis* but currently do not pose a threat of transmission to cattle due to spatial separation of the two species. African buffalo (*Syncerus caffer*) and several other African wildlife species have serologic evidence of infection to *Brucella* spp but are considered of minor importance as a reservoir for infection in cattle due to infrequent contact.[16]

In North America other species of wildlife in brucellosis-endemic environments have serologic evidence of exposure to or infection with *B abortus*; however, these animals are not considered significant reservoirs. White-tailed deer and mule deer (*O hemionus*) have been extensively surveyed for brucellosis. In a summary of more than 30 surveys of deer in the United States, many conducted when the disease was prevalent in cattle, Davis[17] found 42 of more than 25,000 deer had diagnostically significant serologic reactions and *B abortus* was isolated from a single, free-ranging, white-tailed deer. The low prevalence was attributed, in part, to the browsing rather than grazing behavior of deer. Canids and ursulids have received speculative blame for spread of the disease; surveys of wild coyotes (*Canis latrans*) in Texas when brucellosis was prevalent in cattle[18] and in Canadian wolves (*Canis lupus*) in proximity to infected bison in Canada[19] demonstrated antibodies and *B abortus*–positive tissues. A single survey of coyotes in the GYA did not show serologic evidence of *B abortus* infection.[20] Experimentally infected coyotes transmitted brucellosis to comingled cattle,[21] and wolves were shown to maintain the organism at least a year and shed small numbers of brucellae for up to 50 days in feces.[22] Grizzly (*Ursus horribilis*) and black bears (*U americanus*) in the GYA have serologic evidence of brucellosis (Keith Aune, MS, unpublished data, 2009),[23] and the vaccine strain *B abortus* RB51 was recovered from lymph nodes of one black bear 23 weeks post inoculation.[24] Due to the fecal route of shedding and the small numbers of organisms shed, carnivores are not considered significant vectors of brucellosis in nature. Additionally, the disease has been eradicated from most of North America where carnivores were prevalent without regard for the disease in those species. Currently, there are no known significant wildlife reservoirs of *B abortus* in North America except bison and elk in the GYA and bison in and around Wood Buffalo National Park.

The most notorious wildlife-cattle interface where wildlife serves as a reservoir for infection in cattle is the elk and bison of the GYA. Evidence of infection in bison first occurred in 1917, when animals from the introduced herd in Yellowstone National Park (YNP) tested positive on agglutination tests after the observation of abortions.[25] Elk were found seropositive on the National Elk Refuge (Jackson Hole, Wyoming) in 1930[26] and the organism was isolated from aborted elk fetuses in 1969.[27] Investigators have speculated that infection in GYA bison and elk likely resulted from exposure to cattle.[2,28] Currently, at least two biovars of *B abortus* (biovars 1 and 4) are present in GYA elk indicating at least two introductions of the agent into wildlife.

In recent years brucellosis has emerged as a hot button disease at the wildlife/cattle interface largely due to the recent and nearly total eradication of *B abortus* from cattle in the United States after 70 years of a state-federal cooperative effort. Since 2000, state and federal animal health authorities have been eliminating the disease from the last infected herds in the nation. In 2008, the livestock industry was briefly declared free of brucellosis for the first time. Since 2004, however, positive cattle herds in Idaho, Wyoming, and, most recently, in 2008 in Montana have been discovered resulting in the loss of brucellosis-free status for those states. In each instance, epidemiologic investigations have led to the conclusion that elk were the source of infection for the cattle. Currently, Idaho and Wyoming have regained their class-free status and Montana is in the process of eliminating brucellosis in cattle.

Results of serologic surveys of bison in the GYA have varied but generally average an approximately 50% seroprevalence for the YNP herd. A study of the disease in the Grand Teton bison herd, which uses feedgrounds on the National Elk Refuge for winter feeding, found a seroprevalence of 77%.[29] In a limited study of naturally infected, female bison from YNP, 46% of seropositive animals were culture positive for *B abortus*.[30] The most consistently culture-positive tissues were retropharyngeal, iliac, and superficial inguinal lymph nodes. In bison bull studies, the organism has been isolated from many lymph nodes and genitalia, especially seminal vesicles.[29,31]

Recent studies indicate the pathogenesis and epidemiology of brucellosis in YNP bison is similar to that in a chronically infected herd of cattle.[30,32,33] Specifically, *B abortus*–infected bison usually abort and shed the organism in the first gestation after seroconversion and occasionally in later gestations. Infection significantly affects birth rates of the herd.[32] Among the seronegative bison, positive seroconversion rates are high (approximately 20% per year) in calves and juveniles and lower (approximately 10% per year) in adults.[33]

In Wyoming, on the National Elk Refuge and 22 state-managed feedgrounds, where elk are fed hay during winter months, seroprevalence rates are highly variable but average in the low- to mid-20th percentile range. GYA elk populations remote from feedgrounds have much lower seroprevalence, less than 5%, and outside of the GYA, brucellosis is absent.[2,34] Similar to bison and cattle, the primary means of intra- and interspecies transmission by elk is the late-term abortion event. Infected animals may also bear weak calves or likely healthy calves and still shed organisms in the placental membranes and fluids.

Experimentally[35] and in nature[36] bison have transmitted brucellosis to cattle. The lack of known cases of bison to cattle transmission in the GYA is a testimony to the continuing concerted efforts of GYA wildlife and animal health personnel in keeping a temporal and spatial separation between the two species. This currently involves following a carefully crafted management plan that requires hazing bison that exit YNP during winter back into the Park several weeks before cattle being allowed to graze those lands. *Brucella* persistence and fetal scavenging studies in the GYA have demonstrated persistence of the organism a maximum of 81 days on fetuses placed in the environment in mid-February and 77, 69, and 25 days for fetuses placed in mid-March, mid-April, and mid-May, respectively.[37] Fetuses placed in the environment outside of YNP but in proximity were scavenged between 1 and 78 days (mean 18.23 days). Monitoring naturally occurring, *B abortus*–positive bison birth sites in YNP with weekly sample collection (tissues, vegetation, and soil), showed viability of the organism for 10 to 43 days at April sites (N = 6) and 7 to 26 days for May sites (N = 3). Undoubtedly, climatic conditions in any given year (cool wet spring vs warm dry spring), the location of the abortion site (shade vs sun or dry and windy vs damp and sheltered), and the local density of scavengers have an impact on the persistence of *B abortus* in the environment and the accompanying risk of transmission to cattle.

Ecologic and behavioral factors play a large role for elk-to-elk and elk-to-cattle transmission risks. The use of feedgrounds concentrates elk populations during winter when abortions may occur. Fetuses are sometimes aborted on feedgrounds where one study showed that up to 150 elk may investigate a bovine fetus used as a surrogate[38] and recent work has shown the proximity of a fetus to the feedline correlates with the degree of exposure of at-risk elk.[39] Even when abortions occur off-site, the aborting dam likely visits the feedlines while shedding large numbers of organisms in the vaginal discharge resulting in exposure of other animals. The increased prevalence of brucellosis in feedground elk increases the risk of transmission to cattle in proximity. When elk are allowed to feed on cattle feedlines, the risk of exposure of cattle to infection dramatically increases. One known case of elk-to-cattle transmission occurred at a ranch where elk routinely fed on hay lines with cattle.[40]

In areas of the GYA remote from feedgrounds, changing ecologic factors are influencing intraspecies and ultimately interspecies transmission. One is the recent trend of harboring elk. This is the practice, intentional or not, of some property holders to preserve land for the purpose of providing a sanctuary for elk during winter. Without establishing a true feedground, these landholders are increasing the density of animals at a crucial time of year, which likely facilitates transmission of brucellosis. The recent reintroduction of wolves to the GYA is a second factor of unknown consequence on brucellosis transmission in elk. The presence of this predator has probably had short-term behavioral effects and perhaps long-term demographic effects on elk, both of which might influence brucellosis transmission. Changes in property management for hunting have also caused changes in movement patterns of elk in some areas, resulting in earlier migration to lower private lands and prolonged congregation on lower pastures in the spring. These movement changes, caused in part by decreased hunting pressure on private properties accompanied by continued pressure on public lands, may result in increased exposure of elk and surrounding cattle to *B abortus* in late winter and spring.

Species' behavior at parturition plays a large role in the epidemiology of brucellosis in bison and elk.[41] Groups of bison frequently investigate parturition events, especially early in the calving season. Cows and calves often lick and sniff the presented membranes and neonate during the birthing process. This contrasts with elk parturition behavior, which is private, the dam keeping the neonate hidden and sequestered from the herd for several days after birth. This difference in parturition-related behavior may, in part, account for the disparity in disease prevalence between bison in the GYA not being fed on feedgrounds (approximately 50%) and elk in the GYA not on feedgrounds (< 5%).

Mitigation strategies to prevent transmission of brucellosis at the wildlife/cattle interface focus on separation of the species, especially during late pregnancy through calving. Other mitigations currently used include vaccination of at-risk cattle, remote vaccination of elk on feedgrounds by means of polymer vaccine–containing bullets fired from airguns, fencing in haystacks, and decreasing the time elk are on feedgrounds. Ongoing developmental work includes oral vaccine development for elk (Pouline Nol, DVM, MS, unpublished data, 2009) and nonlethal methods of preventing B abortus transmission in bison and elk by means of immunocontraception.[42–44]

TUBERCULOSIS: HISTORY AND CURRENT STATUS

Bovine TB, caused by M bovis, is another zoonotic disease that originated in cattle, infected wildlife, and now, in some areas, is re-infecting cattle via wildlife reservoirs. Prior to the 1990s, the disease in North America was only rarely recognized in white-tailed deer, mule deer, elk, and moose (Alces alces) in areas in proximity to infected cattle or bison herds, and wildlife was not considered a significant reservoir of the disease. In the 1980s and 1990s, TB was found disseminated in commercial bison and elk herds and disease eradication efforts were conducted in those industries. In 1994, TB was found in a hunter-killed white-tailed deer in Michigan[45] in the same area where it had been observed 19 years before.[46] This find precipitated surveillance activities and ultimately disclosed a significant wildlife reservoir of M bovis in the United States. At approximately the same time, a hunter-killed elk near RMNP in Manitoba was found infected and subsequent surveillance disclosed another wildlife reservoir.[47] In the years since its discovery in Michigan deer and in elk near RMNP, many cattle herds have been infected in both locales. Additionally, a smaller cattle/deer interface situation was recently discovered in Northwestern Minnesota where, after discovery of M bovis infection in cattle herds, surveillance disclosed the infection in white-tailed deer in proximity to the infected premises.[48] In Michigan, several wildlife species besides white-tailed deer have been found positive for the organism,[49] the most notable being coyotes.[50] These species are currently considered to be dead-end hosts for the infection.

Other significant wildlife maintenance hosts of TB around the world include brush-tail possums (Trichosurus vulpecula) and possibly ferrets (Mustelo furo) and wild deer in New Zealand, which serve as hosts of the agent and, at least in the case of brush-tail possums, serve to transmit the infection to cattle and farmed deer; badgers in England with transmission to cattle; and wild boars and red deer (Cervus elaphus elaphus) in Spain[11] and France.[12] Known African maintenance reservoirs include cape buffalo, kafue lechwae (Kobus leche), and greater kudu (Tragelaphus strepsiceros).[51] Other African wildlife species are infected with M bovis, including carnivores, but are considered likely dead-end hosts.[51]

Several factors affect the maintenance M bovis infection in deer and its transmission to cattle. Deer in the TB endemic area in Michigan have historically been maintained at levels above the normal carrying capacity by use of supplemental feeding.[46] Additionally, during hunting season it was long the practice to bait deer to certain sites with feed.[46] These management schemes likely led to concentration of a suitable host for M bovis and behavior that allowed transmission between deer via the feed. As prevalence in deer rose, cattle were more at risk until cattle herds in proximity of the deer began to experience infection, probably by means of indirect contact by ingestion of contaminated feed. M bovis has been shown to persist for a week or longer on feedstuffs used as supplemental feed for deer in Michigan,[52] and deer-to-deer[53] and deer-to-cattle[54] transmission by indirect contact via feed has been demonstrated experimentally. This contrasts with two other wildlife-to-cattle transmission situations in which direct contact may be more of a factor in transmission.

During terminal stages of TB, brushtailed possums in New Zealand[55] and European badgers in England[56] display abnormal behavior, losing fear of cattle and deer. It has been shown that cattle and deer, especially dominant individuals, investigate the abnormally behaving possums and badgers by sniffing, licking, and biting, thereby exposing themselves to animals most likely shedding large numbers of infectious organisms.[1,55] Also, a recent study in England[57] showed that specific individual cattle predominated in interactions with badgers, suggesting these individuals would act as hubs in the interspecific contact network. Other studies have shown different grazing practices[58] and pasture management practices[59] have had an impact on the risk of cattle exposure to M bovis–infected wildlife.

Other factors, including matrilinear social structure and relatedness[5] and male behaviors, have an impact on the epidemiology of TB. A recent study of Michigan white-tailed deer showed that TB-infected deer were significantly more related than noninfected deer.[60] Male behaviors, including increased ranging, dominance, and fighting behavior, may contribute to the higher prevalence of TB in male deer in Michigan[46] and male elk in RMNP.[6,47]

Renwick and colleagues[51] recently reviewed the transmission dynamics of M bovis in wildlife in southern Africa. In large predators and greater kudus, unique mechanisms of transmission occur. Besides gastrointestinal exposure by ingestion of M bovis–infected carcasses, large predators can also become infected by percutaneous inoculation via bite wounds from other predators. This also occurs in European badgers in areas having high badger densities.[1] Percutaneous inoculation is a route of transmission in kudus resulting from scratches and abrasions on the face and ears by contaminated thorn bushes on which kudus browse.[51] Percutaneous inoculation of M bovis results in chronic granulomatous inflammation of the skin, subcutis, and underlying tissues.

Mitigation strategies for TB management usually involve reducing density and exposure of the wildlife reservoir by increased hunting, eliminating supplemental feeding, and preventing contact between infected and at-risk populations. Unlike brucellosis, transmission can occur at any season requiring continuous separation of species. An additional mitigation strategy is, potentially, the use of vaccination in wildlife or at-risk cattle. Developmental work on vaccines is ongoing and results of preliminary studies show promise.[61,62]

The several animal population interfaces at which M bovis is present are characterized by unique population, climatic, ecologic, behavioral, and political factors. For effective interface disease management, each situation must be evaluated individually for risk factors and appropriate mitigations designed and implemented in wild and domestic populations.

BOVINE VIRAL DIARRHEA VIRUS

BVDVs are transmitted horizontally and vertically within cattle populations. Of the two modes of transmission, transfer of BVDV from a susceptible heifer or cow to her fetus is ultimately the most important in maintaining the infection in a population. Infection of fetuses during the first trimester of pregnancy before the development of immune competence leads to the establishment of a PI of a calf.[63,64] If a PI calf is born and survives, the large amounts of infectious virus that it sheds in all secretions serve as the main source of infection for other cattle and susceptible species.[65] In addition, the placenta, fetal fluids, and tissues from abortions contain large quantities of BVDV. The introduction of BVDV infection into a new population regardless of species would most likely occur as a result of exposure to a PI animal, whereas maintenance of infection within the population depends on an overlap in time and space of a PI animal and susceptible females in the early stages of gestation.

Evidence indicating that infection of wild ruminants with BVDV occurs in nature includes (1) BVDV specific antibodies, (2) virus isolates, and (3) immunohistochemical (IHC) staining in skin samples from free-ranging animals compatible with PI status. Serosurveys have detected BVDV antibodies in free-ranging populations worldwide.[66] In general, populations with a high percentage of seropositive animals are found in proximity to cattle,[67–69] whereas populations isolated from cattle are seronegative.[70,71] Other factors that may contribute to high proportion of seropositivity include herding behavior, large herd sizes, and high animal densities characteristic of bison[29,72] and caribou[73] that favor BVDV transmission. Antibodies to BVDV have also been found in moose, however, a solitary species.[74] During winter migration, yarding and feeding behavior may place species, such as mule deer, that normally form small matrilineal groups, into larger herds, a situation conducive for BVDV transmission.[5] Before the use of BVDV vaccines, BVDV-infected cow herds had seropositive percentages of greater than or equal to 60%.[75] Similar seroprevalence data from wildlife suggest that BVDV may also be maintained in these populations.[76]

Pestiviruses have been isolated from several free-ranging and captive wild species in North America, including bison,[77] white-tailed deer,[78,79] mule deer,[76] Rocky Mountain goats,[80] and pronghorn (Antilocapra americana).[81] These viruses fall into two categories based on their genetic sequences and growth in cell culture. Some of the viruses are indistinguishable from BVDVs isolated from cattle based on RNA sequence information, which suggests that BVDVs found in wild ruminants originated in cattle and have the potential to reinfect domestic herds.[76,78–80] Other genetically divergent pestiviruses seem highly adapted to their host species and may not be transmissible to cattle.[81] Finally, evidence for the existence of PI animals in free-ranging populations has been found in the form of IHC staining positive for BVDV of ear notch samples from hunter-killed deer.[78,79,82,83] The distribution of BVDV antigen in dermal and hair follicle epithelium from deer is similar to that described for PI cattle.[84] The prevalence of IHC samples positive for BVDV in surveys is similar to or lower than the prevalence of PI animals in domestic cattle.[79,85] Some of the IHC samples positive for BVDV were obtained from adult deer. The age of these presumptive PI deer has important ramifications for the perpetuation of BVDV infections in these populations and potential risk of transmission to domestic cattle.

Once BVDV infects a population, most infections are acute and transients. Sometimes, a PI animal is born and survives long enough to infect the next generation of fetuses. Experimental infections have established that intranasal inoculation and exposure of white-tailed does to PI cattle result in fetal infections and the birth of PI fawns.[84,86] The reduction in live births relative to expected fawn numbers, the occurrence of stillbirths, and low birth weights observed in these experimental infections suggest that BVDV may have detrimental effects on fetal survival and fawn livability in deer similar to the case in cattle.[84,86] Demonstration of IHC staining positive for BVDV in adult animals in free-ranging populations suggests, however, that prolonged survival of PI deer occurs at least occasionally in nature.

The minimal requirement for perpetuating BVDV infections within a herd or population is the infection of females during the first trimester of pregnancy. Deer are fall breeders and the first trimester of gestation coincides with late fall and winter season during which some deer herds migrate to form larger and more concentrated groups on their winter range.[5] In the western United States, deer winter in valleys where beef cattle are also gathered. For pregnant does to become infected and generate PI fawns, PI calves would have to be present at these locations during the winter. In general, PI calves are unthrifty and unhealthy; few survive their first year.[87] Beef calves from spring-calving herds are weaned in the fall and the majority, with the exception of replacement heifers, are shipped to auctions, feedyards, or stocker operations. The decreased survivability of PI calves combined with these common management practices would decrease the number of young cattle on winter range and the chances of contact between PI cattle and pregnant does. Other variations in beef cattle management that might increase the risk of contact with PI cattle include the practice of bringing weaned calves onto the premises for backgrounding and fall-calving beef herds, which are more likely to have PI calves present during the winter than are spring-calving herds.[14] The availability of hay stacks and other feed on winter pastures entice deer and elk to feed in proximity to cattle and increase the chance for infectious contacts between species.

In spring-calving beef herds, cows are in the first trimester of pregnancy from late May through August. Free-ranging ruminants, such as deer, elk, and bison, give birth in late May and early June. The timing of these events is such that PI fawns, elk, and bison calves would only have to survive for a few weeks in the summer to provide a potential source of BVDV for cattle. In nature, the survival of deer to 1 year of age is low and is correlated with size, nutrition, and health; smaller and unhealthy fawns are more likely to succumb to starvation and predation.[88] Survival rates for PI fawns are suspected to be low based on experimental observations[84,86] but have not been established in free-ranging populations. If PI status affects birth weight and vigor, then PI fawns might be expected to have poorer survival rates than uninfected fawns, thus a minimal risk for transmission of BVDV from deer to cattle. The supposition that PI affects survivorship, however, must be balanced by evidence for survival of PI yearling and adult deer.[76,78,79,82,83] Species-specific behaviors, such as selection of secluded or heavily wooded birthing locations and caching of fawns, would also reduce the chances of PI fawn interactions with cows.

The transmission of BVDV from wild ruminant species to cattle in nature has not yet been demonstrated. BVDV infections in wildlife, however, are a relatively new area of research interest. As the European bovine viral diarrhea eradication programs for domestic cattle are successfully completed, the role of wild species in the ecology of BVDV and other pestiviruses may be illuminated, particularly with respect to the maintenance of the virus within wild populations. To determine if wildlife serve as a reservoir and potential source of BVDV for cattle in North America, field investigations and epidemiologic studies of free-ranging populations are needed.

SUMMARY

After exposure and infection of a potential wildlife reservoir to a disease agent, many factors influence the outcome. These factors are unique for each cattle/wildlife interface situation and may result in one of several outcomes. In addition to the usual factors to be considered (host susceptibility, shedding, environment, and so forth) are behavior and interaction of the wildlife species and cattle and the synchrony or asynchrony of events, such as parturition and susceptibility to infection. With careful study of each interface situation and the epidemiology and pathogenesis of the disease in each species, it may possible to craft mitigation strategies to control or eliminate interspecies transmission or to eradicate the disease completely.

REFERENCES

1. Corner LAL. The role of wild animal populations in the epidemiology of tuberculosis in domestic animals: how to assess the risk. Vet Microbiol 2006;112:303–12.

2. Cheville NF, McCullough DR, Paulson LR. Brucellosis in the Greater Yellowstone Area. National Research Council, National Academy of Sciences 1998 National Academy of Sciences. Washington, DC: National Academy Press; 1998. p. 186.
3. Etter RP, Drew ML. Brucellosis in elk of eastern Idaho. J Wildl Dis 2006;42(2):271–8.
4. Aguirre AA, Hansen DE, Starkey EE, et al. Serologic survey of wild cervids for potential disease agents in selected national parks in the United States. Prev Vet Med 1995;21:313–22.
5. Conner MM, Ebinger MR, Blanchong JA, et al. Infectious disease in cervids of North America. Ann N Y Acad Sci 2008;1134:146–72.
6. Nishi JS, Shury T, Elkin BT. Wildlife reservoirs for bovine tuberculosis (*Mycobacterium bovis*) in Canada: strategies for management and research. Vet Microbiol 2006;112:325–38.
7. Corner LA, Barrett RH, Lepper AW, et al. A survey of mycobacteriosis of feral pigs in the Northern Territory. Aust Vet J 1981;57(12):537–42.
8. McInerney J, Small KJ, Caley P. Prevalence of *Mycobacterium bovis* infection in feral pigs in the Northern Territory. Aust Vet J 1995;72(12):448–51.
9. Essey MA, Payne RL, Himes EM, et al. Bovine tuberculosis surveys of axis deer and feral swine on the Hawaiian island of Molokai. In: Proceedings of the 85th Annual Meeting of the United States Animal Health Association. St Louis, MO, October 11–6, 1981. p. 538–49.
10. Essey MA, Stallknecht DE, Himes EM, et al. Follow-up survey of feral swine for Mycobacterium bovis infection ont the Hawaiian island of Molokai. In: Proceedings of the 87th Annual Meeting of the United States Animal Health Association. Las Vegas, NV, October 16–21, 1983. p. 589–95.
11. Naranjo V, Gortazar C, Vicente J, et al. Evidence of the role of European wild boar as a reservoir of *Mycobacterium tuberculosis* complex. Vet Microbiol 2008;127:1–9.
12. Zanella G, Durand B, Hars J, et al. *Mycobacterium bovis* in wildlife in France. J Wildl Dis 2008;44(1):99–108.
13. USDA. Dairy 2007, part I: reference of dairy cattle health and management practices in the United States, 2007. USDA–APHIS–VS. #N482.0608, Available at: http://www.aphis.usda.gov/vs/ceah/ncahs/nahms/dairy/index.htm. Accessed 2007.
14. USDA. Beef 2007-08, part I and II: reference of beef cow-calf management practices in the United States, 2007-08. USDA-APHIS-VS. Fort Collins (CO): CEAH; #N512-1008 and #N512.0209.
15. Foster G, Osterman BS, Godfroid J, et al. *Brucella ceti* sp. nov. and *Brucella pinnipedialis* sp. nov. for *Brucella* strains with cetaceans and seals as their preferred hosts. Int J Syst Evol Microbiol 2007;57:2688–93.
16. Godfroid J. Brucellosis in wildlife. Rev Sci Tech 2002;21(2):277–86.
17. Davis DS. Brucellosis in wildlife. In: Neilsen K, Duncan JR, editors. Animal brucellosis. Boca Raton (FL): CRC Press; 1990. p. 322–34.
18. Davis DS, Boer WJ, Mims JP, et al. *Brucella abortus* in coyotes. I. Serologic and bacteriologic survey in eastern Texas. J Wildl Dis 1979;15(3):367–72.
19. Tessaro SV. A descriptive and epizootiologic study of brucellosis and tuberculosis in bison in northern Canada [PhD dissertation]. University of Saskatchewan, Saskatoon, Saskatchewan, Canada; 1988. p. 320.
20. Gese EM, Schultz RD, Johnson MR, et al. Serological survey for diseases in free-ranging coyotes (*Canis latrans*) in Yellowstone National Park, Wyoming. J Wildl Dis 1997;33(1):47–56.
21. Davis DS, Heck FC, Williams JD, et al. Interspecific transmission of *Brucella abortus* from experimentally infected coyotes (*Canis latrans*) to parturient cattle. J Wildl Dis 1988;24(3):533–7.

22. Tessaro SV, Forbes LB. Experimental *Brucella abortus* infection in wolves. J Wildl Dis 2004;40(1):60–5.
23. Benninger CE, Beecham JJ, Thomas LA, et al. A serologic survey for selected infectious diseases of black bears in Idaho. J Wildl Dis 1980;16(3):423–30.
24. Olsen SC, Rhyan J, Gidlewski T, et al. Safety of *Brucella abortus* strain RB51 in black bears. J Wildl Dis 2004;40(3):429–33.
25. Mohler JR. Abortion disease. In: Annual reports of the department of agriculture. Washington, DC: US Department of Agriculture; 1917. p. 105–6.
26. Creech GT. *Brucella abortus* infection in a male bison. N Am Vet 1930;11:35–6.
27. Thorne ET, Morton JK, Thomas GM. Brucellosis in elk I. Serologic and bacteriologic survey in Wyoming. J Wildl Dis 1978;14(1):74–81.
28. Meagher M, Meyer ME. On the origin of brucellosis in bison of Yellowstone National Park: a review. Conserv Biol 1994;8:645–53.
29. Williams ES, Thorne ET, Anderson SL, et al. Brucellosis in free-ranging bison (*Bison bison*) from Teton County, Wyoming. J Wildl Dis 1993;29(1):118–22.
30. Rhyan JC, Gidlewski T, Roffe TJ, et al. Pathology of brucellosis in bison from Yellowstone National Park. J Wildl Dis 2001;37(1):101–9.
31. Rhyan JC, Holland SD, Gidlewski T, et al. Seminal vesiculitis and orchitis caused by *Brucella abortus* biovar 1 in young bison bulls from South Dakota. J Vet Diagn Invest 1997;9:368–74.
32. Fuller JA, Garrott RA, White PJ. Reproduction and survival of Yellowstone bison. J Wildl Manage 2007;71:2365–72.
33. Rhyan JC, Aune K, Roffe T, et al. Pathogenesis and epidemiology of brucellosis in Yellowstone bison: serologic and culture results from adult females and their progeny. J Wildl Dis 2009;45:729–39.
34. Smith SG, Kilpatrick S, Reese AD, et al. Wildlife habitat, feedgrounds, and brucellosis in the Greater Yellowstone Area. In: Thorne ET, Boyce MS, Nicoletti P, et al, editors. Brucellosis, bison, elk, and cattle in the Greater Yellowstone Area: defining the problem, exploring solutions. Cheyenne (WY): Wyoming Game and Fish Department; 1997. p. 65–76.
35. Davis DS, Templeton JW, Ficht TA, et al. *Brucella abortus* in captive bison. I. Serology, bacteriology, pathogenesis, and transmission to cattle. J Wildl Dis 1990;26(3):360–71.
36. Flagg DE. A case history of a brucellosis outbreak in a brucellosis free state which originated in bison. In: Proceedings of the 87th Annual Meeting of the United States Animal Health Association. Las Vegas, NV, October 16–21, 1983. p. 171–2.
37. Aune, K, Rhyan J, Corso B, et al. Environmental persistance of Brucella organisms in natural environments of the Greater Yellowstone Area—a preliminary analysis. In Proceedings of the 110th Annual Meeting of the United States Animal Health Association. Minneapolis, MN, October 12–18, 2007. p. 205–12.
38. Cook WE, Williams ES, Dubay SA. Disappearance of bovine fetuses in northwestern Wyoming. Wildl Soc Bull 2004;32:254–9.
39. Maichak EJ, Scurlock BM, Rogerson JD, et al. Effects of management, behavior, and scavenging on risk of brucellosis transmission in elk of western Wyoming. J Wildl Dis 2009;45(2):398–410.
40. Hillman B. Brucellosis in eastern Idaho. In: Proceedings of the 106th Annual Meeting of the United States Animal Health Association. St Louis, MO, October 17–24, 2003. p. 189–92.
41. Rhyan JC. Brucellosis in terrestrial wildlife and marine mammals. In: Brown C, Bolin C, editors. Emerging diseases of animals. Washington, DC: ASM Press; 2000. p. 161–84.

42. Rhyan JC, Drew M. Contraception: a possible means of decreasing transmission of brucellosis in bison. In: Kreeger TJ, editor. Brucellosis in elk and bison in the Greater Yellowstone Area. Cheyenne (WY): Wyoming Game and Fish Department; 2002. p. 99–108.

43. Miller LA, Rhyan JC, Drew M. Contraception of bison by GnRH vaccine: a possible means of decreasing transmission of brucellosis in bison. J Wildl Dis 2004;40(4):725–30.

44. Killian G, Kreeger TJ, Rhyan J, et al. Observation of the use of Gonacon in captive female elk (Cervus elaphus). J Wildl Dis 2009;45(1):184–8.

45. Schmitt SM, Fitzgerald SD, Cooley TM, et al. Bovine tuberculosis in free-ranging white-tailed deer from Michigan. J Wildl Dis 1997;33(4):749–58.

46. O'Brien DJ, Schmitt SM, Fitzgerald SD, et al. Managing the wildlife reservoir of Mycobacterium bovis: the Michigan, USA, experience. Vet Microbiol 2006;112:313–23.

47. Lees VW, Copeland S, Rousseau P, et al. Bovine tuberculosis in elk (Cervus elaphus manitobensis) near Riding Mountain National Park, Manitoba, from 1992 to 2002. Can Vet J 2003;44:830–1.

48. Connell KM. Report of the committee on tuberculosis. In: Proceedings of the 111th Annual Meeting of the United States Animal Health Association. Reno, NV, October 18–24, 2007. p. 738–69.

49. Bruning-Fann CS, Schmitt SM, Fitzgerald SD, et al. Bovine tuberculosis in free-ranging carnivores from Michigan. J Wildl Dis 2001;37(1):58–64.

50. Bruning-Fann CS, Schmitt SM, Fitzgerald SD, et al. Mycobacterium bovis in coyotes from Michigan. J Wildl Dis 1998;34(3):632–6.

51. Renwick AR, White PCL, Bengis RG. Bovine tuberculosis in southern African wildlife: a multi-species host-pathogen system. Epidemiol Infect 2007;135:529–40.

52. Palmer MV, Whipple DL. Survival of Mycobacterium bovis on feedstuffs commonly used as supplemental feed for white-tailed deer (Odocoileus virginianus). J Wildl Dis 2006;42(4):853–8.

53. Palmer MV, Waters WR, Whipple DL. Shared feed as a means of deer-to-deer transmission of Mycobacterium bovis. J Wildl Dis 2004;40(1):87–91.

54. Palmer MV, Waters WR, Whipple DL. Investigation of the transmission of Mycobacterium bovis from deer to cattle through indirect contact. Am J Vet Res 2004;65(11):1483–9.

55. Sauter CM, Morris RS. Dominance hierarchies in cattle and red deer (Cervus elaphus): their possible relationship to transmission of bovine tuberculosis. N Z Vet J 1995;43:301–5.

56. Muirhead RH, Gallagher J, Burn KJ. Tuberculosis in wild badgers in Gloucestershire: epidemiology. Vet Rec 1974;95(24):552–5.

57. Bohm M, Hutchings MR, White PCL. Contact networks in a wildlife-livestock host community: identifying high-risk individuals in the transmission of bovine TB among badgers and cattle. PLoS ONE 2009;4(4):e5016.

58. Munyeme M, Muma JB, Samui KL, et al. Prevalence of bovine tuberculosis and animal level risk factors for indigenous cattle under different grazing strategies in the livestock/wildlife interface areas of Zambia. Trop Anim Health Prod 2009; 41:345–52.

59. Scantlebury M, Hutchings MR, Allcroft DJ, et al. Risk of disease from wildlife reservoirs: badgers, cattle, and bovine tuberculosis. J Dairy Sci 2004;87:330–9.

60. Blanchong JA, Scribner KT, Kravchenko AN, et al. TB-infected deer are more closely related than non-infected deer. Biol Lett 2007;3(1):103–5.

61. Nol P, Palmer MV, Waters FE, et al. Efficacy of oral and parenteral Mycobacterium bovis bacilli Calmette-Guerin vaccination against experimental bovine

tuberculosis in white-tailed deer (*Odocoileus virginianus*): a feasibility study. J Wildl Dis 2008;44(2):247–59.

62. Palmer MV, Thacker TC, Waters WR. Vaccination of white-tailed deer (*Odocoileus virginianus*) with *Mycobacterium bovis* bacillus Calmette Guerin. Vaccine 2007; 25:2589–97.

63. Brownlie J, Clarke MC, Howard CJ. Experimental production of fatal mucosal disease in cattle. Vet Rec 1984;114:535–6.

64. McClurkin MW, Littledike ET, Cutlip RC, et al. Production of cattle immunotolerant to bovine viral diarrhea virus (BVDV). Can J Comp Med 1984;48:156–61.

65. Coria MF, McClurkin AW. Specific immune tolerance in an apparently healthy bull persistently infected with bovine viral diarrhea virus. J Am Vet Med Assoc 1978; 172:449–51.

66. Van Campen H, Frolich K, Hofmann M. Pestivirus infections. In: Williams ES, Barker IK, editors. Infectious diseases of wild mammals. 3rd edition. Ames (IA): Iowa State University Press; 2001. p. 232–44.

67. Stauber E, Nellis CH, Magonigle RA, et al. Prevalence of selected livestock pathogens in Idaho mule deer. J Wildl Manage 1977;41:515–9.

68. Kingscote BF, Yates WDG, Tiffin GB. Diseases of wapiti utilizing cattle range in southwestern Alberta. J Wildl Dis 1987;23(1):86–91.

69. Wolf K, DePerno CS, Jenks JA, et al. Selenium status and antibodies to selected pathogens in while-tailed deer (*Odocoileus virginianus*) in southern Minnesota. J Wildl Dis 2008;44(1):181–7.

70. Zarnke RL. Serologic survey for selected microbial pathogens in Alaskan wildlife. J Wildl Dis 1983;19:324–9.

71. Sadi L, Joyal R, St.-Georges M, et al. Serologic survey of white-tailed deer on Anticosti Island, Quebec for bovine herpesvirus 1, bovine viral diarrhea, and parainfluenza 3. J Wildl Dis 1991;27:569–77.

72. Taylor SK, Lane VM, Hunter DL, et al. Serologic survey for infectious pathogens in free-ranging American bison. J Wildl Dis 1997;33:308–11.

73. Elazhary MASY, Frechette JL, Silim A, et al. Serological evidence of some bovine viruses in the caribou (*Rangifer tarandus caribou*) in Quebec. J Wildl Dis 1981;17: 609–12.

74. Van Campen H, Williams ES. Wildlife and bovine viral diarrhea virus. In: Proceedings for the International Symposium: bovine viral diarrhea virus, a 50 year review. Ithaca (NY); 1996. p. 167–75.

75. Malmquist WA. Bovine viral diarrhea-mucosal disease: etiology, pathogenesis, and applied immunity. J Am Vet Med Assoc 1968;152(6):763–8.

76. Van Campen H, Ridpath J, Williams E, et al. Isolation of bovine viral diarrhea virus from a free-ranging mule deer (*Odocoileus hemionus*). J Wildl Dis 2001;37(2): 306–11.

77. Deregt D, Tessaro SV, Baxi MK, et al. Isolation of bovine viral diarrhea viruses from bison. Vet Rec 2005;157:448–50.

78. Chase C, Braun LJ, Leslie-Steen P, et al. Bovine viral diarrhea virus multiorgan infection in two white-tailed deer in southeastern South Dakota. J Wildl Dis 2008;44(3):753–9.

79. Pogranichniy RM, Raizman E, Thacker HL, et al. Prevalence and characterization of bovine viral diarrhea virus in the white-tailed deer population in Indiana. J Vet Diagn Invest 2008;20:71–4.

80. Nelson DD, Dark MJ, Bradway DS, et al. Evidence for persistent bovine viral diarrhea virus infection in a captive mountain goat (*Oreamnos americanus*). J Vet Diagn Invest 2008;20:752–9.

81. Vilcek S, Ridpath J, Van Campen H, et al. Characterization of a novel pestivirus originating from a pronghorn antelope. Virus Res 2005;108(1–2):187–93.
82. Duncan C, Ridpath J, Palmer MV, et al. Histopathologic and immunohistochemical findings in two white-tailed deer fawns persistently infected with bovine viral diarrhea virus. J Vet Diagn Invest 2008;20:289–96.
83. Passler T, Walz PH, Ditchkoff SS, et al. Evaluation of hunter-harvested white-tailed deer for evidence of bovine viral diarrhea virus infection in Alabama. J Vet Diagn Invest 2008;20:79–82.
84. Njaa BL, Clark EG, Janzen E, et al. Diagnosis of persistent bovine viral diarrhea virus infection by immunohistochemical staining of formalin-fixed skin biopsy specimens. J Vet Diagn Invest 2000;12:393–9.
85. Duncan C, Van Campen H, Soto S, et al. Persistent bovine viral diarrhea virus infection in wild cervids of Colorado. J Vet Diagn Invest 2008;20(5):650–3.
86. Passler T, Walz PH, Ditchkoff SS, et al. Cohabitation of pregnant white-tailed deer and cattle persistently infected with bovine viral diarrhea virus results in persistently infected fawns. Vet Microbiol 2009;134(3-4):362–7.
87. Taylor LF, Janzen ED, Ellis JA, et al. Performance, survival necropsy, and virological findings from calves persistently infected with the bovine viral diarrhea virus from a single Saskatchewan beef herd. Can Vet J 1997;38(1):29–37.
88. Bishop CJ, White GC, Freddy DJ, et al. Effect of enhanced nutrition on mule deer population rate of change. Wildl Monogr 2009;172:1–28.

Global Implications of the Recent Emergence of Bluetongue Virus in Europe

N. James Maclachlan, BVSc, MS, PhD

KEYWORDS

• Bluetongue • Virus • Arbovirus • Climate change

The process and potential consequences of global climate change were recently summarized by Tim Flannery[1] who posed the provocative question, "So great are the changes scientists are detecting in our atmosphere that time's gates appear once again to be opening. Will the Anthropocene become the shortest geological period on record?" With increasing acceptance of the implied reality of climate change, it has been proposed that this process will favor emergence of arthropod-transmitted virus (arbovirus) diseases because, in part, the tropical insects and the agents they transmit will expand their habitat as the planet warms.[2–5] However, the emergence and spread of arbovirus infections is a complex, multifactorial process, and concrete examples of such events where the role of global warming has been unambiguously defined are lacking.[6]

Chikungunya, dengue, and certain other mosquito-transmitted viruses have recently expanded their respective geographic ranges, consistent with the premise that climate change will favor emergence of arbovirus diseases. However, the direct role of global warming in dispersion of these diseases is uncertain as their spread appears to be most correlated with anthropogenic and social factors, or the movement of virus-infected vectors or their hosts.[7–10] Furthermore, contrary to the predicted emergence of arbovirus infections with climate change, the incidence of other mosquito-transmitted diseases such as those caused by western equine and Saint Louis encephalitis viruses has decreased markedly in western North America in recent years.[11,12] Further complicating interpretation of the impact of climate change on emergence of arbovirus infections is the fact that climate change will itself continue to precipitate adaptive social and economic changes, which, in turn, may contribute directly to emergence and re-emergence of insect-transmitted diseases.

Department of Pathology, Microbiology and Immunology, School of Veterinary Medicine, University of California, One Shields Avenue, Davis, CA 95616, USA
E-mail address: njmaclachlan@ucdavis.edu

Vet Clin Food Anim 26 (2010) 163–171
doi:10.1016/j.cvfa.2009.10.012
0749-0720/10/$ – see front matter © 2010 Elsevier Inc. All rights reserved.

Thus, there is much conjecture and debate regarding the impact of climate change on emergence of arbovirus diseases, and to predicting what might be in store in the future for all residents of the planet, including humans and their livestock.

Bluetongue (BT) is an insect-transmitted disease of ruminants that has recently spread throughout much of Europe leading to an unprecedented pandemic in regions where BT has never been previously documented.[13] Several studies have concluded that climate change is responsible for the emergence of BT in Europe,[14–16] raising the question of whether BT might be the "point of the spear" in terms of global emergence of arbovirus diseases driven by climate change. However, the processes that lead to the recent emergence of BT virus (BTV) infection in northern Europe would appear to be distinct from those that resulted in the earlier spread of multiple BTV serotypes throughout the Mediterranean Basin. The objective of this article, therefore, is to summarize these recent events in Europe in the context of potential global emergence of BTV infection and BT disease of ruminants.

BT

BTV is the prototype virus of the genus *Orbivirus*, family Reoviridae.[17] There are currently 24 recognized serotypes of BTV worldwide, with a probable 25th recently identified amongst goats in Switzerland.[18] BT occurs most commonly in sheep of certain breeds, non-African wild ungulates, and very sporadically in cattle, South American camelids, and even carnivores.[19] Symptoms include conjunctivitis, rhinitis with nasal exudate, and ulceration of the nares (**Fig. 1**A, B), as well as coronitis, facial edema, oral ulceration, muscle necrosis and pulmonary edema.

Biting (hematophagous) insects of the genus *Culicoides* serve as true biologic vectors that transmit BTV infection between susceptible ruminants and, once infected,

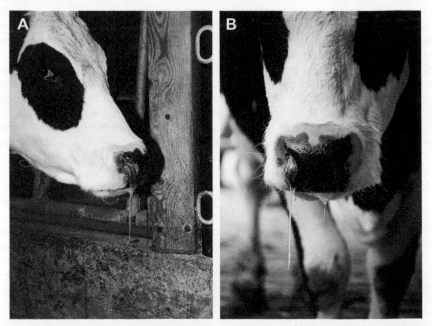

Fig. 1. (*A, B*) Conjunctivitis, rhinitis with nasal exudate, and ulceration of the nares in cattle affected with bluetongue. (*Courtesy of* Christian Griot, Dr med vet, and Gabriella Worwa, Dr med vet, Mittelhäusern, Switzerland.)

competent insects remain persistently infected with BTV throughout their lives.[20] These insects occur on all continents except Antarctica, often in remarkable population densities. However, of the more than one thousand species of *Culicoides* that occur worldwide, only about 30 have been incriminated as likely vectors of BTV infection.[21,22] The species of vector insects that transmit BTV differ between regions of the world, as do the constellations of BTV serotypes that exist in each ecosystem.[23–25]

Appropriate climatic conditions are important to the regional maintenance of BTV infection, thus the virus exists throughout much of the world between latitudes of approximately 40° to 50° north and 35° south.[23–25] However, the virus has spread recently in portions of Europe far beyond the upper limits of this traditional range.[26] Similarly, multiple novel serotypes of BTV have been identified recently in the southeastern United States where they were not detected previously,[27,28] and additional novel serotypes of BTV were also identified recently in the north of Australia and Israel. This profound and simultaneous change in the nature or distribution of BTV infection on at least three continents suggests that the epidemiology of BTV infection is changing. The essential question now becomes—what is the role of climate change in mediating this apparent global emergence of BTV?

THE ONGOING BT PANDEMIC IN EUROPE

BTV has recently spread throughout most of Europe where, until approximately 1998, only sporadic and transient epizootics of BTV infection occurred.[13,26,29,30] Furthermore, there were marked differences in the epidemiologic features of the virus incursions into northern Europe and the Mediterranean Basin. Indeed, different BTV serotypes initially were involved in the incursions of BTV into northern Europe (serotypes 6, 8, and 11) and the Mediterranean Basin (serotypes 1, 2, 4, 9, and 16). However, these two ecosystems are now rapidly merging so that common virus serotypes occur within each (in particular, serotype 8 from northern Europe into the Mediterranean Basin and serotype 1 from the Mediterranean Basin into northern Europe) (**Fig. 2**).

The Mediterranean Basin

BTV has historically been enzootic throughout sub-Saharan Africa, extensive portions of Asia, and much of the Middle East including Israel. Prior outbreaks of BT that occurred in Cyprus, the Iberian Peninsula, and Greece were caused by a single BTV serotype, suggesting that these were transient incursional events from adjacent enzootic regions. Since 1998, however, five different serotypes of BTV (serotypes 1, 2, 4, 9, and16) have invaded the Mediterranean Basin, including Italy, France, Greece, Spain, Portugal, and the Balkan countries.[13–16,26,29,30] Subsequent molecular analyses have confirmed unequivocally that these viruses invaded the region using two different paths: a western pathway through North Africa and an eastern pathway via the Middle East.[15,31] The initial incursions of these viruses have been attributed to the long distance, wind-borne spread of virus-infected vector insects, which then infected naïve ruminants in these areas. These animals were, in turn, the source of infection to resident "local" vector insects. Although *Culicoides imicola*, a major Asian-African vector of BTV is present in the Mediterranean Basin, it was quickly recognized that other species[13,16,21,22] were important in regional transmission of the virus, including *C obsoletus* and *C pulicaris*.

Analysis of available data has strongly linked the unprecedented emergence of BTV throughout the Mediterranean Basin to climate change, which is a rare example where the impact of climate change on emergence of an arbovirus disease is clearly

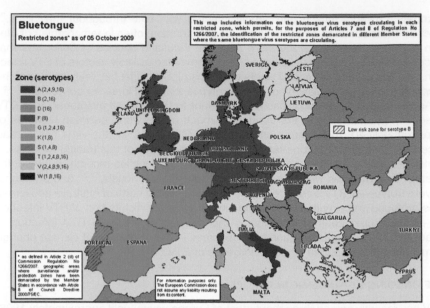

Fig. 2. Restricted zones (serotypes) for bluetongue virus in Europe as of October 5, 2009. *From* European Commission. Restriction zones established by the Member States. Available at: http://ec.europa.eu/food/animal/diseases/controlmeasures/bt_restrictedzones-map.jpg. Copyright © European Communities, 1995–2009. Accessed October 20, 2009.

evident.[14–16] It is abundantly clear that temperature profoundly affects the replication of BTV within vector insects, thus increased ambient temperature would be expected to increase the ability of potential vectors to transmit BTV on a population basis (vectorial capacity).[32] However, the various impacts of climate change that resulted in the emergence of BTV in the Mediterranean Basin are likely to be complex and multifactorial. Nevertheless, the central conclusion remains that five serotypes of BTV have recently invaded and persisted in extensive portions of the Mediterranean Basin where only transient incursions of single BTV serotypes had been documented previously, and that there is an impressive body of evidence linking this unprecedented event to climate change.[14–16]

Individual countries responded differently to the appearance of BTV, and live-attenuated vaccines were widely used in some but certainly not all affected areas. Until very recently, the five BTV serotypes that invaded the Mediterranean Basin all remained confined to the northern rim of the region and did not extend further than approximately 44° north. In Italy, for example, the virus did not extend beyond the Po Valley despite the presence of apparently competent vector insects further north. Similarly, BTV spread throughout much of the Balkan countries but not beyond. There is clear evidence that the strain of BTV serotype 16 that spread through the Balkans is related closely to a live-attenuated vaccine strain of BTV serotype 16 used elsewhere in the Mediterranean Basin,[33] which raises concerns regarding the potential of vaccines to contribute to the regional emergence of BTV. Although initially confined to the immediate region of the Mediterranean Basin, BTV serotype 1 has recently moved progressively northward on the Iberian Peninsula and into southwestern France. Late in 2008, the virus was identified for the first time in Normandy from where it is spreading into adjacent regions. The ecological factors that previously restricted the northern movement of the five serotypes of BTV that invaded the Mediterranean Basin are not yet well understood, nor is it clear what factors lead to the northern spread of serotype 1.

Northern Europe

The unexpected appearance and subsequent rapid spread of BTV serotype 8 that began in northern Europe in 2006[34–37] is especially remarkable because this virus has spread farther north than natural BTV infection of animals and insects has been reported previously, reaching Scandinavia and the United Kingdom. Furthermore, the virus is spread by Palearctic species of *Culicoides* insects and not *C imicola*, which is a major vector of BTV in Africa and Asia.[22] The strain of BTV 8 that invaded northern Europe is highly virulent, not only for sheep but also cattle, free-ranging and captive species of non-African ungulates, South American camelids, and even zoo carnivores fed aborted, virus-infected fetal ruminants.[19,34–41] This strain of BTV serotype 8 also crosses the ruminant placenta to cause fetal infections with remarkable frequency, which is unusual compared with other "field" strains of BTV that occur elsewhere in the world.[19] Indeed, transplacental transmission of BTV previously was considered to be largely or exclusively a property of laboratory-adapted strains of BTV, particularly certain live-attenuated vaccine viruses.[19,42] These properties have raised questions regarding the history and origin of this virus, although it is genetically distinct from the live-attenuated serotype 8 vaccine virus used in South Africa. In 2008, BTV serotype 6 emerged in the same general area in which BTV serotype 8 had emerged 2 years before, and BTV serotype 11 very recently was reported in Belgium.

The route of introduction of BTV serotypes 6, 8, and 11 into Northern Europe is uncertain as these BTV serotypes did not first invade the Mediterranean Basin and then spread northward, as serotype 1 has done recently. Furthermore, the strains of BTV serotypes 6 and 11 apparently include gene segments derived from either South African laboratory prototype viruses or live-attenuated vaccine viruses derived from them, which further accentuates the potential for human activities to contribute to the regional emergence of BTV infection. Regardless of the route or routes of entry of the serotypes of BTV that have invaded northern Europe, once present in the region these viruses have been efficiently spread by Palearctic species of *Culicoides* insects, even in relatively wet, cool, and even cold regions. Several species of *Culicoides* insects resident in the region, including *C obsoletus*, *C dewulffi*, and *C chiopterus*, that were not previously considered as likely vectors are now efficient at transmitting BTV.

Why the Palearctic *Culicoides* species of northern Europe have recently become such efficient vectors of BTV remains uncertain. It would seem highly probable that these insects were exposed to BTV infected livestock or wild ungulates imported into the region in the past, but apparently without subsequent spread of the virus. Indirectly, this might suggest that environmental changes in general, and climate change in particular, have altered the vectorial capacity of these insect populations that have long been resident in northern Europe. The fact that some of these species apparently exist throughout the entire Holarctic region, which includes North America, indicates there is an as yet undefined potential for this virus to continue to spread throughout the world. Unfortunately, these insects have been largely unstudied and it is increasingly apparent that they constitute a broad genetic spectrum.[43] Thus, *Culicoides* insects within a specific taxonomic group likely vary in their efficiency as virus vectors, and potentially in their individual responses to environmental influences such as those induced by climate change. Without better characterization of these critical vector species, it will be difficult to logically define the risk posed by Palearctic *Culicoides* species already resident elsewhere in the world and to accurately predict the potential of highly virulent strains of BTV, such as the European strain of BTV serotype 8, to spread very widely.

CURRENT STATUS OF BTV IN THE AMERICAS AND ELSEWHERE

Until recently, at least two distinct and apparently stable BTV ecosystems existed in the Americas.[23–25] C sonorensis is the predominant, if not exclusive, vector of BTV serotypes 10, 11, 13, and 17 throughout much of the United States, south of the so-called Sonorensis Line that extends from approximately Washington in the west to Maryland in the east. The virus periodically and transiently incurs into a limited portion of Canada (the Okanagan Valley). Although C sonorensis is established even further north than the Sonorensis Line, including portions of Canada, ongoing sero-logic evaluation of ruminants in the region over many years has confirmed that climatic factors preclude significant virus transmission to livestock. BTV serotype 2 was first identified in Florida in the 1980s but has never been identified outside of the south-eastern portion of the United States.

In Central and South America and the Caribbean Basin, C insignis is the predomi-nant vector of a substantial number of different serotypes of BTV.[23–25] The two Amer-ican BTV ecosystems interface adjacent to the southeastern United States but, despite the lack of significant geographic barriers most BTV serotypes within the Caribbean Basin, apparently did not incur previously into the southeastern United States or did not persist if they did so. In recent years (since 1999), however, at least 10 novel (in addition to the previously enzootic serotypes 2, 10, 11, 13, and 17) BTV serotypes have been isolated from animals in the southeastern United States, including BTV serotypes 1, 3, 5, 6, 9, 12, 14, 19, 22, and 24.[27,28] Available information suggests that these viruses have not spread beyond the southeastern United States but, in light of recent experiences in Europe, it would be imprudent to ignore the possi-bility that these viruses might spread far beyond their original site of incursion and potentially use additional species of Culicoides insects as vectors to facilitate their spread. The temperature effects of climate change are especially pronounced in the southeastern United States,[14] thus there is a very real possibility that species of Culi-coides that previously were not considered as vectors of BTV could become so. A central conclusion is that any change in the epidemiology of BTV infection in the United States equivalent to that which recently has occurred in Europe will most quickly and efficiently be detected through prospective serologic and virological surveillance of sentinel ruminants in key regions throughout the United States.

The recent emergence of BTV in Europe is unique because of the associated occur-rence of severe disease in susceptible animal species. Similarly, the recent emergence in Israel of BTV serotypes 8, 15, and 24 was associated with outbreaks of BT disease that was often severe. Only BTV serotypes 2, 4, 6, 10, and 16 were recognized in Israel before 2006. In contrast, the appearance of additional novel serotypes of BTV in the southeastern United States was not associated with any dramatically obvious increased expression of disease in domestic ruminants. Similarly, additional novel serotypes of BTV were isolated recently in northern Australia without any associated occurrence of clinical disease. Specifically, BTV serotypes 2 and 7 were identified in 2007 to 2008. Australia has long maintained an intensive prospective surveillance program using sentinel cattle that previously has identified BTV serotypes 1, 3, 9, 15, 16, 20, 21, and 23 in the continent. This surveillance system rapidly can identify the incursion of new viruses, either new serotypes or novel genotypes of BTV. Given recent events in Europe and the unmistakable impact of climate change, it would seem very appropriate that all countries at the incursional margins of the global range of BTV adopt and institute similar global surveillance strategies.

SUMMARY

The disconcerting warning to the global community provided by the events that lead to the recent emergence of BTV throughout much of Europe is self-evident. Although it is not yet clear just how far the highly virulent strain of BTV serotype 8 that appeared in northern Europe in 2008 might eventually spread, the fact that this virus has spread so rapidly in the absence of "traditional" vector species of *Culicoides* insects is disconcerting because the Palearctic species that so efficiently transmit BTV in extensive portions of Europe also occur throughout much of the upper portions of the northern hemisphere, including North America. The rapid spread of BTV serotype 8 into Scandinavia, Eastern Europe, the United Kingdom and the Mediterranean Basin since its initial incursion in 2006 would suggest that this virus has yet to encounter ecological barriers that will determine its range, thus it is difficult to predict what the distribution of this virus ultimately will be.

Although there is substantial evidence linking climate change to the emergence of BT in Europe, both in the Mediterranean Basin and in northern Europe, much remains to be learned regarding specific aspects of this link between climatic factors and the epizootiology of BTV infection. Similarly, the potential involvement of climate change in mediating the emergence of novel serotypes of the virus into the southeastern United States and northern Australia is highly disconcerting as it suggests that previously stable ecosystems are now expanding. Serious outbreaks of disease can be expected to follow the incursion of BTV into regions where livestock have never been exposed previously to the virus and, coupled with difficulties in controlling spread of the virus, this will lead to substantial economic disruption potentially of the magnitude recently encountered in Europe. It is critical that the mechanisms responsible for the emergence and regional spread of BTV in previously free regions be determined, through identification of anthropogenic and climatic factors that were responsible for the remarkable recent events in Europe. In particular, this will require thorough analysis of the impact of the various aspects of climate change on the populations of *Culicoides* insects that occur within each region. Only through such understanding will the economically devastating impact of such events be prevented or minimized in the future. Ongoing prospective surveillance is essential for rapid identification of any such events in the future.

Despite repeated assertions that climate change will alter the distribution of arboviruses and their vectors, specific examples are lacking wherein the role of global warming alone has been unambiguously defined in the spread of such infections. Thus, the recent emergence of BTV infection throughout extensive portions of Europe has attracted much interest because of the potential role of climate change and, in particular, increased ambient temperature[14] in causing the drastic recent alteration in the global distribution of this virus. Specifically, could this event be the "point of the spear" in terms of global emergence of arbovirus infections driven by climate change? Only certain species of *Culicoides* insects can serve as biologic vectors that transmit BTV infection between ruminants, and ambient temperature exerts profound effects on the vectorial capacity of populations of these insects.

REFERENCES

1. Flannery T. The weather makers. Melbourne (Australia): Text Publishing Co; 2005. p. 68.

2. Gould EA, Higgs S, Buckley A, et al. Potential arbovirus emergence and implications for the United Kingdom. Emerg Infect Dis 2006;12:549–55.
3. MacDonald NE. West Nile virus in the context of climate change. Can J Infect Dis Med Microbiol 2008;19:217–8.
4. Pinto J, Bonacic C, Hamilton-West C, et al. Climate change and animal diseases in South America. Rev Sci Tech 2008;27:599–613.
5. Gould EA, Higgs S. Impact of climate change and other factors on emerging arbovirus diseases. Trans R Soc Trop Med Hyg 2009;103:109–21.
6. Zell R, Krumbholz A, Wutzler P. Impact of global warming on viral diseases: what is the evidence? Curr Opin Biotechnol 2008;19:652–60.
7. Petersen LR, Marfin AA. Shifting epidemiology of Flaviviridae. J Travel Med 2005; 12(Suppl 1):S3–11.
8. Pialoux G, Gauzere BA, Jaurequiberry S, et al. Chikungunya, an epidemic arbovirosis. Lancet Infect Dis 2007;7:319–27.
9. Beebe NW, Cooper RD, Mottran P, et al. Australia's dengue risk driven by human adaption to climate change. PLoS Negl Trop Dis 2009;3:e429.
10. Russell RC, Currie BJ, Lindsay MD, et al. Dengue and climate change in Australia: predictions for the future should incorporate knowledge from the past. Med J Aust 2009;190:265–8.
11. Reisen WK, Carroll BD, Takahashi R, et al. Repeated West Nile virus epidemic transmission in Kern County, California, 2004–2007. J Med Entomol 2009;46:139–57.
12. Forrester NL, Kenney JL, Deardoff E, et al. Western equine encephalitis submergence: lack of evidence for a decline in virus virulence. Virology 2008;380:170–2.
13. Mellor PS, Carpenter S, Harrup L, et al. Bluetongue in Europe and the Mediterranean Basin: history of occurrence prior to 2006. Prev Vet Med 2008;87:4–20.
14. Purse BV, Mellor PS, Roger DJ, et al. Climate change and the recent emergence of bluetongue in Europe. Nature Rev Microbiol 2005;3:171–81.
15. Purse B, Brown HE, Harrup L, et al. Invasion of bluetongue and other orbivirus infections into Europe: the role of biological and climatic processes. Rev Sci Tech 2008;27:427–42.
16. Wilson A, Mellor P. Bluetongue in Europe: vectors, epidemiology and climate change. Parasitol Res 2008;103(Suppl 1):S69–77.
17. Mertens PP, Diprose J, Maan S, et al. Bluetongue virus replication, molecular and structural biology. Vet Italiana 2004;40:426–37.
18. Hoffman MA, Renzullo S, Mader M, et al. Genetic characterization of toggenberg orbivirus, a new bluetongue virus, from goats, Switzerland. Emerg Infect Dis 2008;14:1855–61.
19. Maclachlan NJ, Drew CP, Darpel KE, et al. The pathology and pathogenesis of bluetongue. J Comp Pathol 2009;141:1–16.
20. Mellor PS. Replication of arboviruses in insect vectors. J Comp Pathol 2000;123: 231–47.
21. Meiswinkel R, Gomulski LM, Delecolle JC, et al. The taxonomy of Culicoides vector complexes-unfinished business. Vet Italiana 2004;40:151–9.
22. Meiswinkel R, Baldet T, de Deken R, et al. The 2006 outbreak of bluetongue in northern Europe—the entomological perspective. Prev Vet Med 2008;87:55–63.
23. Gibbs EP, Greiner EC. The epidemiology of bluetongue. Comp Immunol Microbiol Infect Dis 1994;17:207–20.
24. Tabachnick WJ. Culicoides and the global epidemiology of bluetongue virus infection. Vet Italiana 2004;40:145–50.
25. Maclachlan NJ, Osburn BI. Impact of bluetongue virus infection on the international movement and trade of ruminants. J Am Vet Med Assoc 2006;228:1346–9.

26. Saegerman C, Berkvens D, Mellor PS. Bluetongue epidemiology in the European Union. Emerg Infect Dis 2008;14:539–44.
27. Johnson DJ, Ostlund EN, Stallknecht DE, et al. First report of bluetongue virus serotype 1 isolated from a white-tailed deer in the United States. J Vet Diagn Invest 2006;18:398–401.
28. Johnson DJ, Ostlund EN, Mertens PP, et al. Exotic bluetongue viruses identified from ruminants in the Southeastern U.S. from 1999–2006. Proc US Anim Hlth Assoc 2007;111:209–10.
29. Gomez-Trejedor C. Brief overview of the bluetongue situation in Mediterranean Europe. Vet Italiana 2004;40:57–60.
30. Rodriguez-Sanchez B, Iglesias-Martin I, Martinez-Aviles M, et al. Orbiviruses in the Mediterranean basin: updated epidemiological situation of Bluetongue and new methods for the detection of BTV serotype 4. Transbound Emerg Dis 2008;55:205–14.
31. Maan S, Maan NS, Ross-Smith N, et al. Sequence analysis of bluetongue virus serotype 8 from the Netherlands 2006 and comparison to other European strains. Virology 2008;377:308–18.
32. Gerry AC, Mullens BA, Maclachlan NJ, et al. Seasonal transmission of bluetongue virus by *Culicoides sonorensis* (Diptera: Ceratopogonidae) at a southern California dairy and evaluation of vectorial capacity as a predictor of bluetongue virus transmission. J Med Entomol 2001;38:197–209.
33. Listes E, Monaco F, Labrovic A, et al. First evidence of bluetongue virus serotype 16 in Croatia. Vet Microbiol 2009;138:92–7.
34. Enserink M. Emerging infectious diseases: during a hot summer, bluetongue invades northern Europe. Science 2006;313:1218–9.
35. Thiry E, Saegerman C, Guyot H, et al. Bluetongue in northern Europe. Vet Rec 2006;159:327.
36. Elbers AR, Backx A, Meroc E, et al. Field observations during the bluetongue serotype 8 epidemic in 2006. I. Detection of the first outbreaks and clinical signs in sheep and cattle in Belgium, France and the Netherlands. Prev Vet Med 2008; 87:21–30.
37. Elbers AR, Backx A, Mintiens K, et al. Field observations during the Bluetongue serotype 8 epidemic in 2006. II. Morbidity and mortality rate, case fatality and clinical recovery in sheep and cattle in the Netherlands. Prev Vet Med 2008;87: 31–40.
38. Darpel KE, Batten CA, Veronesi E, et al. Clinical signs and pathology shown by British sheep and cattle infected with bluetongue virus serotype 8 derived from the 2006 outbreak in northern Europe. Vet Rec 2007;161:253–61.
39. Dal Pozzo F, De Clercq CA, Guyot H, et al. Experimental reproduction of blue-tongue virus serotype 8 clinical disease in calves. Vet Microbiol 2009;136: 352–8.
40. Henrich M, Reinacher M, Hamann HP. Lethal bluetongue virus infection in an alpaca. Vet Rec 2007;161:764.
41. Jauniaux TP, De Clercq KE, Casssart DE, et al. Bluetongue in Eurasian lynx. Emerg Infect Dis 2008;14:1496–8.
42. Maclachlan NJ, Osburn BI. Induced brain lesions in calves infected with blue-tongue virus. Vet Rec 2008;162:490–1.
43. Kiehl E, Waldorf V, Kimpel D, et al. The European vectors of bluetongue virus: are there species complexes, single species or races in Culicoides obsoletus and C. pullicaris detectable by sequencing ITS-1, ITS-2 and 18S-rDNA. Parasitol Res 2009;105:331–6.

Vaccination Strategies for Emerging Disease Epidemics of Livestock

D. Scott McVey, DVM, PhD[a],*, Jishu Shi, DVM, PhD[b]

KEYWORDS

• Vaccination • Immunization • Livestock immunization
• Foot and mouth disease

INTRODUCTION—TRADITIONAL VACCINATION

Vaccination of susceptible populations has been a successful and relatively safe and efficient means of disease prevention.[1] Smallpox immunization has achieved near-complete prevention of infection and transmission and has led to eradication of the disease from the planet.[2] In the case of smallpox, mass immunization of entire populations coupled with isolation and quarantine practices were effective. The vaccinia virus was used as the primary immunogen in these programs. Live vaccine virus delivered as an intradermal vaccine conferred immunity for up to 20 years. This same basic strategy has been used to vaccinate human and animal populations against many infectious diseases with variable degrees of success.[1] As the incidence of many infectious diseases has been drastically or completely reduced in some regions, immunization strategies have begun to focus on blocking infection and transmission from discrete outbreaks within specific geographic regions.[3] The objective of these control strategies (as a component of integrated outbreak management) would be to limit disease spread from the initial point of disease outbreak. With respect to cattle populations, effective outbreak control would limit animal suffering and the economic impact of direct disease losses and potential trade restrictions.

The traditional and most common method of immunizing cattle populations is to broadly immunize potentially susceptible animals (which may be all animals in

[a] Department of Clinical Microbiology, School of Veterinary Medicine and Biomedical Sciences, University of Nebraska Lincoln, Lincoln, NE
[b] Department of Anatomy and Physiology, College of Veterinary Medicine, Kansas State University, Manhattan, KS
* Corresponding author.
E-mail address: dmcvey2@unlnotes.unl.edu (D.S. McVey).

Vet Clin Food Anim 26 (2010) 173–183
doi:10.1016/j.cvfa.2009.10.004
0749-0720/10/$ – see front matter

a herd setting) with particular emphasis on young animals and new herd additions.[1] The delivery of vaccines may be timed to provide immunity during seasonal periods of vulnerability (before breeding for example) or during times of production-related stress (such as pre- or postweaning periods). The success of immunization depends on the clinical efficacy of the vaccine, the immunologic potency of the vaccine, effective administration of the vaccine, and the use of sound herd management strategies.[4]

There are many factors that must be considered when making decisions regarding immunization strategies. Among these considerations is the most probable nature of the disease threat. If a disease agent is broadly disseminated throughout an animal population, there is little choice but to administer vaccines to large segments of the susceptible population. The decision to immunize, therefore, would be taken with consideration of the probability of disease exposure; health and economic risks of developing disease; the effectiveness, safety, and availability of approved vaccines; and the total costs and feasibility of immunization.[5–7] It is recognized that even vaccines with less-than-perfect efficacy may provide substantial disease protection via herd immunity and disruption of disease agent transmission.[8]

IMMUNIZATION IN THE FACE OF EMERGING DISEASES

Potential outbreaks of newly emerging diseases represent a unique threat to cattle populations. Such outbreaks could occur from multiple types of sources, such as introduction of new infectious disease agents to a geographic region or emergence of unique strains of existing agents. The introduction of such agents could occur accidentally as people and materials frequently cross borders or it could occur intentionally as an act of bioterrorism or biologic warfare.[9] In either case, if the point of introduction is quickly identified and appropriate animal trafficking rules are in place, targeted vaccination programs of susceptible and exposed animals surrounding index case herds may be a useful alternative to mass vaccination.[10] Targeted vaccination programs may have distinct advantages, particularly if the numbers of available vaccine doses and vaccine banks are limited or if there are substantial logistic issues associated with mass vaccination of all animals and a threatened region.[10] Also, if immunization may cause a significant number of adverse events or interfere with serologic investigations of disease spread, targeted vaccination strategies may reduce potential problems after immunization procedures are in place. In cases where disease introduction may be at multiple points or initial restriction of the animal movement fails, there may be no alternative to mass vaccination strategies. Mass vaccination may also be required if initial disease outbreak containment fails.

CHARACTERISTICS OF SUCCESSFUL TARGETED IMMUNIZATION PROGRAMS

North America, Europe, and other regions of the world are concerned with introduction of foot and mouth disease virus (FMDV) to highly susceptible cattle populations. The disease is endemic in many regions of Asia and South America.[11] Introduction of the virus could occur by accidental introduction of infected animals, accidental transfer of virus-contaminated materials, or the deliberate intention to cause harm. In this article, FMDV is discussed as a principle infectious agent as are the following critical components of a potentially successful targeted vaccination program: (1) nature of disease pathogenesis and transmission; (2) likelihood of early diagnosis and containment; (3) efficacy characteristics of vaccines available; (4) field effectiveness of immunization; and (5) alternative immunization strategies.

Nature of Disease Pathogenesis and Transmission

Foot and mouth disease (FMD) is caused by a highly contagious aphthovirus of the family, Picornaviridae.[12–14] There are distinct serotype families that contain multiple strains in distinct geographic regions of the world. The FMDV infects and causes disease in cloven-footed animals, such as swine, cattle, sheep, and goats, and the virus may infect deer if exposed. The FMDV is typically spread by aerosols that contain high virus concentrations. The infection spreads through close-contact exposure of comingled animals, as can occur in livestock markets and with introduction of new animals to a herd.[15] The virus can be transferred via contaminated fomites, such as clothing, boots, instruments, people, or vehicles. Also, transmission via windborne spread of droplets can occur over land up to 60 km distance from point of original infection and up to twice as far spread over water.[12,16] Many of the epidemiologic analyses of disease outbreaks and potential interventions have been reported.[10,17,18]

Once an animal is infected with FMDV, a typical incubation period is approximately 3 to 4 days but may be up to 14 days. Infected cattle may shed virus 1 to 2 days before the onset of clinical signs.[12–14] Clinical signs include moderate to overt lameness, milk drop, severe salivation and mastication. Animals may be febrile and are reluctant to stand or walk. Direct mortality is low but permanent production losses are associated with any recovery. In the 2001 FMD outbreak in Great Britain, it was observed that herds close to known infected farms were at the highest risk for acquiring new cases of FMD.[17,18] Slaughter of all animals on infected farms was an effective control measure although eliminating all animal movement (especially cattle, sheep, and hogs) and closing all livestock markets contributed to the success.[17] These combined measures effectively reduce the transmission potential of FMDV.[10] Retrospective analysis of FMDV and smallpox outbreaks strongly support the high probability of infection in close case contacts (such as herd mates). This supports the practice of depopulation of all animals and infected herds because it reduces the sources of infection and sources of susceptible animals in close contact to infected animals on farms.[17,19] Even though it was the goal of government authorities to initiate slaughter of animals on infected farms within 24 hours of case reports (without laboratory confirmation), depopulation alone could not reduce the transmission potential to completely block the spread of FMDV.[10] Therefore, additional intervention measures, such as enhanced movement restrictions and aggressive culling of at-risk premises, may be required to effectively reduce transmission of FMDV. Any other measures chosen, however, must have the ability to rapidly and substantially reduce the number of susceptible animals in close contact with infected animals on farms.

Likelihood of Early Diagnosis and Containment

With regard to FMD epidemics, the magnitude of disease spread depends on critical time intervals. These intervals include the time from initial exposure to the observations of lesions, the time to report suspected disease to authorities, laboratory confirmation of disease, and implementation of effective control measures on the index farms.[20] Similar conclusions hold for other contagious diseases of livestock.[21] Unfortunately, especially among the first cases of the disease outbreak, the time from the initial examination of lesions to reporting to authorities may be prolonged by as much as 2.5 days.[17] This time interval is generally reduced throughout an outbreak. As producers become aware of the disease possibility, reporting times decrease.

The logistics of specimen collection from suspect cases along with transportation logistics and laboratory capacity and availability may also contribute to delays in taking further control decisions.[20] Once an outbreak is diagnosed, however, many control measures (barring movement and marketing) would be in place and decisions to depopulate likely initiated on presumptive diagnosis on the farms. The time intervals between field detection of suspect cases, reporting, and confirmation of FMD would be critical. Because the onset of immunity of vaccines for the prevention of FMDV infection is 3 to 4 days, identification and isolation of index farms would be critical to the success of any immunization scheme.[22–24] If there were substantial delays between infection and confirmation of where disease spread had begun, vaccination would likely have minimal impact on the ultimate spread of disease.

Efficacy Characteristics of Vaccines Available

Vaccines for the prevention of FMDV infection typically contain inactivated, concentrated antigens derived from multiple serotypes. These antigens are mixed with adjuvants to achieve high potency (as described for use in epidemics). The onset of immunity is 3 to 4 days in cattle and sheep.[22–24] Standard potency formulations may require 10 days for onset of immunity. The diversity of the naturally occurring strains limits efficacy and the duration of immunity for the vaccine (4 to 6 months). Protective fractions are approximately 80% to 90% but vaccinated animals may develop productive, subclinical infections and shed virus. Immunity is considered to be limited to the serotype of the vaccine antigens although some cross-type protection may occur. Vaccinated animals are seropositive to FMDV after vaccination and this response characteristic could interfere with some epidemiologic studies and severely limit any commercial utility of the vaccinated animals.[23–25]

The desirable characteristics of any vaccine formulation used for FMD control are

1. Rapid onset of immunity
2. Efficacy in multiple species against multiple serotypes and subtypes with the ability to
   a. Block or significantly reduce viral shedding
   b. Prevent persistent infection
   c. Provide an extended duration of immunity
   d. Be compatible with vaccinate to live strategies
3. Robustness and availability of global manufacturing methodologies to enhance availability
4. Stability of in-use formulations, including potential short-term stability at temperatures of 10°C to 40°C, allowing storage in readily deployable vaccine banks
5. Efficacy against broad sets of serotypes
6. Efficacy in animals incubating FMDV
7. Acceptable safety profiles in young and pregnant animals

These characteristics were reported by Gay (The 5th International Veterinary Vaccines and Diagnostic Conference. Madison, WI, June 19–23, 2009).[26]

Most current FMD vaccines are formulated using inactivated viral antigen produced in baby hamster kidney cells.[27] The FMDV used is fully virulent and inactivated with binary ethylenimine. A downstream processing includes combinations of ultrafiltration or chemical concentration with ultrafiltration.[27] These processed antigens may be further purified by chromatography. The fully processed antigens are stored frozen until formulated.[27] Adjuvants commonly used include oil-in-water emulsions or aluminum hydroxide/saponin emulsions.[27] The viral serotypes used to formulate vaccines are selected based on the prevalent strains of a given geographic region and the vaccines are usually bivalent or trivalent. For example, South American vaccines typically contain types C, O, and A strains. African formulations may contain

South African Territory 1 (SAT1), SAT2, SAT3, type A, and type O strains.[28] Typical antigen doses are 1.0 to 10 μg. Vaccine serial or batch potency testing is completed according to the OIE Manual using direct challenge of immunized cattle (OIE. Foot and mouth disease. In: *Manual of Standards for Diagnostic Tests and Vaccines.* 6th edition. Vol. 1. Paris: World Organization for Animal Health; 2008).[29,30] Indirect potency measurements may be established by determination of virus-neutralizing titers in serum obtained from vaccinated animals, however.[31]

The application of FMD vaccines has been reviewed by Parida.[28] Vaccination of cattle with high potency vaccines will likely produce protection from clinical FMD within 1 week and reduce viral shedding.[22,25] Vaccination is ultimately associated with decreased numbers and persistently infected animals, reducing transmission efficiency.[32–34] The efficacy of the vaccines in this regard, however, may vary depending on the serotypes of the antigen in the vaccine and the serotype of the outbreak virus.

Immunization of cattle produces measurable neutralizing antibody within 4 to 7 days after vaccine administration.[35] The IgG titers peek at approximately 14 days after immunization.[36] Immunity to FMD infection also depends on T-lymphocyte responses, however, as T-helper lymphocytes and probably as cytotoxic T lymphocytes.[37–40] The generation of stimulation of class II restricted CD4 cells is important for two reasons: (1) these helper cells stimulate the expansion at differentiation of B-lymphocytes that eventually produce high affinity, neutralizing antibody (IgG)[39,41] and (2) the CD4 helper cells produce interferon-γ that promotes natural killer cell and macrophage activation to limit FMDV replication and spread.[42,43] A more complete understanding of FMDV epitopes (present in capsid and nonstructural proteins) could lead to cross-reactivity and cross-protective immunity.[39,44] There is a need to develop vaccines to improve serotype coverage, reduce the time to the onset of immunity, increase the duration of immunity, reduce the number of persistently infected animals, and further reduce viral shedding and transmission. A review of experimental vaccines for FMD outbreak emergency use has recently been published.[45] There are new technologies available that may enhance the effectiveness of FMDV vaccines.

Estimations of the Effectiveness of Specific Immunization Strategies

For any vaccine to have an impact on the reduction of FMDV transmission, the rapid onset of solid and heterogeneous immunity would be advantageous. There are additional considerations and desirable characteristics of vaccines used depending on how the vaccines may be applied within control programs. These have been described and reviewed in depth by Keeling and colleagues[10] and are discussed in the following sections describing potential immunization strategies.

Prophylactic immunization
Prophylactic immunization is the general vaccination of select random production units before any known infection. This approach would require considerable risk analysis to determine the strains of FMDV that would represent the greatest risks to that particular animal population. The approach would require only the standard potency vaccines and immunization plans would likely allow multiple doses of vaccines. This approach to immunization would not depend on an exceptionally short onset of immunity. Analytic estimates predict substantial reduction of the numbers of infected farms (approximately 80%) and reduction of the duration of any epidemic (by 50% to 60%) with as few as 15% to 25% of random farms vaccinated or as few as 5% to 10% of the largest cattle farms vaccinated.[10] The same models also predict an efficacy reduction estimate of 90% to 50% has little effect on the overall impact of prophylactic immunization. Similar estimations also predict that immunization enhances the effectiveness

of culling of infected premises and dangerous contacts if as few as one third of herds are immunized.

There are significant disadvantages to prophylactic vaccination. One disadvantage is the expense of vaccination for prevention of a disease that may not occur (including the actual cost of the vaccination program and losses associated with adverse events of vaccination). An additional issue is the serologic status of animals and the problems associated with determination of most favored trade status. The development of robust marker strategies could alleviate this problem but such strategies incur further expenses of vaccine development and field testing.[46] The required capability and capacity to maintain marker-associated serologic testing may place an increased burden on diagnostic laboratories.

The implementation of specific prophylactic vaccination programs also depends on the regional distribution of animal populations. In the 2001 Great Britain outbreak of FMD, only 1% of initial reported cases were in swine. Thus, immunization of only cattle or only the largest cattle farms would have resulted in significantly reducing the extent and duration of the outbreak.[17,18] If the population density of swine had been greater, however, a much greater epidemic could have occurred if only cattle had been vaccinated. These estimations assume that the strain of FMDV in the outbreak would have spread efficiently by aerosol transmission between pigs.

Reactive immunization

There are several approaches and strategies of immunization that could be applied after an infectious outbreak has been established. These include mass vaccination of all susceptible animals, ring vaccination around identified infected premises or zones, or other forms of predictive vaccination of select premises of greatest infection risk or of progressive transmission risk.[10] The degree of success for all of these reactive strategies depends on the time interval between the beginning of the outbreak and the beginning of immunization and the number of animals vaccinated per day.[10]

When all susceptible animals are targeted for immunization, the magnitude of an epidemic can potentially be drastically reduced as the number of animals vaccinated per day increase over time. A significant reduction of the epidemic (up to an 85% reduction of case numbers and a 75% reduction of duration) may occur as the rate of vaccinations approaches 100,000 per day and then plateaus at approximately 300,000 per day (calculations based on Great Britain populations in population densities). These estimates depend on of the effects of culling and an initiation of vaccination between 14 to 24 days after the initial infection reports.[10]

Ring vaccination[25] would likely have less impact on the magnitude of an FMD epidemic. The models reviewed almost all predict that the magnitude of FMD spread is correlated to the number of vaccinated premises. This would hold true with the highly contagious disease, such as FMD, where the reproduction ratio of uncontrolled infection approaches a 5.0.[17,18] As estimated, vaccination of a ring of 10 km around infected premises reduces the total number of infected farms in an epidemic only by approximately 20%. There are several reasons for this relative lack of effect. It is likely that vaccine efficacy is compromised in infected herds (infected during the delays associated with reporting and vaccinating and the time required for the onset of immunity). It is also possible that windborne infected aerosols may extend beyond the vaccination ring into highly susceptible populations.[17] Also, because the neighborhood approach to immunization bypasses a substantial number of susceptible premises, the tail, or duration, of an epidemic may be extended and secondary outbreaks could occur once culling and movement restrictions are removed.[10] The role or significance of asymptomatic carriers (possibly present and increased numbers and vaccinated animals) could also contribute to extended or secondary outbreaks. Assuming that vaccine formulations or the concurrent use of immunostimulants could be developed with a much reduced and effective onset of immunity, improved ring vaccination strategies could be developed[28] allowing "vaccinate to live" strategies to be used where fewer animals would be included in initial stamp out depopulation efforts.

FOOT AND MOUTH DISEASE CONTROL

It is believed that only aggressive culling with or without mass vaccination would control an FMD outbreak. Further, even optimistic estimates of ring vaccination effectiveness are limited. The immunization of "predictive horizon" farms among the latter generations of premises may have much greater impact, however.[10] This approach could be useful when mass immunization is not logistically or economically feasible or when complete and aggressive culling is delayed. Such delays could occur because of logistic and economic considerations or because of political opposition to mass depopulation of infected premises. In any outbreak, the index farms and the dangerous contact farms more likely have established or incubating infections at the time diagnostic examinations, reporting and laboratory confirmation occur. These are the primary premises of an outbreak. With regard to predictive immunization, success is likely achieved due to the aggressive culling of primary premises and immunizations of at risk premises with sufficient time to achieve onset of effective immunity. Predictive vaccination of as few as 50 to 500 farms per day could substantially reduce the magnitude of an epidemic (as well as or better than ring vaccination). The greatest impact of the predictive vaccination, however, would be a truncation of the epidemic even though fewer total premises would be vaccinated. This approach immunization as a component of outbreak control is interesting and promising as it offers effectiveness, even with some delays in reporting and confirmation of the disease and delays in the initiation of vaccination. Although perhaps not as effective as complete mass immunization and aggressive, complete depopulation—strategic predictive vaccination may specifically reduce the duration of an outbreak and drastically reduce the probability of secondary outbreaks.

ANTHRAX AND OTHER INFECTIOUS DISEASE OUTBREAKS IN CATTLE

In a recent North American outbreak of anthrax in 2005 in the North Dakota Red River basin, proper vaccination of cattle had a protective effect.[47] Cattle that had been vaccinated multiple times (more than once per year and before the onset of the outbreak period) were likely to be on a protected premise (odds ratio of 0.12).[47] Also, premises that vaccinated only during the outbreak (with or without concurrent use of antibiotics) were seven times more likely to be an infected premise (odds ratio of 7.14).[47] The duration of immunity of this vaccine is generally less than 1 year. The manufacturer (Colorado Serum Company, Denver, Colorado) recommends an initial immunization series with annual boosters. In endemic regions, two doses 2 to 3 weeks apart are recommended. Annual vaccination would be required in endemic regions with possible booster doses in the face of actual disease outbreaks.[48,49] With regard to anthrax, the nature of the source of infection is different from the source of infection with FMD.[49–51] With anthrax, the infectious spores of *Bacillus anthracis* are in the soil and animal to animal transmission among cattle is insignificant. Therefore, in these endemic regions, annual vaccination must be maintained to provide sufficient immunity. Fortunately, in some cases, the immunization can be timed to provide maximum immunity at the time of expected disease outbreaks. Further, immunization of cattle against anthrax does not create a major diagnostic dilemma. Immunization with the attenuated Sterne strain vaccine is relatively inexpensive and the immunization can be incorporated into most management practices. Ranch-to-ranch compliance with the need for multiple doses of vaccine will likely never approach 100%, however, and there is need for improved, safe formulations with improvements in onset of immunity and duration of immunity.

During an anthrax outbreak in Australia in 1997, creating a vaccination buffer zone (ring) around infected premises was an effective control method.[52] Again, onset of immunity was limiting in that it took nearly 2 weeks before control could be realized. No specific vector of spread was identified in this outbreak and it was the opinion of experts that significant earthwork and drainage work may have disturbed old anthrax graves. Ongoing, annual vaccination of cattle in high-risk endemic areas is necessary for protection because of the rest of the community and the time required for onset of effective impunity are less than ideal.

Immunization for many other diseases is common in cattle. For the most part, these infections are endemic within populations (bovine viral diarrhea virus, respiratory syncytial virus, *Mannheimia haemolytica*, and so forth) or pathogens present in the environment (black leg, malignant edema, tetanus, and so forth). In most of these situations where the relative risk of disease exposure is inherently high, immunization practices and vaccine selections focus on absolute efficacy and safety. That is, strong preferences are exercised to maximize protection of individuals (and collectively the herd) and minimize risk of adverse reactions. Small increments of increased efficacy will generally not overcome real or perceived safety risks, such as anaphylaxis, injection site reactions, virulence reversion, abortions, persistent infections, or immunosuppression. Therefore, the likelihood of significant losses due to disease and the effectiveness of the vaccine are important considerations in the process of creating vaccination programs for individual herds. In these situations, the return on investment must be determined and the return depends on the total cost of the immunization program, the vaccine, labor, and handling.

SUMMARY

Well-designed immunization programs have an important role in the control of disease outbreaks in cattle. The success of these immunization programs depends on the coordinated and effective use of an efficacious vaccine along with other required control measures. Efforts to improve key characteristics of vaccines (such as onset of immunity, duration of immunity, and basic safety and efficacy) will allow greater utility of the vaccines for outbreak control.

REFERENCES

1. Lombard M, Pastoret PP, Moulin AM. A brief history of vaccines and vaccination. Rev Sci Tech 2007;26:29–48.
2. Wehrle PF. A reality in our time—certification of the global eradication of smallpox. J Infect dis 1980;142:636–8.
3. Kretzschmar M, van den Hof S, Wallinga J, et al. Ring vaccination and smallpox control. Emerg Infect Dis 2004;10:832–41.
4. McVey DS, Galvin JE, Olson SC. A review of the effectiveness of vaccine potency control testing. Int J Parasitol 2003;33:507–16.
5. MacIntyre CR, Seccull A, Lane JM, et al. Development of a risk-priority score for category A bioterrorism agents as an aid for public health policy. Mil med 2006; 171:589–94.

6. Wildman BK, Perrett T, Abutarbush SM, et al. A comparison of 2 vaccination programs in feedlot calves at ultra-high risk of developing undifferentiated fever/bovine respiratory disease. La revue vétérinaire canadienne. Can Vet J 2008;49:463–72.
7. Plummer PJ, Rohrbach BW, Daugherty RA, et al. Effect of intranasal vaccination against bovine enteric coronavirus on the occurrence of respiratory tract disease in a commercial backgrounding feedlot. J Am Vet Med Assoc 2004; 225:726–31.
8. Schat KA, Baranowski E. Animal vaccination and the evolution of viral pathogens. Rev Sci Tech 2007;26:327–38.
9. Elsken LA, Carr MY, Frana TS, et al. Regulations for vaccines against emerging infections and agrobioterrorism in the United States of America. Rev Sci Tech 2007;26:429–41.
10. Keeling MJ, Woolhouse ME, May RM, et al. Modelling vaccination strategies against foot-and-mouth disease. Nature 2003;421:136–42.
11. Kitching P, Hammond J, Jeggo M, et al. Global FMD control—is it an option? Vaccine 2007;25:5660–4.
12. Woolhouse M, Donaldson A. Managing foot-and-mouth. Nature 2001;410:515–6.
13. Gloster J, Blackall RM, Sellers RF, et al. Forecasting the airborne spread of foot-and-mouth disease. Vet Rec 1981;108:370–4.
14. Hugh-Jones ME, Wright PB. Studies on the 1967–8 foot-and-mouth disease epidemic. The relation of weather to the spread of disease. J hyg (Lond) 1970; 68:253–71.
15. Donaldson AI, Doel TR. Foot-and-mouth disease: the risk for Great Britain after 1992. Vet Rec 1992;131:114–20.
16. Gibbens JC, Sharpe CE, Wilesmith JW, et al. Descriptive epidemiology of the 2001 foot-and-mouth disease epidemic in Great Britain: the first five months. Vet Rec 2001;149:729–43.
17. Ferguson NM, Donnelly CA, Anderson RM. The foot-and-mouth epidemic in Great Britain: pattern of spread and impact of interventions. Science 2001;292: 1155–60.
18. Ferguson NM, Donnelly CA, Anderson RM. Transmission intensity and impact of control policies on the foot and mouth epidemic in Great Britain. Nature 2001;413: 542–8.
19. Woolhouse M, Chase-Topping M, Haydon D, et al. Epidemiology. Foot-and-mouth disease under control in the UK. Nature 2001;411:258–9.
20. Howard SC, Donnelly CA. The importance of immediate destruction in epidemics of foot and mouth disease. Res Vet Sci 2000;69:189–96.
21. Howard SC, Donnelly CA. Estimation of a time-varying force of infection and basic reproduction number with application to an outbreak of classical swine fever. J Epidemiol Biostat 2000;5:161–8.
22. Doel TR, Williams L, Barnett PV. Emergency vaccination against foot-and-mouth disease: rate of development of immunity and its implications for the carrier state. Vaccine 1994;12:592–600.
23. Cox SJ, Barnett PV, Dani P, et al. Emergency vaccination of sheep against foot-and-mouth disease: protection against disease and reduction in contact transmission. Vaccine 1999;17:1858–68.
24. Sanz-Parra A, Vázquez B, Sobrino F, et al. Evidence of partial protection against foot-and-mouth disease in cattle immunized with a recombinant adenovirus vector expressing the precursor polypeptide (P1) of foot-and-mouth disease virus capsid proteins. J Gen Virol 1999;80:671–9.

25. Salt JS, Barnett PV, Dani P, et al. Emergency vaccination of pigs against foot-and-mouth disease: protection against disease and reduction in contact transmission. Vaccine 1998;16:746–54.
26. Gay C. Presented at The 5th International Veterinary Vaccines and Diagnostic Conference. Madison, June 19–23, 2009.
27. Doel TR. FMD vaccines. Virus Res 2003;91:81–99.
28. Parida S. Vaccination against foot-and-mouth disease virus: strategies and effectiveness. Expert Rev Vaccines 2009;8:347–65.
29. De Clercq K, Goris N, Barnett PV, et al. FMD vaccines: reflections on quality aspects for applicability in European disease control policy. Transbound Emerg Dis 2008;55:46–56.
30. World Organisation for Animal Health (OIE) Foot and mouth disease. In: Manual of diagnostic tests and vacanies for terrestrial animals 2008: mammals, birds, and bees. Vol. 1. 6th edition. Paris: Office International des Epizooties; 2008.
31. Goris N, Willems T, Diev VI, et al. Indirect foot-and-mouth disease vaccine potency testing based on a serological alternative. Vaccine 2008;26:3870–9.
32. Parida S, Fleming L, Oh Y, et al. Reduction of foot-and-mouth disease (FMD) virus load in nasal excretions, saliva and exhaled air of vaccinated pigs following direct contact challenge. Vaccine 2007;25:7806–17.
33. Parida S, Fleming L, Oh Y, et al. Emergency vaccination of sheep against foot-and-mouth disease: significance and detection of subsequent sub-clinical infection. Vaccine 2008;26:3469–79.
34. Cox SJ, Parida S, Voyce C, et al. Further evaluation of higher potency vaccines for early protection of cattle against FMDV direct contact challenge. Vaccine 2007;25:7687–95.
35. Salt JS. The carrier state in foot and mouth disease—an immunological review. Br Vet J 1993;149:207–23.
36. Salt JS, Mulcahy G, Kitching RP. Isotype-specific antibody responses to foot-and-mouth disease virus in sera and secretions of "carrier" and "non-carrier" cattle. Epidemiol infect 1996;117:349–60.
37. Sobrino F, Sáiz M, Jiménez-Clavero MA, et al. Foot-and-mouth disease virus: a long known virus, but a current threat. Vet Res 2001;32(1):1–30.
38. Blanco E, Garcia-Briones M, Sanz-Parra A, et al. Identification of T-cell epitopes in nonstructural proteins of foot-and-mouth disease virus. J Virol 2001;75(7): 3164–74.
39. Collen T, Baron J, Childerstone A, et al. Heterotypic recognition of recombinant FMDV proteins by bovine T-cells: the polymerase (P3Dpol) as an immunodominant T-cell immunogen. Virus Res 1998;56:125–33.
40. Childerstone AJ, Cedillo-Baron L, Foster-Cuevas M, et al. Demonstration of bovine CD8+ T-cell responses to foot-and-mouth disease virus. J Gen Virol 1999;80:663–9.
41. Foster M, Cook A, Cedillo L, et al. Serological and cellular immune responses to non-structural proteins in animals infected with FMDV. Vet Q 1998;20(Suppl 2): S28–30.
42. García-Briones MM, Russell GC, Oliver RA, et al. Association of bovine DRB3 alleles with immune response to FMDV peptides and protection against viral challenge. Vaccine 2000;19:1167–71.
43. Zhang ZD, Hutching G, Kitching P, et al. The effects of gamma interferon on replication of foot-and-mouth disease virus in persistently infected bovine cells. Arch Virol 2002;147:2157–67.

44. van Lierop MJ, van Maanen K, Meloen RH, et al. Proliferative lymphocyte responses to foot-and-mouth disease virus and three FMDV peptides after vaccination or immunization with these peptides in cattle. Immunology 1992;75:406–13.
45. Cox SJ, Barnett PV. Experimental evaluation of foot-and-mouth disease vaccines for emergency use in ruminants and pigs: a review. Vet Res 2009;40:13.
46. Dong XN, Chen YH. Marker vaccine strategies and candidate CSFV marker vaccines. Vaccine 2007;25:205–30.
47. Mongoh MN, Dyer NW, Stoltenow CL, et al. Risk factors associated with anthrax outbreak in animals in North Dakota, 2005: a retrospective case-control study. Public Health Rep 2008;123:352–9.
48. Kaufmann AF, Fox MD, Kolb RC. Anthrax in Louisiana, 1971: an evaluation of the Sterne strain anthrax vaccine. J Am Vet Med Assoc 1973;163:442–5.
49. Fox MD, Kaufmann AF, Zendel SA, et al. Anthrax in Louisiana, 1971: epizootiologic study. J Am Vet Med Assoc 1973;163:446–51.
50. Dragon DC, Rennie RP. The ecology of anthrax spores: tough but not invincible. La revue vétérinaire canadienne. Can Vet J 1995;36:295–301.
51. Dragon DC, Bader DE, Mitchell J, et al. Natural dissemination of Bacillus anthracis spores in northern Canada. Appl Environ Microbiol 2005;71:1610–5.
52. Turner AJ, Galvin JW, Rubira RJ, et al. Experiences with vaccination and epidemiological investigations on an anthrax outbreak in Australia in 1997. J Appl Microbiol 1999;87:294–7.

Index

Note: Page numbers of article titles are in **boldface** type.

A

Abdominal viscera, examination of, in investigation of emerging infectious diseases of food animals, 6

American Veterinary Medical Association, Guidelines on Euthanasia of (2007), 2

Animal and Plant Health Inspection Service, of US Department of Agriculture, 15

Anthrax, vaccination strategies for, 179–180

Antimicrobial resistance, to BRD pathogens, **79–88.** See also *Bovine respiratory disease (BRD), pathogens of, antimicrobial resistance to.*

Attaching-effacing *Escherichia coli* infections, in cattle, **29–56.** See also *Escherichia coli infections, attaching-effacing, in cattle.*

B

Bacterial infections, of respiratory tract, in cattle
  Histophilus somni, 60–61
  management of, 63–67
    pathogen treatment in, 65–66
    risk-related, 66–67
    vaccines in, 63–65
  Mannheimia haemolytica, 59–60
  Mycoplasma bovis, 61–62
  Pasteurella multocida, 57–59
  pathology related to, 62–63

BCoV. See *Bovine coronavirus (BCoV).*

Biotype(s), variations in, 108–110

Bison, brucellosis in, 21–22

Bluetongue virus
  described, 164–165
  in Europe
    Mediterranean Basin, 165–167
    Northern Europe, 167–168
    ongoing nature of, 165–168
    recent emergence of, global implications of, described, 163–164
  in the Americas, current status of, 168–169

Bluetongue virus (BTV), in Europe, recent emergence of, global implications of, **163–171**

Bovine brucellosis, **15–27.** See also *Brucellosis, bovine.*

Bovine coronavirus (BCoV)
  clinical manifestation of, 127
  described, 124
  diagnosis of, 131–132
  diarrhea in calves and, 128–129
  economic impact of, 127

Vet Clin Food Anim 26 (2010) 185–190
doi:10.1016/S0749-0720(09)00119-4
0749-0720/10/$ – see front matter © 2010 Elsevier Inc. All rights reserved.

vetfood.theclinics.com

Moving?

Make sure your subscription moves with you!

To notify us of your new address, find your **Clinics Account Number** (located on your mailing label above your name), and contact customer service at:

Email: journalscustomerservice-usa@elsevier.com

800-654-2452 (subscribers in the U.S. & Canada)
314-447-8871 (subscribers outside of the U.S. & Canada)

Fax number: 314-447-8029

Elsevier Health Sciences Division
Subscription Customer Service
3251 Riverport Lane
Maryland Heights, MO 63043

*To ensure uninterrupted delivery of your subscription, please notify us at least 4 weeks in advance of move.

Printed and bound by CPI Group (UK) Ltd, Croydon, CR0 4YY

03/10/2024

01040454-0018